NursetoNurse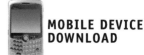

MOBILE DEVICE DOWNLOAD

TRAUMA CARE

FOLLOW THESE INSTRUCTIONS TO DOWNLOAD:

1) Use your Web browser to go to:
http://www.mhnursetonurse.com

2) Register now

3) Fill in the required fields

4) Enter your unique registration code below

5) Download the software and sync into your handheld device

Code Listed Here

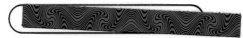

NOTE: BOOK IS NOT RETURNABLE ONCE SCRATCH-OFF IS REMOVED

Scratch off coating above to reveal your unique code to download your mobile device software.

See above for complete directions.

If you have any problems accessing your download, please email: techsolutions@mhedu.com

CARD P/N
9780071596794 • 0071596798
part of set
ISBN 978-0-07-159677-0
MHID 0-07-159677-1

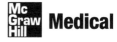

mcgraw-hillmedical.com

Nurse to Nurse
TRAUMA CARE

Nurse to Nurse
TRAUMA CARE

Donna Nayduch, RN, MSN, ACNP, CAISS
Trauma Consultant
Evans, Colorado

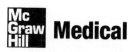 **Medical**

New York Chicago San Francisco Lisbon London Madrid Mexico City
Milan New Delhi San Juan Seoul Singapore Sydney Toronto

BP45

Nurse to Nurse: Trauma Care

1 2 3 4 5 6 7 8 9 0   DOC/DOC   12 11 10 9

Set ISBN 978-0-07-159677-0; MHID 0-07-159677-1
Book ISBN 978-0-07-159678-7; MHID 0-07-159678-X
Card ISBN 978-0-07-159679-4; MHID 0-07-159679-8

This book was set in Berkeley Book by International Typesetting and Composition.
The editors were Joseph Morita and Karen Davis.
The production supervisor was Catherine H. Saggese.
Production management was provided by Somya Rustagi, International Typesetting and Composition.
The book designer was Eve Siegel; the cover designer was David Dell'Accio.
RR Donnelley was printer and binder.

This book is printed on acid-free paper.

Library of Congress Cataloging-in-Publication Data

Nayduch, Donna.
    Nurse to nurse. Trauma Care / Donna Nayduch.
        p. ; cm.
    Includes index.
    ISBN-13: 978-0-07-159677-0 (set)
    ISBN-10: 0-07-159677-1 (set)
    SBN-13: 978-0-07-159678-7 (pbk. : alk. paper)
    ISBN-10: 0-07-159678-X (pbk. : alk. paper)
    1. Emergency nursing—Handbooks, manuals, etc.   2. Emergency medicine—Handbooks, manuals, etc.   I. Title.   II. Title: Trauma.
    [DNLM: 1. Wounds and Injuries—nursing—Handbooks.   2. Emergency Nursing—methods—Handbooks.   WY 49 N331n 2009]
    RT120.E4N39 2009
    616.02'5—dc22
                                                    2009016413

1/12/10

I dedicate this book to Michael J. Rhodes, MD, FACS, Chair, Department of Surgery, Christiana Care Health System, Wilmington, Delaware. He was my mentor in trauma care who spent endless nights with us in the shock trauma ICU in Allentown, Pennsylvania. His dedication and knowledge of trauma was the inspiration for me. Like a doting father, he sent me off to my first trauma coordinator position with confidence. The passion in this book mirrors the passion for the trauma patient that he demonstrated every day. It is that foundation upon which my trauma knowledge is built and for which I am forever grateful to him.

Contents

Preface

When I was asked to write this book on trauma nursing, I found the opportunity not only exciting, but a chance to share 26 years of trauma nursing experience. As I have watched the staff and participated in the care of the trauma patient, I have wanted to produce a manual that would provide the information needed in a rapid, quick-find method. I have been a trauma nurse all of my career, from student nurse through trauma regional director positions. The faces, names, injuries, smells, and everything that comes with caring for trauma patients have remained embedded in memory all of my life. I can to this day name certain patients who had an impact on my career, knowledge, or for whom I have shed tears with the family. I have had the honor of saving lives and sitting with others as they make the transition. I have been a staff nurse, trauma nurse coordinator (as we were called back then), trauma registrar, trauma consultant/site surveyor, and trauma acute care nurse practitioner.

I was taught to be an active part of the trauma team, participating in patient assessment and identifying actions necessary to manage the patient. We were expected to interpret data and be ready to act without instructions. The team was completely collaborative and for that I am very grateful. Therefore you will find that this text is written with the understanding that the nurse is working side by side with the physicians and processing the same input. It is assumed that the nurse knows the limitations of his or her practice and will apply the knowledge in this book appropriately. There are occasions when the nurse will need to act independently and the goal of this book is to provide the information needed for the optimal care of the trauma patient.

In addition, I hope that the support services so necessary to the functional outcome of the trauma patient will also find this reference useful to their understanding of trauma care. To all those in the trauma nursing roles and all the staff supporting the trauma patient through to rehabilitation, I offer this text as your quick reference guide to rapid decision making and outstanding patient outcomes.

The book was extensively researched; however, due to the size, only references cited in the text will appear. All of the standard references including *Advanced Trauma Life Support* (ATLS), *Trauma Nursing Core Course* (TNCC), *McQuillan's Trauma Nursing from Resuscitation through Rehabilitation,* and the *Eastern Association for the Surgery of Trauma (EAST) Practice Management Guidelines* were used in every chapter. In addition, many other references provided insight and knowledge. Trust that these resources were exhausted in search of the most current and accurate data. I hope to find *Nurse to Nurse: Trauma Care* in many lab coat pockets as I round on trauma patients and survey trauma centers throughout the country.

To my colleagues who have been reading along with me throughout this year, I cannot express enough thanks for your time, expertise, gentle guidance, and friendship. To the friends and family who have patiently listened to me through this process and provided chocolate (and champagne when I was done), mahalo nui loa!

Acknowledgments

Linda Laskowski-Jones, RN, MS, ACNS-BC, CCRN, CEN, Vice President: Emergency, Trauma and Aeromedical Services, Christiana Care Health System, Wilmington, Delaware.

Fred Luchette, MD, MS, Director of Cardiothoracic Critical Care Services; Professor of Surgery, Loyola University Hospital, Maywood, Illinois.

William Richardson, MD, Professor of Orthopaedic Surgery, Duke University Medical Center, Durham, North Carolina.

Suzanne Buchanan, RN, BS, CCRN, Arizona Burn Center Outreach Educator, Maricopa Medical Center, Phoenix, Arizona.

Jill Pleban, MLT, ASCP, Laboratory Information System Coordinator, Doylestown Hospital, Doylestown, Pennsylvania

Maggie Reynard, Illustrator/Artist, Half Moon Bay, California.

Heidi DeLeon, RN, BSN, Staff Nurse, St Joseph's Medical Center, Phoenix, Arizona.

Vicki Bennett, RN, MSN, Trauma Program Manager, Scottsdale Healthcare-Osborn, Scottsdale, Arizona.

Harry Teter, Esquire, Executive Director, American Trauma Society, Upper Marlboro, Maryland.

Kevin Foster, MD, Burn Surgery, Arizona Burn Center, Maricopa Medical Center, Phoenix, Arizona.

Acronyms

ABC	Airway, breathing, circulation
ABG	Arterial blood gas
A/C	Assist-control (ventilation)
ACL	Anterior cruciate ligament
ACS	Abdominal compartment syndrome
ACS-COT	American College of Surgeons-Committee on Trauma
AD	Autonomic dysreflexia
ADH	Antidiuretic hormone
ADL	Activities of daily living
AHS	Autonomic hyperexcitability/dysfunction syndrome
AIDS	Acquired immunodeficiency syndrome
AIS	Abbreviated injury scale
ALI	Acute lung injury
ALS	Advanced life support
AMS	Acute mountain sickness
A-O	Atlanto-occipital
A-P	Anteroposterior
APP	Abdominal perfusion pressure
aPTT	Activated partial thromboplastin time
ARDS	Acute respiratory distress syndrome
ARS	Acute radiation syndrome
ASIA	American Spinal Injury Association
ATA	Atmosphere absolute
ATLS	Advanced trauma life support
ATS	American Trauma Society
ATV	All-terrain vehicle
AVN	Avascular necrosis
BIS	Bispectral index
BMR	Basal metabolic rate
BP	Blood pressure
BSF	Basilar skull fracture

BUN	Blood urea nitrogen
CAVR	Continuous arteriovenous rewarming
CBC	Complete blood count
CCF	Carotid cavernous fistula
CDC	Centers for Disease Control and Prevention
CHF	Congestive heart failure
CISM	Critical incident stress management
CMV	Controlled mechanical ventilation
CO	Carbon monoxide
COPD	Chronic obstructive pulmonary disease
CPAP	Continuous positive airway pressure
CPK	Creatine phosphokinase
CPP	Cerebral perfusion pressure
CPR	Cardiopulmonary resuscitation
CRIF	Closed reduction with internal fixation
CRRT	Continuous renal replacement therapy
CSF	Cerebrospinal fluid
CSW	Cerebral salt wasting
CT	Computed tomography
CVA	Costovertebral angle
CVP	Central venous pressure
CVVR	Continuous venovenous rewarming
CXR	Chest x-ray
DAI	Diffuse axonal injury
DI	Diabetes insipidus
DIC	Disseminated intravascular coagulation
DNR	Do not resusitate
DPL	Diagnostic peritoneal lavage
DVT	Deep vein thrombosis
EAC	External auditory canal
ECA	External carotid artery
ECG	Electrocardiogram
ED	Emergency department
EDH	Epidural hematoma
EEG	Electroencephalogram

EMS	Emergency medical services
EOC	Emergency operations center
EOP	Emergency operations plan
ERCP	Endoscopic retrograde cholangiopancreatography
ETT	Endotracheal tube
FAST	Focused assessment with sonography for trauma
FES	Fat embolism syndrome
FFP	Fresh frozen plasma
FHT	Fetal heart tone
FTSG	Full thickness skin graft
FWB	Full weight bearing
GCS	Glasgow coma scale
GI	Gastrointestinal
GLF	Ground level fall
GOS	Glasgow outcome score
GSW	Gunshot wound
HACE	High-altitude cerebral edema
HAPE	High-altitude pulmonary edema
HBO	Hyperbaric oxygen
HBOC	Hemoglobin-based oxygen carrier
HIT	Heparin-induced thrombocytopenia
HIV	Human immunodeficiency virus
HO	Heterotrophic ossification
HR	Heart rate
ICA	Internal carotid artery
ICBG	Iliac crest bone graft
ICP	Intracranial pressure
ICS	Incident command system
ICU	Intensive care unit
I:E ratio	Inspiratory/expiratory ratio
IED	Improvised explosive device
IICP	Increased intracranial pressure
IMN	Intramedullary nail
INR	International normalized ratio
IO	Intraosseous line

IS	Incentive spirometry
ISS	Injury severity score
IV	Intravenous
IVC	Inferior vena cava
IVC-F	Inferior vena cava filter
LCL	Lateral collateral ligament
LLE	Left lower extremity
LMA	Laryngeal mask airway
LMP	Last menstrual period
LMWH	Low molecular weight heparin
LOC	Loss of consciousness
LR	Lactated ringer [solution]
LUE	Left upper extremity
MAP	Mean arterial pressure
MASH	Mobile Army surgical hospital
MAST	Military antishock trousers
MCI	Mass casualty incident
MCL	Medial collateral ligament
MI	Myocardial infarction
MMF	Maxillomandibular fixation
MODS	Multiple organ dysfunction syndrome
MOI	Mechanism of injury
MRI	Magnetic resonance imaging
MSOF	Multisystem organ failure
MVC	Motor vehicle collision
NCIPC	National Center for Injury Prevention and Control
NDMS	National Disaster Medical System
N/G	Nasogastric
NHTSA	National Highway Traffic Safety Administration
NIMS	National Incident Management System
NPO	Nothing by mouth
NSAID	Nonsteroidal anti-inflammatory drug
NSS	Normal saline solution
NTDS	National Trauma Data Standard
NWB	Nonweight bearing
OB	Obstetrics

OFR	Oxygen free radical
OOB (fall)	Out of bed
OR	Operating room
ORIF	Open reduction with internal fixation
OT	Occupational therapist/therapy
OU	Both eyes
PASG	Pneumatic antishock garment
PCWP	Pulmonary capillary wedge pressure
PE	Pulmonary embolism
PEEP	Positive end-expiratory pressure
PERRLA	Pupils equal, round, and reactive to light and accommodation
PI	Performance improvement
PICC	Percutaneously introduced central catheter
PMH	Past medical history
PPE	Personal protection equipment
PPI	Proton pump inhibitor
PPN	Peripheral parenteral nutrition
PPV	Positive pressure ventilation
PRBC	Packed red blood cells
PT	Physical therapist/therapy
PT	Prothrombin time
PTSD	Posttraumatic stress disorder
PTT	Partial thromboplastin time
PWB	Partial weight bearing
RBC	Red blood [cell] count
RLE	Right lower extremity
ROM	Range of motion
RR	Respiratory rate
RRT	Renal replacement therapy
RSI	Rapid sequence intubation
RTS	Revised trauma score
RUE	Right upper extremity
RUG	Retrograde urethrogram
SAH	Subarachnoid hemorrhage
SARS	Severe acute respiratory syndrome

SBIR	Screening, brief intervention, and referral
SCD	Sequential compression device
SCI	Spinal cord injury
SCIWORA	Spinal cord injury without radiographic abnormality
SDH	Subdural hematoma
SIADH	Syndrome of inappropriate secretion of antidiuretic hormone
SIRS	Systemic inflammatory response syndrome
SMA	Superior mesenteric artery
STSG	Split thickness skin graft
SVR	Systemic vascular resistance
SVT	Supraventricular tachycardia
TBI	Traumatic brain injury
TBSA	Total burn surface area
TDWB	Touchdown weight bearing
TENS	Transcutaneous electrical nerve stimulation
TLSO	Thoracolumbosacral orthosis
TM	Tympanic membrane
TMJ	Temporomandibular joint
TPN	Total parenteral nutrition
TRISS	Trauma and injury severity score
TTWB	Toe touch weight bearing
U/S	Ultrasound
V fib	Ventricular fibrillation
VAC	Vacuum-assisted closure (device)
VAP	Ventilator-associated pneumonia
VATS	Video-assisted thoracoscopy
V̇/Q̇	Ventilation-perfusion
VTE	Venous thromboembolism
WBAT	Weight bearing as tolerated
WBC	White blood [cell] count
WMD	Weapons of mass destruction

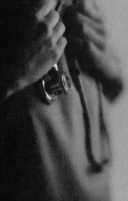

Chapter 1

MECHANISMS OF INJURY

INTRODUCTION

Trauma starts with the transfer of energy to the body from an outside force. The transfer of kinetic energy may be blunt or sharp in nature. In addition to blunt and sharp mechanisms, there is the situation of thermal energy in the form of heat, cold, or chemical agent, which generates the heat or cold. With the event of more frequent war-like situations, blast injuries and other mass casualty events are more common from improvised explosive devices (IED) or other mass disasters and are discussed in Chapter 15. Because the mechanism drives the injury sustained, injury prevention goes hand in hand. Table 1-1 identifies common mechanisms and the appropriate e-code for each (ICD9-CM 2008).

Trauma remains the leading cause of death in individuals aged 1 to 44 years, with the majority of injuries preventable (www.cdc.gov/ncipc/osp/data.htm). Motor vehicle collisions are the leading cause of trauma death in all age groups between 1 to 65 years. In individuals over 65 years, falls become the leading cause of death. The most common causes of nonfatal injuries as reported by the Centers for Disease Control and Prevention (CDC) are the following:

- Falls: 0 to 14 years and 25 years and older
- Unintentionally struck: leading cause of injury 15 to 24 years
- Motor vehicle collisions: second leading cause of injury 15 to 24 years.

Table 1-1   E-codes for Common Mechanisms of Injury (ICD9-CM 2008)

MOI	E-code (ICD9-CM)	Comments
MVC x represents the fourth digit, meaning occupant position		
MV to MV	E812.x	Any two motorized vehicles involved in the collision, even if one is stationary or parked
MV to object in road	E815.x	Any motorized vehicle impact with an on-the-road object, such as an animal, road sign, median, overpass; not an off-road stationary object, such as a tree
MV to object off road	E816.x	See loss of control
MV loss of control	E816.x	Any loss of control on the road including leaving the road and ultimately crashing into an off-road object; rollover
Car surfing	E818.1	Standing on vehicle while moving
MVs to MV off-road	E821.x	MVC in vehicle traveling wholly off streets/roads, ATV
Off-road snow vehicle	E820.x	Snowmobiles
Pedestrian struck	E814.7	Pedestrian struck by any motorized vehicle on the road
Bicycle struck	E813.6	Any pedal cycle struck by any motorized vehicle on the road
Falls		
GLF	E888.8	General GLF without other specifics
GLF struck sharp object	E888.0	GLF in which a sharp object is struck en route to ground

(Continued)

Table 1-1   E-codes for Common Mechanisms of Injury (ICD9-CM 2008) (*Continued*)

MOI	E-code (ICD9-CM)	Comments
Falls		
GLF struck blunt object	E888.1	GLF in which a blunt object is struck en route to ground
Slip, trip fall	E885.9	GLF from slipping, tripping and then falling
Fall from bike	E826.1	Riding bike, then collision on own, fall off
Fall OOB	E884.4	Fall from bed
Fall from chair	E884.2	Fall from chair
Fall while skiing	E885.3	Fall while skiing
Fall from snowboard	E885.4	Fall while snowboarding
Fall from skateboard	E885.2	Fall off roller skates, ice skates, in-line skates
Trip over curb	E880.1	Fall from tripping over a curb
Fall from toilet	E884.6	Fall from toilet
Fall from ladder	E881.0	Fall from ladder any height
Fall from building	E882	Fall from roof, other building, balcony
Fall in sports	E886.0	Collision or other cause of a fall during sports activities
Fall into hole	E883.9	Fall into a hole
Fall down steps	E880.9	Fall down any number of stairs
Fall from other	E884.9	Fall from height other object not found in the list
Struck—unintentional		
Without fall	E917.x	Struck unintentionally by object or persons without a fall

(*Continued*)

Table 1-1   E-codes for Common Mechanisms of Injury (ICD9-CM 2008) (*Continued*)

MOI	E-code (ICD9-CM)	Comments
Struck—unintentional		
In sports, no fall	E917.0	Struck unintentionally in sports activities without subsequent fall
Crushed between objects	E918	Caught between two objects, crushed
By falling object	E916.0	Struck by any falling object
Others		
Lawnmower	E920.0	Injury while using a lawnmower, powered or not
Cut by glass	E920.8	Unintentional cut by glass
Unintentional GSW	E922.x	Gunshot, unintentional
Unintentional stab	E920.3	Injury caused by sharp implement, unintentional
Homicide		
Assault	E960.0	Struck by fists, kicked, assaulted
Assault with object	E968.2	Struck by object during assault, pistol-whipped, baseball bat, concrete block, etc
Assault with vehicle	E968.5	Intentionally struck by vehicle
Rape	E960.1	Rape
GSW	E965.x	Intentional gunshot; fourth digit represents weapon
Stab	E966	Intentional stab with implement
Abuse	E967.x	Abuse of child, adult, elderly; inflicted by another
Set on fire	E968.0	Intentional burning by fire

(*Continued*)

**Table 1-1   E-codes for Common Mechanisms of Injury
(ICD9-CM 2008) (*Continued*)**

MOI	E-code (ICD9-CM)	Comments
Suicide		
Hanging	E953.0	Intentional self-inflicted hanging, suffocation, asphyxiation, not caused by chemicals
GSW	E955.x	Intentional self-inflicted gunshot
Stabbing/cutting	E956	Intentional self-inflicted stab/cutting
Vehicle	E958.5	Intentional injury to self with a vehicle
Burn		
Conflagration	E890.x	Housefire or fire in a building
Conflagration—bed	E898.0	Housefire started in bed occupied by the injured
Jump burning building	E890.8	Jumping from a burning building
Hot water scald	E924.2	Burn from hot water—tap Burn from hot water—heated
Hot substance/liquid scald	E924.0	Burn from other hot substance
Hot object	E924.8	Burn from touching hot object
Frostbite	E901.x	Burn from cold exposure, causing frostbite
Chemical	E924.1	Burn from chemical—acid Burn from chemical—alkali
Electrical	E925.x	Burn from electrical source

(*Continued*)

Table 1-1   E-codes for Common Mechanisms of Injury (ICD9-CM 2008) (*Continued*)

MOI	E-code (ICD9-CM)	Comments
Bites/Animal		
Dog	E906.0	Bite from dog
Kicked by animal	E906.8	Other injury inflicted by animals, such as gored, kicked, fallen upon
Fall off horse	E828.2	Fall off horse being ridden
Venomous snake	E905.0	Bite from venomous snake
Human	E968.7	Bite from human, intentionally inflicted
	E928.3	Bite from human, unintentional

The word "accident" will not be used in this text because of the preventable nature of trauma and the need for professionals to address trauma as a preventable disease, not happenstance, acts of god, and so on (Sisley 2007). Injury prevention activities by healthcare staff are hindered by time, education, and resources (Wilding et al. 2008), although hospital providers have the prime opportunity for these efforts. Every patient presents an injury prevention teaching opportunity. Natural disasters are some of the few "accidental" situations. Trauma is referred to as intentional versus unintentional in order to address the more appropriate nature of the event. For example, drunk driving is preventable, yet the injuries are usually unintentional. C. Everett Koop, former U.S. Surgeon General, made a profound statement regarding trauma: "If a disease were killing our children in the proportions that injuries are, people would be outraged and demand that this killer be stopped."

BLUNT TRAUMA

Blunt trauma occurs when the force applied to the body is not sharp in nature. Forensic medicine refers to blunt versus sharp injuries. Thus gunshot wounds (GSW) are classified as blunt to the medical examiner because the bullet is not a sharp implement. However in the trauma center, trauma is divided into blunt and penetrating, and placing GSW in the penetrating category because of its action on the body.

Principles of physics that operate when trauma, both blunt and penetrating, occurs are

- A body in motion remains in motion until acted upon by an outside force
- Velocity of the load applied determines damage (force = mass × acceleration)
- Tissue is displaced in the direction of the moving object (especially important for forensic evaluation)
- If an object is deformable, the time to impact is increased and thus the damage is increased
- Kinetic energy transferred is additive (both objects moving); $1/2$ mass × velocity^2.

Blunt trauma results in fracture, laceration, and other external wounds, tearing by shear forces, pressure causing "blowout" type injuries, and coup–contrecoup (side to side) injuries that are bilateral caused by the recoil after initial impact. This chapter will discuss common mechanisms and the expected injuries that result.

Motor Vehicle Collisions

Motor vehicle collisions (MVC) are usually unintentional; however some individuals have attempted suicide or homicide through the use of a vehicle. Most collisions begin on a street or highway and end with the collision itself. MVC can also occur in off-road situations, such as snowmobiles, all-terrain vehicles (ATV), and motocross or motorbikes. In addition, the position of the occupant at the time of impact determines injury. Since most collisions are unexpected, it is not uncommon for the occupant to inhale and hold the breath at the moment of impact. The blow to the chest that follows compresses the air-filled lungs resulting in pneumothorax. Car surfing and riding in the back of a pickup truck provide no protection for the occupant and result in the potential for total body injury.

Depending upon the choice of restraint, the individual has several options while in the vehicle. The unrestrained occupant has a greater chance of ejection from the seat through the "up and over" mechanism or entrapment under the dashboard via the "down and under" path. Restraints worn properly (lap and shoulder) hold the occupant in place with minimal movement as well as minimal injury. The airbag has room to deploy (at approximately 200 mph) without severe injury to the occupant. However, lap-only belts (that includes the shoulder belt placed behind the shoulder) result in the upper body coming in contact with objects in front of them (steering wheel, airbag) and shoulder-only results in the pelvis sliding downward and the neck becoming entrapped by the shoulder belt. Table 1-2 describes injuries associated with these pathways. The table includes the injuries to children improperly restrained. Restraint requirements for pregnant women and children are discussed below in injury prevention. Occupants in reclined seats have demonstrated severe torso injury while wearing the seat belt, lower extremity injury, and an increased mortality (Dissanaike et al. 2008). Serious injuries sustained while properly restrained would likely have resulted in death if unrestrained.

Head-on or rear-end collision

Most commonly involves the up and over or down and under pathways unless restrained. An impact with the steering wheel at 30 mph is comparable to standing against a wall and having a telephone pole rammed into the chest. Organs with ligamentous attachments (eg, aorta, liver, spleen) are particularly susceptible to injury. In the down and under path, the femur

Table 1-2   MVC-related Mechanisms of Injury

Pathway	Potential Injuries
Unrestrained— "up and over"	Head, face, and neck injuries from impact with windshield or sunroof Chest injuries—steering wheel impact Abdominal injuries—steering wheel impact (dependent upon body habitus) Airbag injury to face, neck, chest Lower extremity injury if tangled under dash/gas-brake pedals
Unrestrained— "down and under"	Lower extremity injuries—crush mechanism; entrapped in pedals, knee fracture/dislocation, hip fracture/dislocation Pelvis injury impact Abdominal injury—crush, impalement, body habitus affects Possible chest injury, neck injury
Lap-only belt	Head, neck, face injury from steering wheel impact, especially larynx/trachea; airbag injury Chest injury—steering wheel impact Potential for ejection or partial ejection and windshield impact
Shoulder-only belt	Neck vascular injury, head injury Abdominal injury—steering wheel impact
Improperly worn restraints	Lap belt too high: abdominal hollow viscus injury, thoracic and lumbar spine injury Lap belt too loose: hyperflexion injury at T12- L1 vertebrae Lap belt too high in pregnant passenger: abdominal injury as above in addition to injury to the fetus, placenta, uterus (determined by the age of the fetus)
Car seat not tethered to vehicle	Ejection; becomes a missile to other passengers All injuries, especially atlantooccipital dislocation with spinal cord injury from large head and inevitability of landing face down

(Continued)

Table 1-2   MVC-related Mechanisms of Injury (*Continued*)

Pathway	Potential Injuries
Child <12 years, front seat	Airbag impact to chest, abdomen, head, face Broad cadre of injury if unrestrained
Rear-facing car seat, front seat	Airbag impact to the car seat results in severe head, neck injury
Child <4′8″ or 60 lb in adult restraint	Slides under the seat belt as above "down and under," or If lap only, folds in half resulting in hollow viscus abdominal injury and chance fracture with spinal cord injury at L1-L2 vertebrae
Airbag Injuries	Airbags require a collision >35 mph to deploy and unless lateral airbags present, no deployment in lateral collisions Injuries to upper extremities, face, neck, corneal abrasions, chest Burns or abrasions may occur Seated too close (<10-14 in) can result in cervical hyperflexion injury Airbag only—54% increase in cervical spine injury in drivers (Donaldson et al. 2008)

strikes the dashboard ramming the bone into and through the acetabulum and causes pelvic fracture as well as posterior dislocation. Particularly in rear-end collisions, the position of the headrest can result in either injury to the neck or protection of the neck. Cervical ligamentous injury can result after hyperextension of the neck over the headrest. The headrest should be positioned properly at the midposterior skull.

Lateral impact (T-bone)

Injury occurs in a lateral impact determined by the degree of intrusion and any car components striking the occupant. For example, the control panel on the driver's door will impact the hip if it protrudes into the passenger compartment and the body habitus of the driver in relation to its position. Common injuries in lateral impact are determined by the position in the vehicle as well as restrained and reclined seats. The driver should be observed for aortic injury, spleen, rib fractures, pelvis fracture, left upper extremity injury. For the front passenger struck on the passenger side, anticipate liver, rib, pelvis, and right upper extremity injury. Unrestrained occupants will be pushed toward the opposite side, either into the door or other passengers and have a significant increase in mortality (Ryb et al. 2007).

Motorcycle and bicycle crashes

Head-on collision frequently results in the rider ejecting or partially ejecting over the handlebars. Common injuries include

- Head and neck injury if no helmet in place
- Thoracoabdominal injury from handlebar impact (common in children)
- "Open book" pelvic fracture—a splaying open (like a book) of the anterior and posterior pelvis from striking the handlebars
- Bilateral femur fracture
- Skin abrasions, lacerations

Injuries are decreased when a helmet is in place in proper position and if protective clothing is worn. Angular collisions or collisions with a vehicle result in multiple overall injuries and are dependent upon the site of impact. There is no demonstrated relationship between cervical spine injury and the use of a helmet (Goslar et al. 2008). Helmets are known to be protective of the head.

Pedestrian struck by vehicle

Pedestrian injuries are injuries sustained when an individual is struck by a vehicle but is not traveling in or on a motorized conveyance. For example, the wheelchair, skateboard, in-line skates, walking individual struck by a vehicle are pedestrian situations. Small children struck by vehicles are usually knocked over by the bumper and then run over by the tires. This is not due to driver intention, but rather the child's low center of gravity that causes him or her to fall over. The child not seen is now under the tire and run over before the driver can realize that the car has struck something.

School-age children and short adults are struck by the bumper in the femur/distal femur. When the pedestrian is taller, the impact is lower on the leg, most commonly the tibia. If the individual is facing toward or away from impact, bilateral tibia will be involved. If the individual is struck while walking, one side will take the impact. The victim is then either thrown away from the vehicle causing extremity, pelvis, thoracoabdominal, head/neck injuries, or flips up onto the hood of the vehicle and strikes the windshield increasing the potential for head, neck, and face injury.

A larger vehicle, such as a truck or SUV that has a higher bumper will strike the pedestrian at a higher site, such as the pelvis or abdomen, or perhaps the chest in a child. If the driver realizes an impact may occur and applies the brakes, the pedestrian will be struck lower on the body as the braking drops the bumper slightly lower.

Other Transport

The human body can be transported by multiple means. Other than MVC, the most common conveyances resulting in injury are bicycles and animals being ridden, such as horses and bull-riding. There are other conveyances, such as skateboards, skis/snowboards, and in-line skates, which have a fall event or if struck by a car, are similar to a pedestrian injury. Boating injuries occur and the clinician must consider the mechanism and identify if immersion or submersion was involved as well as exposure to other environmental issues, such as cold. Airplane/helicopter crashes are usually severe because of the velocities achieved during the fall or the severity of the crash (in air or on the ground). Vehicle-type injuries occur with or without burns if the passenger survives the event. This includes, of course, ultralight and other such craft falling from flight.

Bicycle and ATV

Because these vehicles transport a rider in the same unprotected way as a motorcycle, the mechanisms causing injury are the same as for motorcycles. Speed and place of injury may determine different circumstances of injury. Attention to the details of the event will provide the clues to suspected injuries.

Animal being ridden

A rider thrown from an animal being ridden is similar to a pedestrian struck by a vehicle. The impact is increased by the height of the fall and the degree to which the animal throws the rider.

Falls

Falls remain one of the most common mechanisms across the age groups, with the highest occurrence in children and the elderly. Falls can be as simple as tripping or slipping on a wet surface to falls from significant height, like parachutes and bungee jumping, that result in severe injuries. Diving injuries may not be caused by a high fall; however they involve the striking of the head/neck on the bottom surface resulting in hyperflexion. Other falls include falling downstairs, off playground equipment, or simply off a curb, or more serious intentional injuries, like jumping from a balcony or bridge. The mechanics of the fall and the position of landing give clues to the injuries sustained. In the case of intentional injury, psychiatric support must be anticipated in addition to identifying and managing the injuries.

Ground level

Simple ground level falls (GLF) happen to all age groups, however injury occurs more often in the elderly as the bones are more fragile. It is not uncommon for a ground level fall with a hip fracture to progress to a serious decrease in function and possibly death. Lumbar vertebra injuries are common as well as cervical spine injury from hyperflexion of the neck. Most GLF result in fractures or head injury dependent upon the surface and if a sharp or blunt object is struck on the way to the ground. In the elderly, a subdural hematoma is not uncommon, but normally progresses slowly. The patient and family may not remember the fall by the time symptoms occur from a slow hemorrhage.

Axial load

Falls from a height result in an axial load. It is important to identify the body part on which the victim landed. For example, landing on the feet can result in calcaneus and long bones fractures and possibly lumbar or thoracic spine fractures as the force travels up the body. Sometimes the victim has struck something on the way down resulting in injury to other body parts. The thoracic aorta due to its ligamentous attachments is particularly susceptible. Solid organs also do not tolerate the stress of the axial load and will fracture. The force of impact must be understood, for example, a fall of 10 ft is like catching a 200 lb bag of cement thrown out of a first story window.

Other

Other blunt trauma mechanisms include windsurfing, machinery crush mechanisms, falling objects, or sports injuries. Injuries are dependent upon the site of impact, transfer of energy, and environment.

PENETRATING TRAUMA

Penetrating injuries result from an object entering the body and sometimes exiting the body causing damage along the path. The object may not penetrate the fascia resulting in an external injury only. More commonly the object penetrates the fascia and injures underlying structures resulting in "open" injuries. On occasion the implement may still be present in the body. The velocity, size of the implement, and direction of entry and path determine the injuries.

Gunshot Wounds

Gunshot wounds (GSW) are usually intentional (suicide, homicide) but can be unintentional (hunting, gun not in holster, gun cleaning). Handguns are usually low-velocity weapons whereas rifles are high-velocity that inflict greater damage. However, not all handguns are low-velocity. The bullet forms a cavity that is a permanent hole and due to compression during entry, the surrounding tissue is pushed out of the way and deformed resulting in surrounding damage. There is also a shock wave present ahead of the bullet, which has a concussive effect. This wave causes serious injury in air- and fluid-filled spaces, like the lung. Other mechanisms at work with gunshots include

- Yaw: vertical and horizontal oscillation about the axis of the bullet; can result in a larger surface area on impact with the body depending on the position of the bullet on the axis at time of impact.
- Tumbling: rotation of the bullet upon impact resulting in some parts of the cavity larger than others as the bullet rotates along the path.
- Rifling: spiraling grooves within the barrel of the weapon put spin on the bullet as it exits the barrel; provides stability in flight along the axis.
- Hollow-point bullets: deform on impact causing a larger surface area to inflict damage.
- Shotgun: multiple pellets within the cartridge; also possible to have one large projectile, such as a "pumpkin ball," both air resistance and gravity spread the pellets over distance; closer shotgun wounds result in serious large wounds as the pellets remain clumped together.

The bullet does not usually travel in a straight path. This results in the need for exploration as multiple injuries can occur although the path appears to be in a straight line. Intentional injuries may require either psychiatric support (suicide attempts) or safety (homicide attempts).

Stabbing

Stabbings are also usually intentional (suicide, homicide) but can be unintentional, (eg, a slip on wet floor and landing on open dishwasher with knives pointing upward). A stabbing most often follows a direct path, is low velocity resulting mostly in damage along the line of the path itself, and are of varying depth. The type of blade affects the wound inflicted, such as straight blade versus a serrated edge. From a forensic medicine perspective, a stab is deeper than it is long and a cut is longer than deep. A cut differs from a blunt laceration in that the edges are clean and the direction of the wound inflicted indicates the direction of the force.

Stabs to the chest and abdomen are particularly important to investigate as the angle of the penetration may indicate that the wound crosses both cavities injuring the diaphragm in between the two.

Other

Impalement on objects (see Chapter 8, Figures 8-3 and 8-4) is another means of causing a penetrating injury. As with a typical stabbing by knife, the wound must be investigated and a determination made regarding both surgery and/or repair. Impalements have occurred on fences during rollover MVC, pieces of wood ejected from a saw, and various other and sometimes surprising mechanisms. The anticipated injuries are approached in the same manner as a knife stabbing.

Other "sharp" or penetrating injuries can occur from tools and machinery, fan blades, and other objects with a sharp edge. Any penetrating event results in "open" injuries in which the underlying injury has a direct communication with the external world via the wound path. Be aware that all penetrating events cause open injuries but not all open injuries are from penetrating mechanisms. An open fracture during an MVC is blunt trauma with an open fracture caused by the bone connecting with the environment from the inside-out.

BURNS

Thermal

Thermal burns are caused by extreme cold or long cold exposure with or without humidity or exposure to heat/direct flame. Exposure to heat can be in the form of hot air, hot water, chemicals with an exothermic reaction, or other hot substance. For example, water temperature of 140°F (60°C) causes a deep partial thickness to full thickness burn in 3 seconds of exposure (Auerbach 2007). Conflagration is the most common form of burn injury and is preventable by early warning from a smoke detector, not smoking in bed, and proper positioning of heating devices. Over 40% of house fires involve drug and alcohol use. Up to 25% of residential fires involve smoking (ENA 2007). Details on burn events and care are found in Chapter 10.

Other

Chemical burns can result from direct injury of the chemical and the skin interaction or indirect injury when the chemical results in an exothermic reaction producing heat. Some antidotes for chemicals produce the exothermic reaction of the chemical causing more injury than the chemical exposure itself.

Radiation exposure can also result in burn with the depth of burn varying with the type of radiation and length of exposure. The types of injury resulting from radiation exposure are discussed in Chapter 15.

Lightning causes up to 100 deaths per year in the United States. However, overall mortality is low due to a more common "flashover" burn rather than a high-voltage electrical injury. The flashover burn resulting from a lightning exposure is very superficial. The electrical and sound impact is more serious resulting in arrest, tympanic membrane rupture, and cataracts. Retinal detachment occurs with telephone-mediated lightning strikes.

Electrical, particularly high voltage, exposure results in serious burns from the inside out. The voltage travels along the nerves burning and coagulating tissue along the path to the exit from the body.

SPECIAL SITUATIONS—RISKS

Women

Overall, trauma in women spans all possible mechanisms, both blunt and penetrating. The risk for injuries to the genitourinary tract in women is actually low due to the safe positioning within the pelvis and the short length of the urethra. Pelvic fractures however, can result in vaginal lacerations with associated open, and now contaminated, pelvic fractures.

For women of childbearing age (10–50 years), 1 in every 12 pregnant women will sustain some injury with 4 in 1000 requiring medical admission for management (Hoyt and Selfridge-Thomas 2007, Mattox et al. 2000, ATLS 2008). A pregnant trauma patient also has a nearly 2 times increased risk of preterm delivery (Shah and Kilcline 2003).

In the pregnant woman, trauma is the leading cause of nonobstetrical maternal death (Ikossi et al. 2005, Shah et al. 1998, ENA 2007). The majority of these maternal deaths occur in the third trimester (Hoyt and Selfridge-Thomas 2007, ENA 2007). Head injury and shock are the leading causes of death for the mother although fetal survival is directly related to maternal shock (80%) and death (Hoyt and Selfridge-Thomas 2007, Patteson et al. 2007, Ziglar et al. 2004). Fetal death exceeds maternal death by a three-to-one ratio (Ikossi et al. 2005). The age of the fetus increases susceptibility to trauma especially after 24 weeks when the fetus is fully within the abdomen and is no longer protected by the pelvis. Gestational age at the time of delivery also affects fetal outcome (El-Kady et al. 2004, Shah and Kilcline 2003). Risk factors for fetal death include ejection from a vehicle, motorcycle crash, pedestrian struck by vehicle, and unrestrained in a MVC (Curet et al. 2000).

Blunt trauma is the most common mechanism of injury. In the pregnant trauma patient, the placenta is susceptible to the shear forces of blunt trauma caused by its inherent inelasticity resulting in abruptio placenta (Ziglar et al. 2004, ENA 2007, ATLS 2008). In pregnancy, MVC are the most common cause of injury (Ziglar et al. 2004, Patteson et al. 2007, Minow 1999, Metz and Abbott 2006, Mattox and Goetzi 2005, Baerga-Varela et al. 2000). Domestic violence during pregnancy occurs in at least 17% to 20% of women with up to 60% suffering repeated episodes of violence (Hoyt and Selfridge-Thomas 2007, Ziglar et al. 2004, ATLS 2008). These statistics are likely underestimated and are poorly documented because women do not report the cause or do not seek medical attention. Domestic violence frequently increases as delivery approaches.

The pregnant woman is also susceptible to falls caused by changes in her center of gravity that result in an altered gait, laxity of the pelvic joints, and fatigue (Ziglar et al. 2004, ENA 2007). If burns occur to the pregnant trauma patient there is an increased morbidity of up to 65% with burns of 20% to 50% TBSA (Ziglar et al. 2004). Delivery is recommended if TBSA exceeds 50%. It is essential to monitor the pregnant burn patient for carbon monoxide (CO) poisoning. Fetal hemoglobin has a much higher affinity for CO, which impairs the release of oxygen to the fetus.

Pediatrics

Over 10 million visits to the emergency department by children are due to injury. More than 10,000 of these children die (ATLS 2008). Approximately 11% of all pediatric intensive care unit admissions are trauma patients (Ponsky et al. 2005). Trauma remains the leading cause of death for children over 1 year and the second leading cause of death for those under 1 year (CDC-NCIPC 2008; Ziglar et al. 2004). The leading mechanism of injury resulting in death is MVC. In children under 10 years, unintentional drowning and burns are the second leading cause of death. The second leading cause of death for children over 10 years is homicide by firearms and suicide events. Falls are the leading cause of emergency department visits and admissions (Stewart et al. 2004). The mechanism shifts to recreational injuries in children aged 10 to 14 years. As the mechanisms become MVC, there is an increase in injury severity score (ISS) as well.

One would expect mechanisms of injury in children to be primarily focused on play. However the leading causes of injury involve motor vehicles with children as passengers or pedestrians. The body of a child is not strong enough or made to fit the design of seat belts until 8 years and therefore requires a car seat or booster seat.

Falls are frequent among children under 10 years. The awkward gait of the toddler as well as the large head leads to falls. In addition, as children mobilize, they are also curious and begin to investigate home hazards, like cords, hot water, sharp objects, etc. Falls are the most frequent mechanism under age 5 years, but the least frequent cause of death. As children reach school age, bicycles and sports injuries become more frequent. In children over 10 years, firearms play an increased role.

The majority of pediatric trauma deaths result from head injury. The anatomy of the small child lends itself to head injury. The head consists of 20% total body surface area of the body in the first year. The higher center of gravity also leads to loss of balance and head injury. The small size of the body experiences an increased applied force as it is distributed over the relatively larger body surface area. Muscle mass is less and therefore provides less protection. Penetrating wounds may also be deeper because of the thinner muscle wall.

Risk-taking behaviors increase as children participate in school activities and begin to drive. Bicycles, pedestrians struck, and MVC are leading mechanisms in which children make risk-taking decisions. In these instances they must choose to buckle up, wear a helmet, not drink and drive, choose their speed, look both ways, watch traffic, and more.

Geriatrics

Unintentional falls are the leading cause of trauma death in individuals 65 years and older (www.cdc.gov/ncipc). It is followed closely by MVC as the second leading cause of death. Trauma is the fifth overall leading cause of death for the elderly (Ziglar et al. 2004). Burns are also frequent for the elderly usually related to alcohol use, smoking in bed, or a building fire. With decreased touch sensation and pain receptors, the elderly are also susceptible to burns from scalds and touching hot objects, for example a stove or oven.

Geriatric patients are at risk for falls caused by postural instability, decreased coordination and motor strength, and balance difficulties. Other factors include past medical history, medications, and decreased physical reserve. Overall, the elderly are less likely to be injured than younger people but more likely to have a fatal outcome. Geriatric trauma patients are less likely to die at the scene than younger trauma patients but more likely to die in hospital with lower injury severity. Geriatric trauma patients have increased mortality and morbidity with lower severity of injury and less apparent instability (higher revised trauma scores). Comorbidities present their influence on outcome with previous myocardial infarction and pulmonary disease leading to an increased mortality after trauma. On the positive side, 80% of elderly trauma patients return to their previous state of health (ATLS 2004).

Obesity

The obese patient is particularly at risk in vehicular crashes because of the improper or lack of use of safety equipment. Most individuals require an extension on the seat belt. In addition, the placement of the belt itself may be too high across the abdomen instead of across the hips or the shoulder belt may be too close to the neck. Airbag deployment can result in increased incidence of chest injury. There is increased renal injury in abdominal trauma but less liver injury. Pelvic and lower extremity fractures are more likely. There is less facial injury. Because of a relatively unstable gait, the likelihood of falls is increased.

There is controversy regarding increased or similar mortality in obese patients versus average patients. Some studies identify obesity as an independent risk factor for mortality after trauma (Duane et al. 2006, Neville et al. 2004) and increased morbidity for bacteremia, urinary tract and respiratory infections (Bochicchio et al. 2006). Still others hold that age and injury severity are more closely associated with mortality than obesity (Alban et al. 2006).

Substance Abuse

Injury associated with substance abuse has been documented since 1500 BC in Egypt when people were warned that drinking beer could result in falling and breaking bones (Soderstrom et al. 2001). Alcohol has been associated with up to 10% of trauma deaths, in which 40% to 50% were MVC, and up to 67% of work- and home-related incidents. Intoxication is also associated with an increased prevalence of violent acts. In situations of domestic violence, intoxication is indicated in 66% of the situations and in 33% of violence to strangers. Intoxication is also present in 58% of suicides.

Intoxicated patients have a mortality two times that of those not intoxicated (Dischinger et al. 2001). The chronic drug user has significantly more serious injuries especially in males.

INJURY PREVENTION

With the degree of injury that is preventable, trauma centers need to focus on prevention programs and healthy communities. Although sometimes difficult to measure, a program is effective if even one injury is prevented. Programs should focus on local common causes of injury. The data is obtainable through the trauma registry and local databases, such as the medical examiner and police crash database. The American College of Surgeons Committee on Trauma requires an injury prevention coordinator at Levels I and II trauma centers to demonstrate the importance of these programs in the community (ACS-COT 2006).

Methods

Injury prevention programs use the interaction of factors that result in injury as the means to investigate as well as to prevent these injuries. Factors include the following:

- Human: predisposition to injury or choices that place the person at risk
- Energy transfer: the mechanism itself and the interaction of the kinetic energy with the body
- Environment: factors within the environment that enhance or inhibit the mechanism.

Analysis of local data provides the most common mechanisms as well as the use of safety mechanisms, such as seat belts and helmets. In addition to an analysis of common injury mechanisms, a community analysis of age, cultures, home and work environments provides insight into potential mechanisms as well. Injury prevention programs should focus on common mechanisms as well as potential mechanisms, such as drinking and driving on prom night. Prevention programs can be staged into three types of programs:

- Primary: focuses on preventing the injury before it happens by means of education (eg, road edge rumble strips, turn signals on traffic lights)
- Secondary: focuses on high-risk groups and is often accomplished through manipulation of the environment (eg, softer auto interiors, antilock brakes)
- Tertiary: focuses on injury prevention intervention after trauma to decrease recidivism (eg, home safety evaluation after an elder has fallen).

Programs are developed in three venues to affect the outcomes of various mechanisms. The three methods of prevention programs include the following:

- Education
  — Most commonly offered program
  — Lecture format, brochures, ads on television or newspaper/billboards
  — Common topics include
    - Motor vehicle safety (seat belts, car seats, airbags, drinking and driving, speed, elder driving training)
    - Playground safety (structure, surface, architecture)
    - Home safety (burn, fire prevention, fall prevention/exercise)
    - Gun safety (proper handling, locks/safes)
  — Messages should be simple, clear statements
  — Multiple programs already available; research programs before developing from scratch (Table 1-3)

Table 1-3   Injury Prevention Reference

Organization	Phone/Web site	Programs
American Trauma Society	1-800-556-7890 www.amtrauma.org	Traumaroo, fall prevention, home safety, second trauma, trauma survivors network
Emergency Nurses Association	www.ena.org	ENCare
National Highway Traffic Safety Administration	202-366-1836 www.nhtsa.gov	Brochures: traffic safety; red light running; school bus safety
CDC/NCIPC	404-639-3311 www.cdc.gov/ ncipc	Multiple areas of injury prevention and statistics
Consumer Product Safety Commission	1-800-638-2772 www.cpsc.gov	Baby safety showers; reports on consumer product safety and recalls
National Rifle Association	1-800-672-3888 www.nra.org	Gun safety, Eddie Eagle
National Fire Protection Agency	1-800-344-3555 www.nfpa.org	Burn safety programs; Sparky the Dog
American Burn Association	www.ameriburn.org	Burn safety programs
National Crime Prevention Council	518-842-4388 www.ncpc.org	Safety and crime prevention programs; McGruff the Dog
SafeKids	www.usa. safekids.org	Multiple safety programs for children
National Safety Commission	www. nationalsafety- commission.com	General safety information

- Environment (includes engineering in the public health model)
  - Automatic protection provided in which the consumer does not need to make many decisions
  - Examples include
    - Airbags
    - Antilock
    - Brakes
    - Road engineering
    - Automatic shut-off on electrical appliances
  - As common mechanisms are researched, means of protection are developed without human intervention that can provide safety. Primarily the realm of the engineers
- Enforcement
  - An effective means of prevention, however uses the threat of legal intervention if noncompliant
  - Examples include
    - Seat belt and child restraint laws
    - Drinking and driving laws and penalties
    - Red light running cameras at intersections
    - Graduated licensing
  - Although associated with fines or loss of license, in some situations the only method of increasing compliance is through enforcement.

Programs

Programs are directed to the appropriate audience and provided in a way to effect change. Not every program needs to be developed from scratch. There are programs on the market that can be adapted to the local region. Programs must include analysis of the community, distribution of the program appropriate for the community involved and in the appropriate language, and followed by an evaluation of the program for effectiveness. A program that provides even a 10% reduction in injury would demonstrate effectiveness (Stewart 2007). The removal of even one predisposing factor, such as intoxication, speed, and lesser use of seat belt or helmet, would decrease the severity of injury (Stewart 2007). Table 1-3 lists resources for available programs.

Injury Prevention Issues

Pregnancy

As with all injury prevention, during pregnancy it is essential for the safety of the mother and the fetus. Studies show that 33 to 50% of pregnant women in MVC were not using seat belts (Ikossi et al. 2005, Metz and Abbott 2006, Minow 1999, ATLS 2008). Worn improperly, the seat belt across the abdomen can result in uterine rupture. Lap-only belts can compress the uterus and bladder. Proper use should position the lap portion of the seat belt below the "belly." Instruction in proper seat belt use as well as its importance at all times is essential during pre-natal visits (Figure 1-1). Drug and alcohol abuse has also been evident in 20% to 50% of the incidences of trauma (Ikossi et al. 2005, Minow 1999). Prenatal education should consistently include the risks of substance abuse effects on the fetus as well as increased risk of injury. Fall prevention through awareness of the awkward gait will also assist the mother safely through the pregnancy period. For domestic violence, identification of the occurrence along with providing safe housing availability through social services and the legal system is the key to break-ing the cycle. The National Domestic Violence Hotline is 1-800-799-SAFE (www.ndvh.org, www.CDC.gov/ncipc)

Pediatrics

Injury prevention efforts focus on the most common areas of potential injury for the age group. All age groups require motor vehicle safety. Infants up to 1 year of age and 20 lb must be in a rear-facing child seat and placed in the rear seat (NHTSA 2008). Infant car seats placed in the front can result in death from airbag deployment. The infant then graduates to a forward-facing

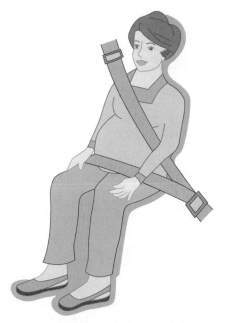

Figure 1-1   Proper seat belt use in the pregnant patient. (Illustration by Maggie Reynard.)

car seat until they are approximately 4 years or 40 lb. A booster seat is then required until approximately 8 years old. No child should be seated in the front seat until 12 years when the bones are strong enough to tolerate an impact while restrained in a seat belt. Car seat clinics with trained technicians are one of the best ways to teach car seat safety. As adolescents begin to drive, injury prevention focused on the operation of the vehicle is essential as peer pressure will test them otherwise.

Every aspect of the child's life is injury focused. Baby safety showers teach parents how to prepare the house to keep the baby safe through the early stages of mobility. Home safety protects children as they become curious and mobile. Crossing the street safely and not chasing toys into the street prevent pedestrian events. Bicycle helmets are essential from the tricycle and on to larger vehicles even if children stay on the sidewalk. Playground safety prevents serious injury from falls. Gun safety keeps weapons away from children and locked. Bicycle rodeos and helmet give-a-ways reach out to children who may not be able to afford a helmet. Safety towns provide a means to learn traffic safety. Prom night and preprom programs provide information for teens about drinking and driving and other risk-taking behaviors.

Geriatrics

Injury prevention programs need to focus on the primary causes of injury for the elderly. There are programs designed to retest drivers older than 55 years to assess reflexes and driving skills. Seat belt education is always necessary especially since a large population of the elderly drove for many years before seat belts existed in every vehicle. Fall prevention is the topmost priority. These programs involve topics from home evaluations for safety hazards to exercise programs to maintain healthy muscles, bone, and balance. Exercise can decrease the incidence of hip fractures by up to 20% (Ziglar et al. 2004). Overall, injury prevention needs to include programs for healthy nutrition with calcium and vitamin D, and exercise to maintain a strong body with good balance and gait, as well as programs to enhance alertness and memory. Increased awareness of the most common causes of injury may decrease incidence of injury and include the following:

- Changes in medications
- Vision changes, changes to prescription of eyewear
- Decreased judgment and reaction time, especially when deciding to wear a seat belt, changing traffic lanes, and merging

Burns

Burn centers have extensive injury prevention programs and should include the elderly. Burn prevention activities have been the most effective programs as evidenced by the decreasing number of burn admissions. The local burn center is a resource for assistance with burn prevention programs.

Substance abuse

From trauma's perspective, a patient with alcoholism is three and a half times more likely to experience a second trauma. If these patients can be identified early in their trauma care, there is a perfect opportunity for intervention and prevention of recidivism. The best injury prevention is to encourage a designated driver and moderation of intake. Drug use has multiple other risks as well. Drug prevention programs with complete abstinence are the only program for these substances. As noted in Chapter 12, substance abuse screening and intervention are required by the ACS-COT (2006).

REFERENCES

Alban RF, Lyass S, Marqulies DZ, et al. Obesity does not affect mortality after trauma. *Ann Surg.* 2006;72(10):966-969.

American College of Surgeons. *Advanced Trauma Life Support* (ATLS). 7th ed. Chicago, IL: American College of Surgeons, 2004.

American College of Surgeons. *Advanced Trauma Life Support* (ATLS). 8th ed. Chicago, IL: American College of Surgeons, 2008.

American College of Surgeons Committee on Trauma (ACS-COT). *Resources for Optimal Care of the Injured Patient.* Chicago, IL: American College of Surgeons, 2006.

Auerbach P. *Wilderness Medicine.* 5th ed. St Louis, MO: CV Mosby, 2007.

Baerga-Varela Y, Zietlow SP, Bannon MP, et al. Trauma in pregnancy. *Mayo Clin Proc.* 2000;75(12):1243-1248.

Bochicchio GV, Joshi M, Bochicchio K, et al. Impact of obesity in the critically ill trauma patient: a prospective study. *J Am Coll Surg.* 2006;203(4):533-538.

CDC. Injury prevention. www.cdc.gov/ncipc/osp/data.htm/. Accessed November 10, 2008.

Curet MJ, Schermer CR, Demarest GB, et al. Predictors of outcome in trauma during pregnancy: identification of patients who can be monitored for less than 6 hours. *J Trauma.* 2000;49(2):18-24.

Dischinger P, Mitchell KA, Kufera JA, et al. A longitudinal study of former trauma center patients: the association between toxicology status and subsequent injury mortality. *J Trauma.* 2001;51(5): 877-886.

Dissanaike S, Kaufman R, Mack CD, et al. The effect of reclined seats on mortality in motor vehicle collisions. *J Trauma.* 2008;64(3): 614-619.

Donaldson W, Hanks S, Nassr A, et al. Cervical spine injuries associated with the incorrect use of airbags in motor vehicle collisions. *Spine.* 2008;33(6):631-634.

Duane TM, Dechert T, Aboutanos MB, et al. Obesity and outcomes after blunt trauma. *J Trauma.* 2006;61(5):1218-1221.

El-Kady D, Gilbert WM, Anderson J, et al. Trauma during pregnancy: an analysis of maternal and fetal outcomes in a large population. *Am J Obstet Gynecol.* 2004;190(6):1661-1668.

Emergency Nurses Association (ENA). *Trauma Nursing Core Curriculum.* 6th ed. Des Plaines, IL: Emergency Nurses Association; 2007.

Goslar PW, Crawford NR, Petersen SR, et al. Helmet use and associated spinal fractures in motorcycle crash victims. *J Trauma.* 2008;64(1):190-196.

Hoyt KS, Selfridge-Thomas J. *Emergency Nursing Core Curriculum.* 6th ed. St Louis, MO: Saunders Elsevier; 2007.

2009 Ingenix ICD9-CM Expert-Hospitals Vol 1, 2, & 3. Eden Prairie, MN: Ingenix, 2008.

Ikossi DG, Lazar AA, Morabito D, et al. Profile of mothers at risk: an analysis of injury and pregnancy loss in 1195 trauma patients. *J Am Coll Surg.* 2005;200(1):49-56.

Mattox KL, Feliciano DV, Moore EE. *Trauma.* 4th ed. New York, NY: McGraw-Hill; 2000.

Mattox KL, Goetzi L. Trauma in pregnancy. *Crit Care Med.* 2005;33(10)(suppl):S385-S389.

Metz TD, Abbott JT. Uterine trauma in pregnancy after MVCs with airbag deployment: a 30 case series. *J Trauma.* 2006;61(3): 658-661.

Minow M. Violence against women: a challenge to the supreme court. *N Engl J Med.* 1999;341(25):1927-1929.

National Committee for Injury Prevention and Control (CDC-NCIPC). *Injury Prevention: Meeting the Challenge.* Newton, MA: Educational Development Center; 1989.

NDVH. Domestic violence hotline. www.ndvh.org/. Accessed November 10, 2008.

Neville AL, Brown CV, Weng J, et al. Obesity is an independent risk factor of mortality in severely injured blunt trauma patients. *Arch Surg.* 2004;139(9):983-987.

NHTSA. Automotive safety. www.NHTSA.gov/. Accessed November 10, 2008.

Patteson SK, Snider CC, Meyer DS, et al. The consequences of high risk behavior in trauma during pregnancy. *J Trauma.* 2007;62(4): 1015-1020.

Ponsky TA, Eichelberger MR, Cardozo E, et al. Analysis of head injury admission trends in an urban American pediatric trauma center. *J Trauma.* 2005;59(6):1292-1297.

Ryb GE, Dischinger PC, Kufera JA, et al. Principal direction of force, and restraint use contributions to motor vehicle collision mortality. *J Trauma.* 2007;63(5):1000-1005.

Shah AJ, Kilcline BA. Trauma in pregnancy. *Emerg Med Clin North Am.* 2003;21(3):615-629.

Shah KH, Simons RK, Holbrook T, et al. Trauma in pregnancy: maternal and fetal outcomes. *J Trauma.* 1998;45(1):83-86.

Sisley AC. Preventing motor vehicle collisions (no accidents please!). *J Trauma.* 2007;62(6):849-850.

Soderstrom CA, Cole FJ, Porter JM. Injury in America: the role of alcohol and other drugs; an EAST position paper prepared by the injury control and violence prevention committee. *J Trauma.* 2001;50(1):1-12.

Stewart RM. Trauma systems and prevention summary for injury prevention. *J Trauma.* 2007;62(6):S46.

Stewart TC, Grant K, Singh R, et al. Pediatric trauma in Southwest Ontario: linking data with injury prevention initiatives. *J Trauma.* 2004;57(4):787-794.

Wilding L, O'Brien J, Pagliarello G, et al. Survey of current injury prevention practices by registered nurses in the emergency department. *J Emerg Nurs.* 2008;34(2):106-111.

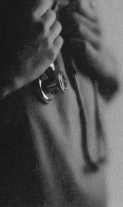

Chapter 2

TRAUMA RESUSCITATION AND STABILIZATION

INTRODUCTION

Trauma care begins at the scene with appropriate bystander and prehospital care and extends through resuscitation and rehabilitation. The foundation for the trauma patient's survival is based upon this care. Clear and rapid decisions are made during this phase of trauma, as well as immediate actions to manage identified injuries.

ASSESSMENT

Assessment of the trauma patient begins at the scene. Based upon the patient's anatomical injuries, physiologic response, and the mechanism, triage decisions are made. Triage from the scene determines the destination as well as the interventions needed immediately. Where there is no trauma center, transport to the closest facility is necessary. The facility may then transfer the patient to the appropriate level of trauma center in a timely manner. Transport to a trauma center is the optimal choice. Within the trauma center, the decision to activate the highest level trauma team is based upon physiology and/or site of anatomical injury. Mechanism of injury may activate a lower level of trauma team response in anticipation of potential injury.

Triage recommendations for trauma center destination include (ACS-COT 2006, Barraco et al. 2008)

Physiology:

- Glasgow coma scale (GCS) score <10; deterioration of level of consciousness
- Systolic blood pressure (BP) <90 mm Hg
- Respiratory rate (RR) <10 or >29 breaths per minute

Anatomy:

- Spinal cord injury
- Penetrating head, neck, torso, proximal extremity injuries
- Proximal amputations (proximal to wrist or ankle), mangled extremity
- Flail chest
- Pelvic fractures, two or more long bone fractures, open fractures
- Fracture with vascular injury or ischemia
- Open or depressed skull fracture

Mechanism:

- Motor vehicle collision with fatality, ejection, intrusion more than one foot
- Fall >20 feet or >2 times child's height
- Pedestrian or cyclist thrown or impact >20 mph
- Motorcycle crash >20 mph

Comorbidities:

- Anticoagulation
- Age >55 years, or children
- Burns with trauma
- Dialysis
- Pregnancy >20 weeks
- Prehospital provider decision

History

During the call from prehospital or on arrival of the patient by emergency medical services (EMS), police, or private vehicle, the story of the mechanism is essential to understand the potential injuries. The patient's personal history will also impact survival as well as the response to treatment. Collection of the history includes the following:

- Mechanism of injury
  - Safety equipment: seat belts, car seat, airbags, helmet, protective clothing
  - Speed, ejection, extrication
  - Collision: two vehicles, single vehicle, point of impact
  - Fatality, intrusion, degree of damage of vehicle
  - Weapon used if known, assault with object or fists/kicked
  - Height of fall, intent, surface, position of landing
  - Submersion, immersion
  - Impaled object
- Scene information
  - Responsiveness, GCS, pupils
  - Vital signs: BP, RR, pulse
  - Capillary refill, especially if pulse not available
  - Environment: temperature, rain/dry, length of exposure
  - Interventions: intravenous (IV) line, oxygen, spinal immobilization, medications, splinting
- Comorbidities
  - Allergies: medications, foods, latex
  - Medications: especially antiplatelets and anticoagulants
  - Past medical and surgical history: especially diabetes, cardiac disease, renal disease
    - Alcohol and drug use
  - Last menstrual period/pregnancy
  - Last meal

Trauma Team Preparation

In preparation for or on arrival of the trauma patient several activities occur. A trauma team activation is called to move the necessary members of the trauma team to the trauma resuscitation bay.

The team members include the trauma surgeon, emergency physician, nurses, anesthetist, laboratory technician, and blood bank, respiratory therapy, and radiology technicians. The response varies according to the level of trauma center and the level of activation. As the members arrive, documentation of the mechanism is initiated and the team prepares as follows:

- Don personal protective equipment (PPE) for universal pre-cautions
  — Gloves
  — Gowns and/or aprons
  — Booties, head covers
  — Masks and goggles or masks with face shields
- Warm the trauma room
- Warm IV fluids available, blood products available
- Activate trauma team
  — If level III, IV trauma center or nontrauma center, may already anticipate transfer and prepare transport for stand-by as well as trauma center communication
  — Perform the interventions necessary to stabilize the patient for transport but do not spend time obtaining computed tomography (CT) scans if there is no one present who can treat the injuries identified
  — CT and magnetic resonance imaging (MRI) scanners put the patient in a situation of risk with minimal access until the studies are complete; only stable patients should travel to the CT or MRI scanner with staff present and on cardiac and BP monitors
  — Sign in each member upon arrival
- Anticipate injuries and prepare equipment accordingly, such as cricothyrotomy or chest tube trays

When the patient arrives, the assessment and management follow in order to determine the most life-threatening injuries first. During the primary survey, interventions are performed as the issues are identified. There is no delay in the performance of these procedures. The following discussion includes both assessment and simultaneous management.

Primary Survey and Interventions

As with all life-threatening conditions, resuscitation begins with airway. Do not move forward in the assessment until the immediate issues are under control. A primary survey should take no longer than 60 seconds, and longer only when interventions are necessary. The trauma team is present to make the interventions happen as quickly as possible. Airway is the absolute first priority and loss of the airway is the leading cause of preventable death in trauma.

Signs and Symptoms of Airway Problems

Verbal response, dysphonia, hoarseness, gurgling
Stridor, accessory muscle use, nasal flaring
Altered mental status
Hypoxemia despite oxygen
Facial or oropharyngeal burns, laryngeal edema
Foreign body or tongue prolapse
Facial fractures, bleeding, epistaxis
Secretions, vomiting

Airway assessment
* Airway management
   — Apply 100% O_2 via nonrebreather mask in all trauma patients
   — Open the airway while maintaining cervical spine immobilization
      ▪ Chin lift or jaw thrust maneuver
      ▪ A towel clip may be used to retract the tongue, if necessary

- Apply rigid cervical collar if not present on arrival
  - There is no place for a soft cervical collar; assume cervical injury until proven otherwise
  - Cervical collar remains on until after resuscitation and the cervical spine is cleared (Chapter 5)
- Obstruction may be resolved as easily as suctioning vomitus and blood from the oropharynx
- If vomiting occurs, turn the patient with the backboard to the right
- Always have suction immediately available
— Airway adjunct placement if patient unable to maintain airway
  - Nasopharyngeal airway: do not place if facial fractures present
  - Oropharyngeal airway: place directly, do not rotate
  - Assists with maintaining tongue position and suctioning
— Emergent intubation—endotracheal tube (ETT)
  - Indications: obstruction, apnea or hypoventilation, hypoxemia despite oxygen, GCS < 9, facial injury, hypotension/hemorrhage, severe chest injury, arrest
  - Nasotracheal intubation is contraindicated in facial fractures and apnea
  - Orotracheal best choice for trauma
  - Bag-valve-mask ventilation until intubated
  - Remove the front of the cervical collar while maintaining manual in-line immobilization
    - Figure 2-1 demonstrates an iatrogenic cervical spine injury from an unprotected intubation in a patient where cervical injury was unsuspected but was actually present
  - Apply cricoid pressure to obstruct the esophagus during intubation
  - Preoxygenate with 100% O_2 prior to induction
  - Administer rapid sequence intubation (RSI) consisting of

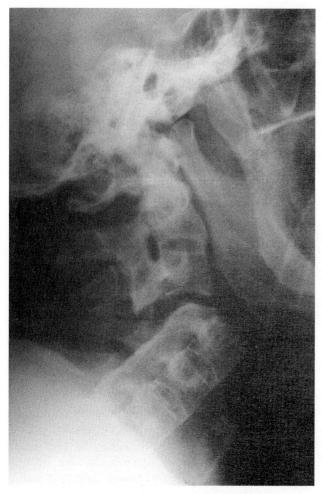

Figure 2-1   Iatrogenic cervical spine injury after intubation.

- o Induction agent—etomidate
- o Neuromuscular blockade—vecuronium, anectine (succinylcholine)
- o Anectine is a depolarizing agent that causes the release of potassium from the cells by opening the sodium channels; fasciculations result; avoid in chronic renal patients and head injury patients
- o Sedation—midazolam, fentanyl
- o Lidocaine may be used in head injury patients to prevent increased intracranial pressure during intubation
- Pass the endotracheal tube
  - o May be facilitated with a flexible bougie as a tracheal tube introducer (Ollerton et al. 2006)
- Check positioning
  - o Listen for bilateral breath sounds and over the epigastrium
  - o Breath sounds on the right only may indicate mainstem intubation; reposition the tube
  - o No breath sounds indicates malpositioned tube; reintubate; oxygenate in between intubations and maintain saturations >90%
  - o End-tidal CO_2 detector or color change colorimeter to determine presence of CO_2 and proper positioning of the tube
  - o It is very difficult to intubate the left mainstem bronchus
  - o Vomitus in the ETT indicates positioning in the esophagus or aspiration; check breath sounds, suction, reposition the tube if esophageal
  - o Chest x-ray
- Prepare a mechanical ventilator and apply to the patient once the airway is secure
  - o Monitor pulse oximetry continuously
- If unable to intubate after two attempts, prepare for a surgical airway (Ollerton et al. 2006)

- Continue bagging the patient manually until the airway is secured
- Monitor the ventilator or bag rate to prevent hyperventilation and dropping PCO_2

— Alternative airways

- If unable to intubate, an alternative airway option must be placed
- Laryngeal mask airway (LMA) serves as a temporary airway (Figures 2-2 and 2-3)
  - Used most often for surgery but can provide oxygenation and ventilation until a definitive ETT or surgical airway is present
  - Requires training for placement
  - Serves as a temporary airway only and intubation must be established as quickly as possible
  - The mask seals the larynx forcing ventilation directly into the trachea
  - Vomiting may occur when removed
- Combitube is another temporary airway used primarily in the prehospital setting
  - Functions to obstruct the esophagus with a balloon; the second balloon seals the pharynx

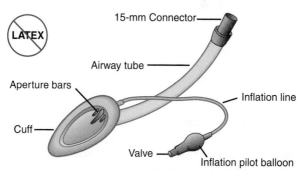

Figure 2-2   LMA. (Courtesy of LMA North America.)

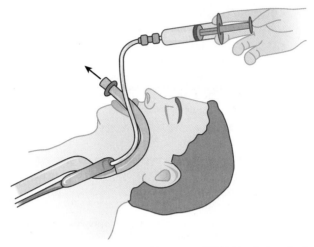

Figure 2-3   LMA in position. (Courtesy of LMA North America.)

- o If the tube is placed into the trachea, the tracheal balloon can be inflated and used as an ETT until exchanged
- o Requires exchange for an ETT or surgical airway
- o High likelihood of vomiting with removal
- Surgical cricothyrotomy
  - o May be necessary for facial fractures or when intubation is unsuccessful
  - o Once entry is made either a tracheostomy tube or an endotracheal tube can be placed through the stoma until a definitive tracheostomy is done

Breathing assessment

Once the airway is established, attention is turned to breathing/ventilation. Respiratory rate should be counted and assessed for quality, symmetry, depth. Observe chest movement for symmetry and palpate the rib cage for a flail segment moving independently of the chest wall and subcutaneous emphysema. Listen to breath sounds for equality, clarity, and presence.

Signs and Symptoms of Breathing Problems

Labored breathing, shallow respirations
Tachypnea
Hypoxia
Decreased breath sounds on the side of injury (hemothorax, pneumothorax)
Distended neck veins (tension pneumothorax)
Tracheal deviation (tension pneumothorax)
Pale, cyanotic
Delayed capillary refill
Dullness to percussion (blood); tympanic to percussion (air)
Paradoxical respirations (flail)
Pain (rib fractures, flail, pneumothorax)

- Breathing management
  — Open "sucking" pneumothorax requires a three-sided dressing that acts as a valve, sealing the hole during inspiration
    ■ Do not use the open wound as the entry point for the chest tube; the wound should be sutured
    ■ Place a large bore chest tube immediately
    ■ If the tube is not placed immediately, a tension pneumothorax may occur
  — Absence or decreased breath sounds with or without subcutaneous emphysema indicates mainstem bronchus intubation, hemothorax, or pneumothorax
    ■ First adjust the ETT position by pulling back and reassess
    ■ If pneumothorax is suspected move on to placement of a chest tube

— Pneumothorax must be identified and treated immediately to prevent progression to a tension pneumothorax and especially in the case of positive pressure ventilation after intubation

- A tension pneumothorax is a life-threatening situation and may present first as sudden hypotension, tracheal deviation, and occasionally jugular vein distention
- Treatment is immediate chest tube placement

— Be prepared with 32 to 36 French chest tubes and a collection device with waterseal

- Chapter 7 discusses chest tube preparation, insertion, and management

— If a chest tube is not immediately available, a large-bore IV catheter can be placed over the third rib, midclavicular line to temporarily relieve the pneumothorax

- Leave the catheter in place until a chest tube can be positioned

— Patients may arrive with a needle thoracostomy done in the field

- Requires chest tube on arrival whether or not a pneumothorax is present

— Continue to monitor the chest as even after chest tube placement, a pneumothorax can reaccumulate and/or cause a tension pneumothorax

- Check that the tubing is secure and connected to 20-cm H_2O suction
- Check that no one or piece of equipment is standing on the suction tubing or drainage tubing; check connections
- Check for tube holes outside the chest wall
- Reassess

— Flail chest results in ineffective breathing

- Splint the chest by using positive end-expiratory pressure (PEEP) on the ventilator and/or pain management
- DO NOT place tape, ace wrap, or a binder as these inhibit full respiration

- Manage pain
- See Chapter 7 for discussion of rib fractures, flail, and pain management

Circulation assessment

Circulation issues are complex and will be managed continuously throughout resuscitation until occult hypoperfusion is resolved and all sources of bleeding are under control. The first BP taken should always be manual and then periodically checked manually thereafter. In the interim automatic BP readings every 5 to 15 minutes are essential. Pulses in all extremities must be assessed to identify possible limb-threatening vascular injury. All obvious bleeding requires pressure to halt the bleeding. Check pulses distal to the site. Table 2-1 lists signs and symptoms of shock. An ECG monitor should be applied for rhythm and rate monitoring.

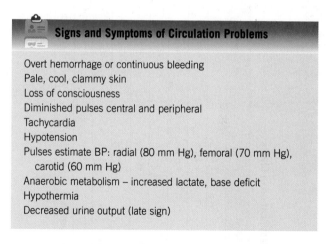

Signs and Symptoms of Circulation Problems

Overt hemorrhage or continuous bleeding
Pale, cool, clammy skin
Loss of consciousness
Diminished pulses central and peripheral
Tachycardia
Hypotension
Pulses estimate BP: radial (80 mm Hg), femoral (70 mm Hg), carotid (60 mm Hg)
Anaerobic metabolism – increased lactate, base deficit
Hypothermia
Decreased urine output (late sign)

- Circulation management

The triad of death includes coagulopathy, hypothermia, and acidosis. Each component feeds the others. Management of airway, breathing, and then circulation should control the three

Table 2-1 Classification of Shock

	I	II	III	IV
Blood loss	<750 mL	750-1500 mL	1500-2000 mL	>2000 mL
Blood loss %	<15%	15-30%	30-40%	>40%
Blood pressure	Normal	Normal	↓	↓
Pulse	<100	>100	>120	>140
Capillary refill	Normal	>3 seconds	>3 seconds	>3 seconds
Skin	Normal	Cool, clammy	Cool, clammy	Cold, pale
Respiratory rate	14-20	20-30	30-40	>35
Urine output	>30 mL/hour	20-30 mL/hour	5-15 mL/hour	<5 mL/hour
Level of consciousness	Slightly anxious	Mildly anxious	Anxious, confused	Confused, lethargic

components. Damage control resuscitation approaches these three issues through normalization of temperature, pH, base deficit, international normalized ratio (INR), and aggressive coagulopathy control (Holcomb 2007, Gonzales et al. 2007). Permissive hypotension (BP 90 mm Hg) through minimization of prehospital fluids prevents rebleeding with resuscitation. In the case of head injury, do not allow the BP to drop <90 mm Hg to prevent secondary brain injury.

— In some urban or suburban situations, it may be appropriate for rapid transport without IV fluids (permissive hypotension) to prevent hemorrhage with volume replacement, as some studies demonstrate improved survival

  ▪ Short transport <20 minutes with BP <100 mm Hg there is little influence of prehospital fluids (Moore 2006)

  ▪ Maintain BP ~90 mm Hg to prevent rebleeding

  ▪ Rapid access to surgical control of hemorrhage is required

— Warm the room and all fluids or blood products administered to the patient to prevent hypothermia

  ▪ Coagulation factors decrease activity by 10% for every degree decrease in temperature (Beckley 2008)

  ▪ Warm fluids to 39°C

— Apply pressure to any obvious bleeding

— If the patient is taking anticoagulants, prepare to administer fresh frozen plasma (FFP) and vitamin K to reverse the effects

  ▪ Note that antiplatlet medications are not reversible and unlike aspirin, administering platelets does not reestablish clotting

— Establish two large-bore IV (12-16 g) with warm fluids (lactated ringers or normal saline)

  ▪ Draw labwork at the same time as placing the IV line (Table 2-2)

    ○ Labs include type and cross, complete blood count (CBC), basic chemistry, lactic acid, blood alcohol level, pregnancy test if not done as point of care testing

Table 2-2 Laboratory Studies

Laboratory Study	Normals	Alterations
Complete blood count (CBC)		
Hemoglobin (Hgb)	Female: 12-16 g/dL Male: 14-18 g/dL	↓ hypovolemia
Hematocrit (Hct)	Female: 37-47% Male: 42-52%	↓ hypovolemia, hemodilution
Erythrocytes (RBC)	Female: 4.2-5.4 mm^6 Male: 4.7-6.1 mm^6	↓ hemorrhage ↑ high altitude, burns, pregnancy, dehydration
Leukocytes (WBC)	4.8-10.8 /mm^3	↓ analgesics ↑ hemorrhage, infection, burns
Lymphocytes Monocytes	20.5-51.1% 1.7-9.3%	↑ TB, lupus, rocky mounted spotted fever
Basophils Neutrophils	0-2% 42.2-75.2%	↓ pregnancy, dehydration, vomiting ↑ postsplenectomy, burn
Eosinophils	0-6%	↑ infection, stress, postsplenectomy, asthma, allergy

Platelets	130,000–400,000/mm^3	↓ postsplenectomy, antipyretics ↑ hemorrhage, pancreatitis
Coagulation		
PT	Same as control (~11.5–14.1 seconds)	↑ vitamin K deficiency, anticoagulant (warfarin), DIC
PTT	23.7–37 seconds	↑ anticoagulant (heparin)
INR	1.0	↑ anticoagulant use
Chemistry		
Potassium	3.5–5.1 mMol/L	↓ diuretics, vomiting or N/G suction, renal injury, alcoholism, heat stroke ↑ dehydration, renal failure
Sodium	135–145 mMol/L	↓ dehydration, diuretics, vomiting, or N/G suction ↑ acidosis, burns
Chloride	98–107 mMol/L	↓ emphysema, diarrhea, diuretics ↑ renal failure, dehydration

(Continued)

Table 2-2 Laboratory Studies (*Continued*)

Laboratory Study	Normals	Alterations
BUN	Female: 7-17 mg/dL Male: 9-20 mg/dL	↓ late pregnancy, malnutrition ↑ hypovolemia, renal failure
Creatinine	Female: 0.6-1.0 mg/dL Male: 0.7-1.3 mg/dL	As for BUN
Glucose	65-99 mg/dL	↓ malnutrition, hepatitis ↑ pancreatitis, DM, dehydration
Magnesium	1.6-2.3 mg/dL	↓ diarrhea, diuretics, toxemia of pregnancy ↑ renal failure, antacids with Mg^{++}, dehydration
Calcium	Total: 8.4-10.2 mg/dL Ionized: 1.15-1.35 mMol/L	↓ pancreatitis, diarrhea, alkalosis ↑ prolonged immobility, respiratory acidosis
Amylase	30-110 units/L	↑ pancreatic injury
Lipase	23-300 units/L	↑ pancreatic injury
Lactic acid	0.7-2.1 mMol/L	↑ occult hypoperfusion, crush injury

Liver studies		
AST (aspartate aminotransferase)	Female: 14-36 units/L Male: 17-59 units/L	↑ cirrhosis, hepatitis, liver injury
ALT (alanine aminotransferase)	Female: 9-52 units/L Male: 21-72 units/L	↑ celiac disease, cirrhosis, hepatitis, liver injury, hypovolemic shock
Arterial blood gas (ABG)		
pH	7.35-7.45	↓ acidosis, diarrhea, hypoventilation, hemorrhage ↑ hyperventilation, alkalosis, N/G suction
PCO_2	35-48 mm Hg	↓ alkalosis, hyperventilation ↑ acidosis, hypoventilation
PO_2	83-108 mm Hg	↓ ARDS, hemorrhage, COPD
Bicarbonate (HCO_3)	18-23 mMol/L	↓ diarrhea, alkalosis ↑ acidosis, bicarbonate administration
Base	−2 to 2 mMol/L	↓ occult hypoperfusion
Saturation	90-100%	↓ hemorrhage, COPD, ARDS, pulmonary injury ↑ CO poisoning demonstrates a false normal or elevation

(Continued)

Table 2-2 Laboratory Studies (*Continued*)

Laboratory Study	Normals	Alterations
Cerebral spinal fluid (CSF)		
Color, clarity	Straw, clear (colorless, xanthochromic)	Cloudy: meningitis/ cerebral infection Pink/red: subarachnoid hemorrhage (SAH)
Glucose	40-70 mg/dL	↓ cerebral infection, meningitis, SAH ↑ cerebral injury, hypothalamic lesions
Protein	12-60 mg/dL	↑ cerebral infection, meningitis, SAH
Total cell count with differential	0-8 mm³	↓ cerebral infarction, inflammation ↑ cerebral infection, SAH
Opening pressure	0-20 mm Hg	↑ meningitis, increased ICP
Diagnostic peritoneal lavage (DPL)		
RBC	Negative	>100,000 RBC/mm³ positive lavage
WBC	Negative	>500 WBC/mm³ positive lavage
Amylase	Negative	>175 units positive lavage
Other	Negative	Presence of bacteria, vegetable, fibers, or fecal matter—positive lavage

- If unable to place peripheral lines, use a large central line or intraosseous line (IO)
  - In children IO are typically placed in the tibia
  - In adults there is a device capable of placing a rapid sternal IO
— Anticipate the need for warm rapid fluid administration
  - Warm the fluids in an appropriately monitored blood warmer or fluid administration unit such as a Level I or Belmont; DO NOT use the microwave
  - Use appropriate IV tubing to prevent resistance to high flow
  - Approximate fluid replacement is 3:1 for crystalloid to blood loss and 1:1 for blood
  - Administer warmed lactated ringer (LR) solution or normal saline wide open rate
    - LR solution is the fluid of choice (Kortbeek et al. 2008); activates the immune system; causes the least variation in thrombin generation (Brommel-Ziedins et al. 2006)
    - Normal saline administration can result in acidosis
    - After 2 L of crystalloid, blood products are necessary if the patient remains a nonresponder or transient responder and the source of bleeding remains without control
    - Assess base deficit or lactate to determine progress towards resuscitation
  - Vasopressors are NOT substitutes for volume restoration and direct hemorrhage control
— Blood products
  - Packed red blood cells (PRBC), FFP, platelets, cryoprecipitate, recombinant factor VIIa (rFVIIa) must be immediately available to the resuscitation area, intensive care unit (ICU), and operating room (OR)
  - Hyperkalemia can occur with PRBC administration
    - Ongoing hemorrhage prevents redistribution of the potassium
    - Blood older than 14 days can result in hyperkalemia (Perkins et al. 2008)

- Aged blood products have been associated with acute lung injury; avoid if possible
- Administer O⁻ blood to women of child-bearing age or O⁺ to men and women older than child-bearing age until type-specific blood is available
  - Type-specific blood may be available before type and crossmatched blood; use this to protect the stock of O blood
- Initiate FFP along with PRBC early to prevent loss of plasma factors and decrease mortality (Spinella et al. 2008)
- Initiate massive transfusion protocol
— Patients respond in various ways dependent upon the degree of hemorrhage and the presence of ongoing hemorrhage
  - Brisk responder: blood loss <35%
    - Stabilizes and remains stable after fluid administration
  - Transient responder: blood loss 35% to 45%
    - Normalizes with fluids but slips back to hypotension quickly requiring continuous fluid replacement, blood products
  - Nonresponder: blood loss >50%
    - Remains hypotensive despite fluids and blood products
    - Anticipate need for OR or angiography with embolization depending upon the source of bleeding
— If there is significant blood loss from the chest, anticipate autotransfusion having the extra sterile collection chamber attached to the chest tube setup
  - Most setups no longer require citrate
  - Follow hospital protocol for administration of autotransfusion
  - Potential for microemboli; use a 140 to 170 micron filter in the IV line

— Identify internal sources of bleeding

- Blood accumulates in the abdomen, pelvis, chest, and retroperitoneum and may not demonstrate any external injury
  - Performing the focused abdominal sonography for trauma (FAST) examination is appropriate at this point in the survey to promptly identify intra-abdominal or intrathoracic bleeding
  - Positive FAST redirects therapeutic intervention to laparotomy instead of CT scan in the fluid nonresponder or transient responder
- Anticipate studies to identify internal injury if the patient is hemodynamically stable; the unstable patient goes directly to the operative suite or interventional radiology
- Other methods of hemorrhage control include
  - Topical sealants through local application of concentrated clotting factors
  - Fibrin impregnated bandages
  - Granular zeolite is a hemostatic agent applied to external wounds through water absorption which concentrates clotting factors and platelets at the wound site; is exothermic and can cause a burn
  - Granular chitosan dressing is similar to zeolite but is not exothermic and functions in hypothermic situations
  - Aprotinin used later to supplement erythropoiesis

— Massive transfusion

- The goal of massive transfusion protocols is to restore circulating blood volume while the site of hemorrhage and coagulopathy are controlled
- From the experience of the Iraqi conflicts, recommendations for changes to transfusion protocols include 1 FFP:1 PRBC or 1.5 FFP:1 PRBC to decrease mortality
  - The 1 FFP:1 PRBC ratio may actually correct coagulopathy earlier rather than decrease mortality (Kashuk et al. 2008)
  - 1:1 ratio mimics whole blood transfusion (Perkins et al. 2008)

- Other ratio recommendations include 2 FFP:3 PRBC with 1 platelet:5 PRBC (Gunter et al. 2008); 1 FFP:1 PRBC:1 platelet (McLaughlin et al. 2008)
- Should be considered for
  - Base deficit > −6
  - INR > 1.5
  - BP < 90 mm Hg
  - Hemoglobin < 11 g/dL
  - Temperature < 35° to 36°C
  - Weak or absent radial pulses (Beckley 2008)
- Massive transfusion has many definitions and includes, for example,
  - >10 units PRBC in 24 hours
  - 6 units PRBC, 6 units FFP, 6 units platelets, 10 units cryoprecipitate
- Use of the massive transfusion protocol should decrease overuse of blood and establish efficient turn-around times for FFP, PRBC, platelets, cryoprecipitate, and rFVIIa
  - Prethawed FFP has a shelf life of 4 to 5 days and allows for more rapid availability

— Recombinant factor VIIa (rFVIIa)
  - Decreases the need for large numbers of PRBC by reversing coagulopathy
  - Least effective if acidosis is present; correct acidosis as quickly as possible
  - Not affected by hypothermia (Beckley 2008)
  - Reduces time to INR correction especially in the head injury patient
  - A suggested protocol for use includes administration with massive transfusion protocol (>10 units PRBC, 8 units FFP, 1 unit platelets) (Dutton et al. 2004)
    - 73% was given within the first 24 hours, averaging 1.23 doses

- o Decreases hemorrhage, develops new clot, decreases PT after the first dose
- o Typical doses are 50 to 100 mcg/kg as a bolus (Stein and Dutton 2004)
— Hemoglobin-based oxygen carrier (HBOC)
  - Nonblood product that is capable of transporting oxygen via a relatively low fluid volume
  - Decreases number of PRBC required to control hemorrhage (Jahr et al. 2008)
  - Associated with adverse events, such as
    - o Increased troponin, angina, myocardial infarction
    - o Transient increase BP especially after the loading dose
  - Provides an alternative to blood transfusion
— Special consideration
  - Patients have the right to refuse blood products, (eg, Jehovah's Witnesses refusal for religious reasons)
  - Mortality increases when hemoglobin drops below 7 g/dL
  - Alternatives to support the patient through the need for blood products include
    - o Recombinant human erythropoietin increases erythropoiesis
    - o Administration of vitamin B_{12}, folate, iron augment red blood cell production
    - o rFVIIa binds tissue factors allowing local coagulation
    - o Autotransfusion
    - o HBOC decreases the need for PRBC through oxygen-carrying capacity
  - Discuss alternatives with the patient
  - Parents cannot refuse blood for their children for religious reasons when the blood administration is warranted (Hughes et al. 2008)

— End points of resuscitation and tools to identify successful resuscitation are discussed under special situations

   ▪ Monitor urine output however do not wait an hour to
   determine that urine output is inadequate (0.5 mL/kg/hour
   adults)

Deficit assessment

A brief neurologic examination is conducted next. By this time,
the patient has either responded or not to verbal and painful
stimuli. The brief neurologic examination should be documented prior to intubation as pharmacologic agents and the
intubation will affect later assessments. For complete description of the neurologic examination, see Chapters 4 and 5. The
brief neurologic classification includes

• Alert
• Responds to verbal stimuli
• Responds to painful stimuli
• Unresponsive

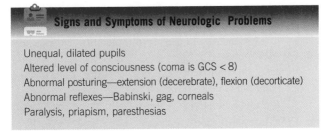

Signs and Symptoms of Neurologic Problems

Unequal, dilated pupils
Altered level of consciousness (coma is GCS < 8)
Abnormal posturing—extension (decerebrate), flexion (decorticate)
Abnormal reflexes—Babinski, gag, corneals
Paralysis, priapism, paresthesias

• Deficit management

Immediate management of neurologic issues is focused on preventing secondary brain or spinal cord injury. At this point in
the primary survey, the neurologic assessment is documented
serially. The GCS should be documented and repeated. If the

patient is already intubated, lightening the patient's sedation and paralytic agents may be necessary to perform an examination.

— Maintain BP to prevent any incidence of hypotension (BP <90 mm Hg)

— Prevent hypoxia through airway and breathing management

— Consider administration of mannitol if evidence of increased intracranial pressure (IICP) and the BP is stable

— Anticipate the need for head CT, although burr holes can be placed if IICP is suspected and emergent laparotomy or thoracotomy is necessary

— Chapters 4 and 5 review the neurologic examination and management of IICP, head and spinal cord injury

Exposure

At the end of the primary survey the patient's body is exposed in a warm room that should be warm enough for the staff to be uncomfortable.

• Expose for visualization of any abnormalities, asymmetry, and skin injuries

— Check posterior scalp

— Stabilize any impaled object to prevent further injury

• Logroll and examine the back palpating for step-offs or tenderness in the spine

• Remove clothing as well as glass and other debris that may be under the patient

• Auscultate posterior lungs

• Any reddened area that may have developed from the presence of the backboard is also noted

• The backboard is removed and the patient is returned to the supine position by logrolling

— Removal of the backboard is required to prevent pressure ulcers

— Any turning of the patient from this point is through logrolling until the spine is cleared of injury

— The cervical collar is maintained
— A rectal temperature can be taken while the patient is turned
  ■ Determines core temperature and is more accurate than oral or axillary
  ■ Up to 60% of trauma patients do not have a temperature measurement (Cohen et al. 2002)
• Cover the patient with warm blankets to prevent hypothermia
  — Limit the exposure time to avoid conductive and radiant heat loss
  — Core temperature <36°C at admission is an independent predictor of death (Wang et al. 2005)
    ■ Hypothermia increases oxygen consumption
    ■ Shivering increases oxygen consumption by up to 400% (Moore 2008)
    ■ Cold diuresis causes further fluid loss
    ■ Hyperglycemia is exacerbated along with decreased insulin production
    ■ Level of consciousness is depressed
    ■ Platelet function is altered causing thrombocytopenia and coagulopathy
  — Forced air warming is an effective means of increasing and maintaining body temperature
    ■ Does make access to the patient more difficult
  — Reflective blankets are also an effective means of maintaining body temperature
    ■ Easier access to the patient (Cohen et al. 2002)

Secondary Survey with Interventions

Secondary survey can now be conducted, incorporating reassessment of the primary survey components. Again, actions are taken to stabilize the injury as issues are identified. After the secondary survey both diagnostics and definitive destination are determined. Consultants may be called during the secondary survey and some bedside diagnostics are performed. Laboratory data may be returned at this point and any actions necessary should be taken.

The secondary survey is the time to obtain the patient's history, particularly allergies to penicillin and iodine. If the patient goes to CT scan, the information regarding allergy to iodine is important before contrast is given. Allergy to penicillin is important as this is the point when a single dose of broad-spectrum antibiotic is usually given. If tetanus is not up to date, it should be provided as well. The secondary survey is a head-to-toe evaluation of the patient to identify injuries and perform procedures as needed.

Head-neck-face assessment and management

Assess the head, neck, and face for injury. Observe, palpate, reassess for any bleeding wounds, and reassess neurologic status. See Chapters 4, 5, and 6 for detailed evaluation.

- Reassess airway and assure patency; if needed, stop and provide for the airway
- Maintain cervical immobilization
  — If the patient is likely to be admitted, clearance of the cervical spine may be reserved until after the initial resuscitation evaluation (see Chapter 5, cervical spine clearance)
- Assess pupils for size, reactivity, extraocular movements
- Reassess GCS and continue to assess serially
- Assess for basilar skull fracture
  — Periorbital ecchymosis; ecchymosis behind the ear (over the mastoid)
  — Clear fluid from the nose or ear
- Anticipate CT scan of the head, face, cervical spine if injury is suspected
- Head injury is managed with prevention of hypotension and hypoxia in the initial resuscitation
- Palpate the skull and face for deformity or depression, including an evaluation of lacerations for open fracture

— Midface fractures present as mobility when the upper teeth are gently "wiggled"

— Mandible fractures and temporal-mandibular joint dislocation may present with an abnormal bite

- Epistaxis may be related to

  — Facial fracture, primarily nasal

  — Bleeding without fracture

  — Anticoagulant and antiplatelet use

- Test sensation to identify any nerve injury to the face/neck

- Remove the front of the cervical collar while holding manual stabilization of the neck

  — Observe asymmetry, jugular vein distention, tracheal deviation

  — Check carotid pulses

  — Assess for cervical spine tenderness to palpation, check for stepoffs

  — Replace the cervical collar

- Insert an orogastric (nasogastric if no facial or head injury) tube and place to low intermittent suction

  — Check placement through auscultation over the gastric area while instilling air into the tube; the bubble of air should be audible

Chest assessment and management

Reassess the chest to assure that earlier interventions are effective or that new interventions are not necessary (see Chapter 7 for specifics of assessment and management)

- Observe for symmetry, equal rise and fall of the chest, paradoxical movement

- Palpate for tenderness, paradoxical movement, subcutaneous emphysema

- Auscultate bilateral breath sounds

  — Check endotracheal tube

  — Check chest tubes

  — If breath sounds have changed, reassess for malpositioned endotracheal tube; need for thoracostomy tube; malpositioned thoracostomy
- Auscultate heart sounds
  — Muffled heart sounds may indicate pericardial tamponade
  — Tamponade may be managed with pericardiocentesis as a temporizing measure
  — Current recommendation for tamponade is to proceed with a pericardial window via thoracotomy (Kortbeek et al. 2008)
- Diagnostic studies
  — The general standard is to perform a plain film of the chest (CXR)
  — If the chest examination is completely normal, there may be no need for this film and radiation exposure (Wisbach et al. 2007)
    - Low yield for injury if the examination is normal per the trauma surgeon (Sears et al. 2005)
  — Chest CT is also performed frequently in conjunction with abdominal/pelvic CT scans and can identify up to 36% of injuries missed on the original CXR
    - With helical CT scanners, a total torso, head, and neck CT takes minutes and provides the most rapid and thorough evaluation of the body
    - Reconstructions can be performed to evaluate the thoracic and lumbar spine from the abdominal and chest CT scans
  — Ultrasound (FAST, see next) may also identify hemothorax, pneumothorax while being used for the abdominal evaluation (Kirkpatrick 2007)

Abdominal assessment and management

The abdomen is evaluated for potential injury through direct examination and diagnostic studies (see Chapter 8 for details of assessment and management)

- Observe the abdomen for distention, wounds, seat belt contusions
- The stomach should already be decompressed with an orogastric tube to prevent vomiting and aspiration
- Auscultate for bowel sounds, although this may be difficult in the trauma room
- Palpate the abdomen for tenderness, rebound tenderness, involuntary guarding
- Assess the pelvis by placing the palm of the hand over the pubic bone and over the iliac spines and apply gentle pressure to elicit pain or instability
  — Do not repeat this examination to prevent the potential for increased bleeding with movement of the pelvic bones
- Assess the perineal area for
  — Blood at the urinary meatus
  — Vaginal blood
  — Perform a rectal examination for any gross blood as well as placement of the prostate
    - A high riding or boggy prostate is indicative of urethral injury
    - Gross blood indicates anal, rectal, or sigmoid injury
    - Assess rectal sphincter tone for spinal cord injury
  — The above signs and symptoms indicate potential urethral injury and a Foley catheter should not be placed
  — A urology consult is necessary for Foley or suprapubic tube placement
  — If negative, a Foley catheter should be placed and a urine sample sent for urinalysis and toxicology screen
- Diagnostic studies (Chapter 8) to evaluate the abdomen include
  — FAST evaluates the liver, spleen, pelvis, and pericardium for blood/fluid and is done at the bedside by the emergency or trauma physician
    - Ultrasound may also be useful to evaluate the inferior vena cava (IVC) after fluid resuscitation; transient

responders have shown a smaller caliber IVC demonstrating insufficient fluid resuscitation (Yanagawa et al. 2007)

— Diagnostic peritoneal lavage (DPL) evaluates the abdomen for blood or bacteria/fecal spillage into the abdominal cavity

- Rarely used, however is a reliable assessment of the need for surgery in the abdomen
- In the situation of multiple casualties, a DPL may be the study available to evaluate multiple patients rapidly to rule out the need for surgery

— Abdominal CT

- Optimal method of evaluation of the abdomen
- Best if done with both oral and IV contrast to see both solid and hollow organs
- If the patient is unstable, has obvious abdominal injury (eg, GSW), or has any peritoneal signs, their place is in the operating suite and never the CT scanner

Extremity assessment and management

Evaluation of the extremities is meant to identify fractures, dislocations, vascular, and soft tissue injuries. Simple measures are taken to stabilize the bony injuries. Loss of pulses requires immediate reduction and immobilization of the extremity. Further evaluation of the vascular injury follows (Chapter 9 discusses specifics of orthopaedic evaluation):

• Evaluate pulses, color, temperature, capillary refill of all extremities

— Note any soft tissue injuries and deformity

— Palpate for crepitus, instability

• Evaluate symmetry between the extremities

— Any deformity should be reduced and splinted until more definitive management by casting or surgical fixation takes place

- Splinting must be placed from one joint above to one joint below the injury

— Reevaluate pulses immediately after reduction and placement of a splint and periodically afterward

— For femur fractures, use a traction splint (eg, hare traction) which reduces the fracture as well as relieves the muscle spasm, decreases pain, and maintains the reduction

■ Do not use for fractures below the midshaft femur

- Further examination includes

  — Plain radiographs of the affected extremity

  — A CT scan may be ordered if the fracture is complex

  — The pelvis and spine usually require both plain films and CT scanning

  — Spine fractures may be evaluated later with MRI scan as well for ligamentous and cord injury evaluation

  — Vascular injury is evaluated with CT angiogram or traditional angiogram; initial management of vascular injury is addressed in the primary survey through immediate reduction, splinting, and hemorrhage control

The secondary survey concludes with diagnostic studies in and outside of the emergency department such as CT scans, ECG, and angiograms, as well as the decision for definitive placement to OR, ICU, or the floor. Some facilities have incorporated a CT scanner into the trauma resuscitation area to decrease the time to scanner as well as eliminate moving the patient onto/off of the scanner table (Jin et al. 2008).

Other facilities have incorporated the operating suite into the trauma resuscitation area to enable instant change from resuscitation to operation without movement of the patient. Surgical trays are usually prepped and ready for surgery and anesthesia is present. This situation is used for hypotension, penetrating torso injuries, multiple long bone fractures, and severe maxillofacial trauma (Rhodes et al. 1989). Of the patients taken to the trauma OR, 58.7% required major operative procedure with a mean time to anesthesia of 8.5 minutes. Survival in this population was greater than the predicted probability of survival via the trauma and injury severity score (TRISS) method.

At the end of the survey, family should be allowed a moment to visit with the patient if instability does not prevent that time. Even with rushing to the operating suite, if a moment can be given to family, it will ease their waiting time and provide a visit with the patient in case he or she does not survive the surgery.

Pain management is also essential during this time and includes

- Early administration of opiates (morphine, fentanyl), which are reversible, to provide some comfort to the patient but not alter the examination process
  - Facilities with pain management protocols note shorter mean time to initial analgesia of <30 minutes (Curtis et al. 2007)
  - Pain medication is also more likely administered if the patient is not disposed to the OR or ICU (Curtis et al. 2007)
  - Monitor BP to prevent hypotension with administration of opiates and benzodiazepines
  - Intubated patients and head injured patients also require pain management
  - Monitor heart rate, grimacing, pallor, tension, diaphoresis, tears as signs of pain in patients unable to express pain sensation
- Alternative means of pain management include
  - Positioning
  - Splinting, traction splints
  - Relaxation techniques and meditation are effective later, but it may be difficult for the patient to focus in the resuscitation area
  - Ice packs to fractures/dislocations
  - Keep the patient warm, decrease/prevent shivering
- Use a pain scale to evaluate the patient's response to treatment
- Document changes in pain and the responses

Tertiary Survey

Prudent management of the trauma patient includes a full examination within 24 hours of arrival. This review includes a recheck of all diagnostic studies as well as the full examination. Any new studies are ordered and completed, hemodynamics are reevaluated, and operative plans organized for nonemergent surgeries. Prophylaxis is initiated if not done on admission as well as plans for initial evaluation by rehabilitative services.

DOCUMENTATION

Documentation of the evaluation and interventions undertaken must be done, usually on a trauma flowsheet. Proper documentation as expected to perform as a trauma center includes

- Mechanism of injury
- Prehospital activities
- Patient history
- Time of arrival of the patient as well as each member of the team
- Arrival set of vital signs, GCS, oxygen saturations, temperature, and full examination
    - In a trauma center the examination is performed first by the physicians and called out to the scribe
    - The nurse should perform and document his or her examination of the patient for comparison with later examinations
- Complete the diagram of external injuries and extremity deformities
- Time all procedures, labs, radiographs
- Travel with the patient to radiology and continue to monitor vital signs while there and traveling
- Provide narrative for any other activities and patient responses not yet documented
- Continue serial vital signs, GCS, pain assessment, oxygen saturations

In addition to the flowsheet documentation, a revised trauma score (RTS) is calculated and assists in identifying patients at risk for death. In the trauma center, the RTS is used within the registry to calculate probability of survival. In the nontrauma centers, an early RTS score can provide data indicating the need for transfer to a higher level facility. The RTS is described in Table 2-3. Initially,

Table 2-3   Revised Trauma Score

Respiratory rate (RR)	10-29/minute	4
	>29/minute	3
	6-9/minute	2
	1-5/minute	1
	None	0
Systolic blood pressure (BP)	≥90 mm Hg	4
	76-89 mm Hg	3
	50-75 mm Hg	2
	1-49 mm Hg	1
	No pulse	0
Glasgow coma scale score (GCS)	13-15	4
	9-12	3
	6–8	2
	4-5	1
	3	0
Total	RR + BP + GCS	0-12

Champion 1989.

the trauma score was designed to include respiratory rate, capillary refill, respiratory effort, BP, and GCS. Because the original trauma score was cumbersome, the capillary refill and respiratory effort were difficult to obtain, and were somewhat subjective, these two components were removed from the revised trauma score. The RTS identified more than 97% of the nonsurvivors (Champion et al. 1989).

SPECIAL SITUATIONS

End Points of Resuscitation

End points of resuscitation serve two purposes: identification of futility of care and identification of successful resuscitation. When measuring resuscitation and occult hypoperfusion, both lactate and base deficit provide markers for complete resuscitation. Failure to achieve normal lactate and/or base deficit results in fatality or an increased likelihood of multiple organ dysfunction syndrome (MODS) or multisystem organ failure (MSOF).

Goals of resuscitation are to increase oxygen delivery, normalize lactic acid, base deficit, and/or pHi within the first 24 hours to prevent complications and increased mortality. Damage control resuscitation as well as surgery is initiated to prevent physiologic exhaustion while focusing on resuscitation.

- Lactic acidosis is a normal result of hypoperfusion and is managed through resuscitation
    — Normal lactic acid level is <2.2 mMol/L
    — Cases with lactic acidosis and low cardiac index have demonstrated MODS, respiratory complications, and death (Blow et al. 1999)
    — Reverse occult hypoperfusion within the first 24 hours to prevent complications
    — Resuscitate until the lactic acid level is <2.5 mMol/L
    — Algorithm 2-1 describes a protocol to reverse occult hypoperfusion
- Base deficit is also a result of hypoperfusion and reflects the body's response; management is through resuscitation
    — Normal base ranges from −2 to 2 mMol/L
    — Table 2-4 describes the relationship of base deficit to resuscitation necessary to correct the value
    — Patients aged >55 years may not generate a base deficit that is outside the normal range
    — Alcohol increases lactate production causing metabolic acidosis, which confounds the base deficit as a predictor or hypoperfusion (Tisherman et al. 2004)
- Gastric tonometry (pHi)
    — Gastric mucosa is vulnerable to hypoperfusion
    — Measured through a nasogastric tube with a saline-filled gas permeable balloon at the tip
    — pHi <7.35 is suggestive of anaerobic metabolism

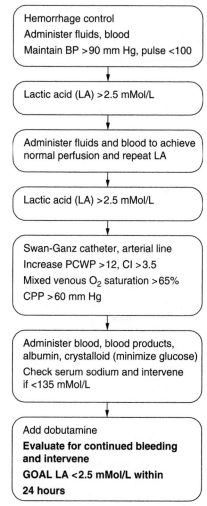

Algorithm 2-1 Lactate resuscitation algorithm. (From University of Virginia Medical Center, Charlottesville, VA, with permission.)

Table 2-4   Base Deficit Reflects Hypoperfusion.

Classification	Base Deficit	Resuscitation Measures
Normal	−2 to 2 mMol/L	
Mild	−5 to −3 mMol/L	Warm fluids
Moderate	−9 to −6 mMol/L	Warm fluids, blood products
Severe	< −9 mMol/L	Warm fluids, blood products, treat source of blood loss in OR or angiography; check for alcohol and other toxins

Ziglar 2000.

— Indicates an increased risk of MODS
— When taking measurements stop tube feedings 30 minutes prior
— Gastric acid suppression and administration of sodium bicarbonate affect pHi readings
— May not reliably describe the state of the entire gut
• Other end points of resuscitation
— Time to normalize/stabilize is predictive of survival
— Blunt trauma patients without signs of life at the scene or on arrival do not survive
— Blunt trauma patients with signs of life on arrival then arrest may have a treatable injury such as pericardial tamponade or tension pneumothorax
— Penetrating trauma patients in arrest on arrival who receive early thoracotomy to relieve tamponade, clamp the aorta, open cardiac massage, control intrathoracic hemorrhage may survive
— Penetrating trauma patients with arrest >5 minutes in the field may not survive
— Trauma patients who receive cardiopulmonary resuscitation without a rhythm do not survive

— Severe brain injury with tissue loss and open skull fracture, GCS = 3 is not survivable

— Consider futility (Coimbra et al. 2007) in trauma patients with

- End-stage renal or liver disease or malignancy
- More than two times the blood volume replacement, hypothermia, and coagulopathy that does not improve over 6 to 8 hours
- Geriatric patients with severe chest and/or abdominal injury, moderate shock, and head injury

Family Presence

The issue of family presence during resuscitation, rounds, and arrest is an area of controversy. The literature holds that the stress may be at the staff level and significantly less so for the family. Walker (2008) identified that staff felt the risk was greater than the benefit for the family. Issues for staff have been identified as

- Fear interference of the family during the procedures
- Feel it is too traumatic for the family to experience
- Feel it interferes with residency teaching
- Feel they cannot keep the professional distance with the family during these events
- Fear liability
- Feel anxiety about performing in front of the family

Families interviewed noted that there are many benefits of family presence for them, including

- Assists with adjustment to the death
- Increases the knowledge of the condition of the patient
- Decrease fear, anxiety, and depression regarding the patient's condition
- Feel they know that everything has been done for their family member
- Feel that the patient was not alone through the experience
- Appreciate the opportunity to say goodbye
- Facilitates grieving

There have been no documented cases of liability issues related to family presence. From the author's experience, one family stated that they did not remember the actual events in the room as much as the mother fixated on the surgeon's cowboy boots. What she remembered most was that he wore cowboy boots, yet the permission to be in the room meant everything, even though the details were obscured.

Family should be involved in daily conferences with the care providers to increase knowledge and consistently reinforce previously shared information. Be truthful. Offer spiritual support. Open, flexible visitation helps the family fit the need to be with the patient into their schedule.

Body Piercing and Tattooing

One of the changes in society that may affect patient care is the increased incidence of tattoos and body piercings. During resuscitation and diagnostic procedures, providers should be aware of these on the patient and take action when necessary to maintain safety.

- Some piercings are safe for MRI scanning (high quality LVM316 or 316L stainless steel, titanium, niobium)
  - Overall radiologic study artifact is dependent on the location of the piercing and the size of the jewelry attached
- Piercings
  - Tongue piercings may obscure cervical spine films
  - Nipple piercings may obscure chest films
  - Perineal piercings may affect pelvic films
  - Make the patient aware that if the films are inadequate, the piercing will need to be removed
  - Ultrasound should not be performed directly over the piercing
- Removal
  - An IV catheter functions very well as a "place holder" when the piercing requires removal and should be in the proper position prior to complete removal of the jewelry

— If the patient is alert and capable, he or she can remove it
— Some require training for removal; be sure to use
  - Ring-opening pliers
  - Nonserrated hemostats
  - Gauze
— Piercings may not stay open after jewelry removal without a place holder

- Tattoos
  — Older and large tattoos may contain inks with iron components
  — Warn the MRI technician, as these may result in a visible burn as the ferrous elements heat
  — If the patient is able, he or she should be instructed to inform the technician if the area feels warm
  — Permanent cosmetics have not shown any evidence of burns with MRI

Evidence Collection

During the trauma resuscitation, care must be taken to preserve evidence when it is present and especially in the case of intentional mechanisms of injury. All evidence needs to be sealed into proper containers and labeled with the identification information of the patient and the name and signature of the person collecting the evidence. Documentation of collection, site, and chain of custody is essential prior to handing the evidence to the police or medical examiner. Evidence must be secure at all times.

- Clothing
  — Wet clothing should be hung to dry before folding and placing each item in a separate paper bag
  — Do not cut through holes made by the weapon, eg, the GSW or stab, as they contain the shape and angle of the penetration
  — Be aware that as clothing is removed bullets or other evidence may fall from it; handle carefully

— Collect dry clothing onto a clean sheet if time does not allow processing immediately
  - Sheet collects evidence that drops off the item
  - Include the sheet when packaging the evidence for delivery to the police
- Foreign bodies
  - Pick up with a gloved hand or rubber-tipped forceps and place in a sterile specimen container with gauze or cotton to prevent damage to the specimen
  - Allow the container to "breathe" especially if the specimen is wet
  - Seal and follow hospital evidence protocols
- Hands/nails
  - If suicide is expected, cover the hands with paper bags to prevent loss of evidence
  - Especially in rape and assault cases, fingernails may contain DNA evidence of the perpetrator; clippings of the nails can be placed in an envelope
  - The thumb and forefinger may be swabbed with a culture tube collection device or a cotton tipped swab to collect gunshot residue and soot
  - The same can be done at the site of the GSW
  - Hands should be covered with paper bags in death cases, especially homicide/suicide
- Exigent evidence
  - Contusions, abrasions, lacerations, and other wounds are exigent evidence because they will disappear as the patient heals, leaving no documentation of themselves in court later
  - Photographs of these wounds allow for the documentation
  - Do not identify wounds as "entrance" or "exit;" simply describe what is seen
- Photographs
  - Follow hospital protocol for patient permission and ensure that documentation is in the medical record

- — Print and label photographs, placing them in the medical record or download them to the electronic record
- — Obtain a full-face, full-body photograph of the patient, followed by photographs of the wounds with and without a sizing device (see Chapter 10 for additional evidence collection)
- After death
  - — Leave all lines in place
  - — Label sites of attempted procedures so that the medical examiner knows the reason for incisions and other marks on the body
  - — All deaths within 24 hours of admission and all trauma-related deaths including simple falls are medical examiner cases and require reporting even if the family does not wish an autopsy
- Legal alcohol
  - — Requires that the site preparation is done with chlorhexidine NOT alcohol swabs
  - — After drawing, label and seal per hospital policy; usually this sample is turned over to the police; do not forget chain of custody

POSTRESUSCITATION MANAGEMENT AND REHABILITATION

Crisis Intervention

Crisis is a sudden unexpected event that threatens everyday life and future goals. Caring for the trauma patient is both stressful to the provider as well as to the family and obviously the patient. All parties may suffer from the crisis and need to recognize when they are in need of assistance. For families, the entire experience is stressful and they should be approached to help them understand the situation, as well as learn new information as needed.

Signs and Symptoms of the Stress Response

Nausea, diarrhea
Tremors
Chills, profuse sweating
Chest pain, tachycardia, tachypnea
Headache, hypertension
Confusion, insomnia, nightmares, pupil dilation
Poor attention, anxiety, fears, memory gaps, slower learning
Guilt, grief, depression, no eye contact
Feeling isolated, irritable, angry
Perceptions become reality
Loud, profanity use
Loss of coping skills

Management during crisis hinges on communication skills. Efforts to decrease stress, provide information, and assist with decision making is part of managing the patient and the family.

- Be honest in all communications for information and answering family questions
- Include all members of the family who are present, however control the number of family members who will contact the staff
  - Designate one family member as the primary contact especially in an emergent or critical situation
  - Other family members should then communicate with the designated member
- Provide information privately, not in the middle of a crowded waiting room
- Sit with the family to talk; do not present information while standing especially if the information is complex or difficult for the family to accept
- Provide short bursts of information rather than prolonged explanations as the family will grasp the data better in that format

- Remind the family that a crisis situation is short-lived and that over time their emotions will settle and subside
- Encourage conversation among the family and with the patient and staff
- Provide support; monitor coping mechanisms among the family
  — Observe for poor coping techniques, such as use of alcohol
  — Provide assistance with finding housing, meals
  — Remind the family to eat, sleep, go home
  — Do not encourage sleeping in the room with the patient except with a child or in unique situations; the family and the patient need rest
  — Be sure to provide social services, case managers, chaplaincy for the family; include financial counseling if needed
- Family support groups
  — American Trauma Society (ATS) (www.amtrauma.org) has developed a Web site for families and patients to provide support and education throughout the hospital stay as well as after discharge
  — Second trauma program (ATS) provides
    ▪ Instruction to the staff on how to assist families
    ▪ Peer visitation program
    ▪ Self-management classes to build on strengths, coping skills
    ▪ Traumapedia informational source
- Staff critical incident stress debriefing
  — Incidents such as child death or severe injury, death or injury of a friend, staff, or family member, a life-threatening situation, media events, mass casualty situations
  — After the event, a debriefing should be held with only the personnel directly involved to allow for discussion of feelings and thoughts
  — A critique is held later to evaluate the events, as well as performance, equipment needs, other technical issues that need resolution or performance improvement

— Further debriefing may be needed and the staff should be free to express the need for further counseling without penalty; they should also be aware of the signs and symptoms of stress to identify them in themselves or fellow staff members

Outcomes After Trauma

Trauma is an ever-growing field of medical care where patients who 20 years ago would have died in the trauma bay, now survive to hopefully return to productive lives. Much time has been spent learning scene care, resuscitation, and follow-up care. The component that is only now receiving attention is what happens after the discharge from the hospital or rehabilitation center. The goal is to return patients to their previous level of function when possible, or to the optimal level of function attainable after the injury.

As more patients survive, the severity of the disability and the longer time to healing increases. Some studies have demonstrated 42% of patients had not yet returned to work at 6 months after injury with only 32% identifying a "good" recovery (Gabbe et al. 2008). The motor disability score at discharge is very predictive of functional recovery. The leading causes of lack of return to work include lower extremity fractures, spinal cord injury, and head injury caused by functional impairment (Zatzick et al. 2008). At 1 year, 20% of patients still had post-traumatic stress disorder (PTSD) with 6% experiencing depression (Zatzick et al. 2008). Patients who were working before injury and subsequently suffered from PTSD or depression afterward had a three-fold increase in the likelihood of no return to work. If both PTSD and depression were present, the likelihood of no return to work increased by five- to six-fold (Zatzick et al. 2008).

Analysis of outcomes is essential to understand the experience of the trauma patient after discharge so that changes can be made during hospitalization to both prepare the patient and perhaps accelerate the healing process. The more the patient understands what is ahead in the healing process, the better prepared he or she will be for the emotions and physical changes that occur during rehabilitation. In-hospital outcomes focus on mortality, morbidity, and length of stay. After discharge, the focus is on regaining independence, return to work and hobbies, reestablishment of relationships with family and friends, and more depending upon the injuries and the patient's situation. As much preparation as can be provided before discharge, the better the patient will face the challenges ahead.

 Critical Lifesavers

- There is no place for a soft cervical collar; assume cervical injury until proven otherwise.
- Apply 100% O_2 via nonrebreather mask in all trauma patients.
- Vasopressors are NO substitute for volume restoration and direct hemorrhage control.

REFERENCES

American College of Surgeons Committee on Trauma (ACS-COT). *Resources for Optimal Care of the Injured Patient 2006.* Chicago, IL: American College of Surgeons; 2006.

Barraco RD, Chiu WC, Bard MR, et al. Practice management guidelines for the appropriate triage of the victim of trauma. Unpublished 2008, www.east.org

Beckley AC. Damage control resuscitation: a sensible approach to the exsanguinating surgical patient. *Crit Care Med.* 2008;6(7): S267-S274.

Blow O, Magliore L, Claridge JA, et al. The golden hour and the silver day: detection and correction of occult hypoperfusion within 24 hours improves outcome from major trauma. *J Trauma.* 1999;47(5):964-974.

Brommel-Ziedins K, Whelihan M, Ziedins E, et al. The resuscitative fluid you choose may potentiate bleeding. *J Trauma.* 2006;61(6):1350-1358.

Champion H, Sacco W, Copes W, et al. A revision of the trauma score. *J Trauma.* 1989;29(5):623-629.

Cohen S, Hayes JS, Tordella T, et al. Thermal efficiency of pre-warmed cotton, reflective blankets in the trauma patients. *Int J Trauma Nurs.* 2002;8(1):4-8.

Coimbra R, Lee J, Bansal V, et al. Recognizing/accepting futility: prehospital, emergency center, operating room, and intensive care unit. *J Trauma Nurs.* 2007;14(2):73-76.

Curtis K, Henriques H, Fanciullo G, et al. A fentanyl-based pain management protocol provides early analgesia for adult trauma patients. *J Trauma.* 2007;63(4):819-826.

Dutton R, McGunn M, Hyder M, et al. Factor VIIa for correction of traumatic coagulopathy. *J Trauma.* 2004;57(4):709-719.

Gabbe B, Simpson P, Sutherland A, et al. Functional measures at discharge: are they useful predictors of longer term outcomes for trauma registries? *Ann Surg.* 2008;247(5):854-859.

Gonzales E, Moore F, Holcomb JB, et al. Fresh frozen plasma should be given earlier to patients requiring massive transfusion. *J Trauma.* 2007;62(1):112-119.

Gunter OL, Au NK, Isbel JM, et al. Optimizing outcomes in damage control resuscitation identifying blood product ratio associated with improved survival. *J Trauma.* 2008;65(3):527-534.

Holcomb JB. Damage control resuscitation. *J Trauma.* 2007;62(6): S36-S37.

Hughes DB, Ullery BW, Barie PS. The contemporary approach to the care of Jehovah's Witnesses. *J Trauma.* 2008;65(1):237-247.

Jahr JS, MacKenzie C, Pearce L, et al. HBOC-201 as an alternative to blood transfusion: efficacy and safety evaluation in a multicenter phase III trial in elective orthopedic surgery. *J Trauma.* 2008;64(6):1484-1497.

Jin P, Gosling J, Ponsen KVC, et al. Assessment of a new trauma workflow concept implementing a sliding CT scanner in the trauma room: the effect on workup time. *J Trauma.* 2008;64(5): 1320-1326.

Kashuk JC, Moore EE, Johnson JL, et al. Postinjury life threatening coagulopathy: is 1:1 fresh frozen plasma:packed red blood cells the answer? *J Trauma.* 2008;65(2):261-271.

Kirkpatrick A. Clinician-performed focused sonography for the resuscitation of trauma. *Crit Care Med.* 2007;35(5):S162-S172.

Kortbeek JB, Al Turki SA, Ali J, et al. Advanced trauma life support, the evidence for change. *J Trauma.* 2008;64(6):1638-1650.

McLaughlin DF, Niles SE, Sulinas J, et al. A predictive model for mass transfusion in combat casualty patients. *J Trauma.* 2008;64(2):S57-S63.

Moore K. Hypothermia in trauma. *J Trauma Nurs.* 2008;15(2):62-64.

Moore KM. Controversies in fluid resuscitation. *J Trauma Nurs.* 2006;13(4):168-172.

Perkins JG, Cap AP, Weiss BM, et al. Mass transfusion and nonsurgical hemostatic agents. *Crit Care Med.* 2008;S325-S339.

Rhodes M, Brader A, Lucke J, et al. Direct transport to the operating room for resuscitation of trauma patients. *J Trauma.* 1989;29(7):907-915.

Sears BN, Luchette F, Esposito TJ, et al. Old fashion clinical judgment in the areas of protocols: is mandatory chest x-ray necessary in injured patients? *J Trauma.* 2005;59(2):324-332.

Spinella PC, Perkins JG, Grathwohl KW, et al. Effect of plasma and red blood cell transfusion in patients with combat related traumatic injuries. *J Trauma.* 2008;64(2):S69-S78.

Stein DM, Dutton RP. Use of recombinant factor VIIa in trauma. *Curr Opin Crit Care.* 2004;10(6):520-528.

Tisherman SA, Barie P, Bokhari F, et al. Practice management guidelines: endpoints of resuscitation. *J Trauma.* 2004;57(4):898-912.

Walker W. Accident and emergency staff opinion on the effects of family presence during adult resuscitation: critical literature review. *J Adv Nurs.* 2008;61(4):348-362.

Wang H, Callaway C, Peitzman A, et al. Admission hypothermia and outcome after major trauma. *Crit Care Med.* 2005;33(6):1296-1301.

Wisbach G, Sise M, Sach D, et al. What is the role of chest x-ray in the initial assessment of stable trauma patients. *J Trauma.* 2007;62(1):74-79.

Yanagawa Y, Sakamoto T, Okaka Y. Hypovolemic shock evaluation by sonographic measurement of the inferior vena cava during resuscitation in trauma patients. *J Trauma.* 2007;63(6):1245-1248.

Zatzick D, Jurkovich G, Rivara FP, et al. A national U.S. study of posttraumatic stress disorder, depression, and work and functional outcomes after hospitalization for traumatic injury. *Ann Surg.* 2008;248(3):429-437.

Ziglar MK. Application of base deficit in resuscitation of trauma patients. *Int J Trauma Nurs.* 2000;6(3):81-84.

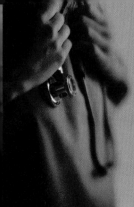

Chapter 3

TRAUMA SYSTEMS

INTRODUCTION

Evidence of trauma exists from the earliest recorded history. Whether it was homicide or just plain clumsiness, humans have injured themselves in one way or another. As vehicles have increased the speed at which we travel and technology offers means of survival for devastating injury, humans have found new ways to be injured and medicine has found ways to save the life of a victim. The number of trauma events continues to rise despite engineering and other technology. In 1966, the white paper, *Accidental Death and Disability: The Neglected Disease of Modern Society*, identified in a formal way that trauma caused death and disability in increasing numbers and required attention. The authors stated that "public apathy to the mounting toll from accidents must be transformed into an action program under strong leadership" (Committee on Trauma 1966).

Currently 38 states are capable of providing level I and level II trauma center care within 60 minutes for 85% of the United States population (Ciesla 2007). Triage to the trauma center should occur from the scene and in rural areas more often from the closest hospital with rapid transfer to higher level trauma centers. Helicopter transport is useful for moderately to severely injured patients (Barraco et al. 2008). In the urban setting, a helicopter may not be useful except in the case of multiple victims, traffic, critical patients and those with long extrication times (Barraco et al. 2008). The most important component of the trauma system is reduction of mortality from all forms of trauma, which should be promoted and developed in every state and country.

HISTORY OF SYSTEM DEVELOPMENT

From the date of the white paper, events have taken place to organize and establish trauma systems and trauma centers. This activity created a flurry of legislative and medical changes; however in 2008, the United States still has communities without designated/verified trauma centers available to the regions. The chronology of development of the current systems includes

- 1966: White paper
- 1973: Emergency Medical Services (EMS) act; first piece of legislation was a 5-year grant program to build an EMS system; the system intended to identify trauma centers and improve EMS resources
  — Access to EMS should be available to all citizens
  — All aspects of trauma and in addition high-risk mothers/ infants, poisonings, and behavioral emergencies
- 1976: American College of Surgeons-Committee on Trauma (ACS-COT) published designation criteria for trauma centers (*Optimal Hospital Resources for Care of the Seriously Injured*)
  — By this time, Illinois (1971) and Maryland (1973) were developing statewide trauma systems
- 1979: ACS-COT published a revision, *Hospital Resources for Optimal Care of the Injured Patient*
  — Stresses hospital commitment
  — Defines the four levels of trauma centers
- 1981: Reconciliation Act
  — Funding from the initial 1973 EMS Act was rolled into a grant for the Centers for Disease Control (CDC)
  — Responsibility for individual programs rests with the states, not a federal program
- 1984: Trauma system reevaluated with the decision to write more legislation

- 1986: General Accounting Office report
  - — 50% of the United States still without 911 access
  - — Rural United States missing advanced life support (ALS) ambulances
- 1990: Trauma Care Systems Planning and Development Act
  - — Poorly funded but initiated the design for inclusive trauma systems
  - — Increased rural trauma care
  - — State plans for trauma
  - — Trauma care standards and model trauma care plan
- 1998: Skamania Conference
  - — Focus on outcomes evaluation
  - — Support from the National Center for Injury Prevention and Control (NCIPC) and National Highway Traffic Safety Administration (NHTSA)
- 1999: ACS-COT revision *Resources for the Optimal Care of the Injured Patient*
  - — Stresses system-wide participation
- 2001 to 2006: Health Resources and Services Administration (HRSA) program with funding to continue trauma system development
- 2006: Most recent revision of ACS-COT *Resources for the Optimal Care of the Injured Patient*

During this time, trauma systems have been shown to decrease overall mortality by 15% and 17% in motor vehicle collisions (MVC) (Dunne 2007, Papa et al. 2006). Voluntary systems have shown a significant effect on preventable death (8%), however in those surviving to treatment, there is still inappropriate care at the prehospital and hospital levels that requires attention (Esposito et al. 2003).

Military Influence

The military experience has been a powerful influence on civilian trauma care. From the time of Florence Nightingale (1854 Crimean War), the mother of nursing, the field of nursing grew out of military care. Clara Barton continued this work during the Civil War and Franco-Prussian War 1869. From this trauma care has developed (Pruitt 2008, Ziglar et al. 2004)

- 1861: Florence Nightingale recommended field hospitals for the Civil War
- 1881: Clara Barton established the American Red Cross
- 1916 (World War I)
  - Development of the National Academy of Sciences Committee on Physiology
  - Laparotomy failed in penetrating trauma when delays to operating room (OR) occurred
  - Subcommittee on traumatic shock
- 1917
  - HW Cushing MD identified the beginning of neurosurgical trauma requirements and believed in the removal of foreign bodies from the cranium
  - H Dakin developed the diluted sodium hypochlorite solution used for dressing changes which decreased the rate of amputation
  - Physiology of hypovolemic shock was understood
- 1943 (World War II)
  - Medical Board for the Study of Severely Wounded established
  - Posttrauma renal failure identified
  - Increased use of blood, blood products, and antibiotics
  - Improved transport decreased delays to OR
  - "Wet lung" (pulmonary edema) identified; perhaps the first cases of acute respiratory distress syndrome (ARDS)
  - Crush syndrome
- 1950 to 1953 (Korean war)
  - Arterial repair by a direct method
  - Mobile army surgical hospital (MASH) unit
  - Rapid transport via helicopter decreased penetrating abdominal mortality dramatically

— Volume resuscitation prevented posttrauma renal failure
— Hemodialysis
- 1967 to 1975 (Vietnam war)
    — Specialists in the field and rapidly available
    — Transport times decreased from 4 to 6 hours to 1.5 hours
    — Value of the arterial blood gas and identification of ARDS
- Current (Iraqi conflict)
    — Damage control surgery in the combat zone
    — Damage control resuscitation with recommendations for 1:1::PRBC:FFP
    — Rapid evacuation to a large level I trauma center after immediate damage control within 72 hours of injury

Trauma System Requirements

A trauma system is the integration of resources within the community, region, state, and nation to afford trauma care to all citizens. System requirements begin with access to EMS using 911 as well as ALS level of care through provision of posttrauma rehabilitative services. Within the system, there are trauma centers. Criteria to provide optimal trauma systems include (Pfohman and Criddle 2004)

- Authority to designate trauma centers with a formal process to perform the designation of trauma centers
- ACS-COT standards are used to designate trauma centers
    — Designation occurs when a state or region has the legal responsibility for evaluation of the trauma center
    — Verification is performed by the ACS and acknowledges completion of all standards by the trauma center
- On-site verification at the time of designation with out-of-state surveyors
- Authority to limit trauma centers based upon need yet remain inclusive
- Prehospital triage protocols for trauma

- Method to monitor trauma center, system, and prehospital performance
- Coverage for trauma that is statewide
- Adequate funding
- Staffing to include trauma program managers at the trauma centers
- Trauma registry both within facilities and statewide

TRAUMA CENTERS

Trauma centers are either designated by a state body or verified by the ACS-COT verification committee. In some state systems, a trauma center may receive both. In state designation, criteria may be exactly the same as the ACS-COT or may vary for regional needs. In states with designation standards of their own, the designation is required and the verification would be supplemental. In other systems, the verification is equivalent to state designation.

Trauma center levels are described in Table 3-1. Viability of trauma centers is affected by funding for indigent care, increasing malpractice insurance, low physician reimbursement, physician specialties, and corporate purchasing of trauma centers that may not be interested in the financial commitment to the trauma center (Pfohman and Criddle 2004, Mann et al. 2005). Costs increase with complications. The majority of trauma patients are without complications (~64%) however, the 25% with serious complications, such as pneumonia lead to increased cost (Hemmila et al. 2008).

The demonstrated 15% decrease in mortality in mature trauma systems strongly favors the presence of a trauma system (Celso et al. 2006). Yet, for example in the state of Florida, 95% of the population has a trauma center within 85 minutes and only 38% of patients are transferred to a trauma center (Durham et al. 2006). Continual systems evaluation is necessary to evaluate the nontransferred patients for appropriate levels of care.

The inclusive trauma system encourages all facilities to participate at the appropriate level of care for their skills. Within an inclusive system, patients are more likely to be transferred to a level I or II trauma center which decreases mortality

Table 3-1   Trauma Centers

Trauma Center	Requirements
Level I	Highest level; provides all specialists and all levels of care; may include pediatrics; includes a research program; may be an academic center or a resident teaching facility
Level II	Provides most levels of trauma care; may transfer complex abdominal injury or pelvic fracture; provides all specialists; may perform research/publication
Level III	Provides most specialists without neurosurgical care; has CT scan available and can provide rapid transport to the operating suite; can provide ICU level care; transfers all complex patients and any specialty patients
Level IV	ACS-COT smallest trauma center to evaluate and provide rapid transfer to a higher level center; provides immediate resuscitation and may keep minor injuries for monitoring; does not usually provide surgery
Level V	In some states, exists as a clinic or small facility that may not be open year round or is located in a remote area, such as ski clinics; this facility enables rapid resuscitation for airway, circulation but immediately moves the patient to a higher level of care

(Utter et al. 2006, Lansink and Leenen 2007). The incorporation of level III trauma centers into a system has clearly demonstrated a decrease in mortality as well as an increase in transfers to the level I facility (Tinkoff et al. 2007). Evaluation of outcomes within the system and trauma center is a significant component of the process, especially for head injuries, penetrating injuries, and the elderly where trauma centers differ in care as well as outcome (Shafi et al. 2008).

The success of trauma centers has demonstrated decreased mortality along with earlier recognition of the need for transfer (Newgard et al. 2007). The mortality rates are significantly lower at trauma centers for patients with severe injuries (MacKenzie et al. 2006, Liberman et al. 2004). For transferred patients, shorter emergency department (ED) stays appear to occur for patients with higher severity of injury and those transferred by helicopter (Svenson 2008). However, ED times at a level III trauma center are longer than at a level IV trauma center, and up to 44% of films taken at the referral hospital are repeated at the trauma center (Svenson 2008).

An analysis of the types of patients referred, a level I trauma center evaluated all consultation calls and noted that 77% are accepted with approximately 4% denied, based on lack of clinical need (Spain et al. 2007). The majority of patients were accepted into the trauma or neurosurgical services with orthopaedic services as the next most frequent reason for transfer (Spain et al. 2007). There was no difference noted in payor status. Most of the patients were operative orthopaedic patients or complex nonoperative trauma service patients.

An evaluation of several trauma systems from different nations noted that one system had a significantly higher mortality (20% vs 11.9%) with concomitant higher comorbidity rates. It was noted that this one system was not utilizing trauma team activations and the intensive care unit (ICU) to the best of its ability thus significantly affecting the probability for survival (Cherry et al. 2008). Another interesting hole in the systems in the United States was the identification of elderly trauma patients as needing transfer to a trauma center. The elderly (>65 years, but may be as early as 50 years) were consistently less likely to be transferred to a trauma center (Chang et al. 2008).

Significantly, it is important for trauma centers to affect not only survival but outcome as well. Nirula and Brasel (2006) noted that there is a higher likelihood of independent functional outcome at discharge from the higher level trauma center with minimal numbers of moderate to severe disability. A definitive improvement in functional outcome is related to trauma centers.

Supporting this, one study identified that 42% of trauma patients from within the trauma system return to work within 24 months of injury (Durham et al. 2006).

TRAUMA CENTER REQUIREMENTS

The foundation of the trauma center is the commitment of the facility, its board of directors, and its medical staff. It can take several years from inception to verification/designation to organize the trauma team and perform to the standards. A full list of standards is available from state offices if designation criteria exist or from the American College of Surgeons resource guide (ACS 2006). A brief list of some requirements for trauma center verification include

- Trauma service staff: trauma medical director, trauma program manager, injury prevention coordinator, trauma registrar
  - Authority to run the program, remove staff from the call rosters
  - Management and organization of the trauma program
  - Responsible for site survey preparation, standards evaluation
  - Develop trauma care protocols/guidelines for management of injury and prevention of complications
  - Trauma medical director is a trauma surgeon in level I, II, III facilities; in smaller level IV and V facilities, it may be a family practice or emergency medicine physician
  - Trauma program manager is a masters prepared nurse with trauma experience and preferably a masters degree in trauma nursing
    - May still be titled Trauma Nurse Coordinator in some facilities
    - Organizes the trauma program and provides oversight of all components including budget, staff, and standards in all departments
    - Oversees the staff of the trauma program and works closely with the medical director for a cohesive program from prehospital through rehabilitation

- Ensures that all requirements of the trauma program for designation/verification are in place and that the commitment of the facility to the program is evident
- Ensures that nursing and support staff are trained in trauma management
- Ensures that the performance improvement (PI) program identifies issues for patients and the system and that an action plan for improvement is enforced
- Staff working for the trauma program manager includes and is not limited to trauma registrar, trauma nurse practitioners, injury prevention coordinator, prehospital coordinator, PI coordinator, trauma clinical nurse specialists, trauma educators

- Medical staff and board of directors commitment
- General surgical (trauma) coverage along with the following specialties determined by level of trauma center
  — Neurosurgery
  — Orthopaedics
  — Plastic surgery
  — Oral-maxillofacial surgery
  — Otorhinolaryngology
  — Critical care medicine
  — Anesthesia
  — Emergency medicine
  — Medical subspecialties
- Pediatric trauma care has standards specifically related to children and must be in place if pediatric verification/designation is to be considered
- Participation in prehospital care to include bypass protocols and disaster planning
- Education
  — Continuing medical education requirements for surgeons including advanced trauma life support (ATLS)
  — Continuing educational units for nursing personnel

— Provision of educational programs for staff as well as pre-hospital personnel and referring facilities

- Injury prevention
  — Provided to the community and based upon common trauma patterns within the community and identified in the trauma registry
  — Evaluation of programs
  — An injury prevention coordinator is required in levels I and II facilities

- Triage and transfer
  — Plans for transfer out to higher level trauma centers or specialty centers (burn, head, or spine injury)
  — Triage protocols developed with EMS
  — Trauma team activation criteria and demonstration of its application at the facility

- Facility services
  — ED 24 hours per day staffed with emergency medicine board-certified physicians
  — Operating room available for trauma 24 hours per day with postanesthesia care unit
  — Intensive care unit 24 hours per day with nursing staffing no greater than two patients per RN
  — Medical surgical floors educated to manage the trauma patient
  — Hemodialysis
  — Laboratory services, blood bank
  — Nutrition services
  — Provision for alcohol and drug screening and brief intervention during the hospital stay
  — Discharge planning
  — Rehabilitative services: occupational, physical, speech, physiatry

- Performance improvement program
  — Identifies audit filter issues, deviations from protocol, staff performance

- — Complication incidence and trends
- — Meets at least monthly
- — Includes case review, all death review, and systems-related issues
- — Communicates regionally for local performance improvement between trauma centers and EMS
- — Receives follow-up on transferred patients; provides follow-up to referral facilities
- — Integrated into the hospital performance improvement program
- Participates in local, regional, and national organizations
  - — Publishes in peer-reviewed journals
  - — Performs trauma-related research (level I)

Trauma Registry

The trauma registry is the repository of trauma-related data for each trauma center. The data should be collected concurrently and entered into the database. Data collected is a short version of the chart to provide the data needed to understand

- Population managed at the trauma center
- Statistics to support the performance improvement program especially related to complications, issues/events, or audit filters
  - — Probability of survival
  - — Comparison to local, regional, state, and national data
- Mechanisms of injury and the use of protective devices to assist with injury prevention program design
- General statistics for program review and description
- Support during site survey

The registry must include all data points required by the local county or state as well as support and download to the National Trauma Data Standard (NTDS). The NTDS provides national data to support standards, survival probability, and benchmarking for trauma center care. Of note, there is variability in reporting to the NTDS as well as data from self-designated trauma centers. Benchmarking should be done with care as not all facilities may be reporting all data or complications with an increased reporting in level I and II trauma centers (Kardooni et al. 2008).

The trauma registrar is the individual who analyzes data, abstracts the medical records, enters and evaluates the data, validates the data, and applies the coding processes to the information received. In addition, reports and statistics are produced from the registry by the registrar. The definition of the trauma patient is a facility, local, state, or national definition. The NTDS trauma inclusion criteria include

- Patient must have sustained a traumatic event (mechanism of injury)
- Have at least one injury within the ICD9-CM codes 800.00 to 959.9
  — Excludes late effects, superficial abrasions and contusions as the only injury, and foreign bodies
- Patient must be admitted, or transferred from/to another hospital, or death in hospital or ED

Coding

In the United States, ICD9-CM is still the standard for coding injuries, environmental codes (e-codes) for mechanisms of injury, and procedure codes. In most of the world, ICD10-CM is already in place and is significantly different from ICD9-CM in its methodology. These codes provide

- 1 to 2 mechanism of injury codes (e-codes)
- A place code (e-code)
- All injury codes (although the number entered is limited for NTDS)
- All trauma-related procedures

Use of the ICD9-CM codes promotes consistency across the trauma centers for data entry and allows for comparisons.

In addition, injury severity codes are also applied by the registrar. The Abbreviated Injury Scale (AIS 2005, update 2008) score is applied to determine how severe the individual injuries are. Each injury receives its own code. From these codes, injuries are categorized into body regions and calculated into the injury severity score (ISS). The ISS is the overall severity of injury for the patient. A score > 16 is a moderately severe injury; a score > 25 is a severe injury. ISS is calculated as the highest score from three separate body regions, each squared ($A^2 + B^2 + C^2$). The value of these calculations is for:

- Comparison of similar patients between facilities and regions
- Calculation of probability of survival through the trauma and injury severity score (TRISS) methodology (revised trauma score vs ISS)
  — Survival in patients with a low probability of survival are "good saves" and should be reviewed for the reasons for success
  — Death in patients with a high probability of survival may identify potentially preventable or preventable deaths
- Defines the severity of the population at the trauma center
- Identifies patients for review at site survey

Rural Trauma

Rural areas across the country differ from areas near urban sites, from lack of resources to the expanses of states like Colorado and Wyoming where there may be more cattle per square mile than people. Most of the rural communities have a small hospital to meet the community's general needs, but do not have higher technology and subspecialists, or necessarily services in house 24 hours each day. The EMS may be at a basic life support level or, if ALS is available, it may only be on certain days or at certain times. Weather becomes an issue in transport especially over distances. If transporting to the trauma center by ground, the only ALS provider in the region may be removed from the area until the transport is concluded. The ED is usually served by family practice physicians or nurse practitioners. The nursing staff is small and in some cases staff may serve multiple roles, ie, the paramedic may be the radiology technician and the CEO the laboratory technician. These facilities are intensely dedicated to the community as they are caring for friends and family.

Participation in the trauma system is essential as these facilities are closest to the incidents and are frequently the first provider. An inclusive system encourages these facilities to commit to appropriate trauma care and the rapid transfer of these patients to higher level centers. With the education and performance improvement programs, overall care is improved as trauma principles are applied to all patients.

Rural trauma data have shown more trauma patients are dead at the scene, longer response times of EMS, and longer scene times. The distance for transport is logically longer as well (Gonzalez et al. 2006). Transfers to trauma centers frequently occur in the evening/night (3 p.m. to 7 a.m.) with orthopaedic or neurosurgical injuries (Esposito et al. 2006).

The trauma system as a whole survives as every member participates fully. From injury prevention programs and safe communities through the provision of rehabilitation services for those who have been injured, the trauma center and the system that provides for the community and trauma patient needs to enable optimal outcomes and functional return.

REFERENCES

American College of Surgeons Committee on Trauma (ACS-COT). *Resources for Optimal Care of the Injured Patient 2006.* Chicago, IL: American College of Surgeons; 2006.

Association for the Advancement of Automotive Medicine. *Abbreviated Injury Scale 2005, Update 2008.* Des Plaines, IL: Association for the Advancement of Automotive Medicine; 2008.

Barraco RD, Chiu WC, Bard MR, et al. Practice management guidelines for the appropriate triage of the victim of trauma. Unpublished 2008, www.east.org

Celso B, Tepas J, Langland-Orban B, et al. A systematic review and meta-analysis comparing outcome of severely injured patients treated in trauma centers following the establishment of trauma systems. *J Trauma.* 2006;60(2):371-378.

Chang D, Bass R, Cornwell E, et al. Undertriage of elderly trauma patients to state-designated trauma centers. *Arch Surg.* 2008; 143(8):776-781.

Cherry C, Graham C, Gabbe B, et al. Trauma care systems: a comparison of trauma care in Victoria, Australia, and Hong Kong, China. *Ann Surg.* 2008;247(2):335-342.

Ciesla DJ. Trauma systems and access to emergency medical care. *J Trauma.* 2007;62(6):S51.

Committee on Trauma, Division of Medical Sciences, National Academy of Sciences, National Research Council. *Accidental Death and Disability: the Neglected Disease of Modern Society.* Washington, DC: Public Health Service Publication; 1966.

Dunne JR. Trauma systems and prevention summary for trauma systems. *J Trauma.* 2007;62(6):S43.

Durham R, Pracht E, Orban B, et al. Evaluation of a mature trauma system. *Ann Surg.* 2006;243(6):775-785.

Esposito T, Sanddal T, Reynolds S, et al. Effect of a voluntary trauma system on preventable death and inappropriate care in a rural state. *J Trauma.* 2003;54(4):663-670.

Esposito, T, Crandall, M, Reed, R, Gamelli, R, Luchette, F. Socioeconomic factors, medicolegal issues, and trauma patient transfer trends: is there a connection? *J Trauma.* 2006;61(6):1380-1388.

Gonzalez R, Cummings G, Mulekar M, et al. Increased mortality in rural vehicular trauma: identifying contributing factors through data linkage. *J Trauma.* 2006;61(2):404-409.

Hemmila M, Jakubus J, Maggio P, et al. Real money: complications and hospital costs in trauma. *Surgery.* 2008;144(2):307-316.

Kardooni S, Haut E, Chang D, et al. Hazards of benchmarking complications with the National Trauma Data Bank: numerators in search of denominators. *J Trauma.* 2008;64(2):273-279.

Lansink KWW, Leenen LPH. Do designated trauma systems improve outcome. *Curr Opin Crit Care.* 2007;13(6):686-690.

Liberman M, Mulder D, Lavoie A, et al. Implementation of a trauma care system: evolution through evaluation. *J Trauma.* 2004; 56(6):1330-1335.

MacKenzie EJ, Rivara FP, Jurkovich GJ, et al. A national evaluation of the effect of trauma center care on mortality. *N Engl J Med.* 2006;354(4): 366-378.

Mann NC, MacKenzie E, Teitelbaum S, et al. Trauma system structure and viability in the current healthcare environment: a state by state assessment. *J Trauma*. 2005;58(1):136-147.

Newgard C, McConnell K, Hedges J, et al. The benefit of higher level of care transfer of injured patients from non-tertiary hospital emergency departments. *J Trauma*. 2007;63(5):965-971.

Nirula R, Brasel K. Do trauma centers improve functional outcomes: a national trauma databank analysis? *J Trauma*. 2006; 61(2):268-271.

Papa L, Langland-Orban B, Kallenborn C, et al. Assessing effectiveness of a mature trauma system: association of trauma center presence with lower injury mortality rates. *J Trauma*. 2006;61(2): 261-267.

Pfohman M, Criddle L. A comparison of five state trauma systems meeting all eight essential ACS criteria: a descriptive survey. *J Emerg Nurs*. 2004;30(6):534-541.

Pruitt B. The symbiosis of combat casualty care and civilian trauma care: 1914-2007. *J Trauma*. 2008;64(2):S4-S8.

Shafi S, Friese R, Gentilello L. Moving beyond personnel and process: a case for incorporating outcome measures in the trauma center designation process. *Arch Surg*. 2008;143(2):115-119.

Spain DA, Bellino M, Kopelman A, et al. Requests for 692 transfers to an academic level I trauma center: implications of the emergency medical treatment and active labor act. *J Trauma*. 2007; 62(1):63-68.

Svenson J. Trauma systems and timing of patient transfer: are we improving? *Am J Emerg Med*. 2008;26(4):465-468.

Tinkoff G, O'Connor R, Alexander E, et al. The Delaware trauma system: impact of level III trauma centers. *J Trauma*. 2007;63(1): 121-127.

Utter G, Maler R, Rivara F, et al. Inclusive trauma systems: do they improve triage or outcomes of the severely injured? *J Trauma*. 2006;60(3):529-537.

Ziglar M, Bennett V, Nayduch D, et al. *The Electronic Library of Trauma Lectures*. Chicago, IL: Society of Trauma Nurses; 2004.

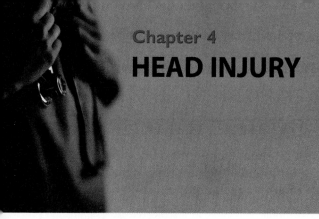

Chapter 4
HEAD INJURY

INTRODUCTION

One of the most devastating events an individual can experience is an injury to the head. Head injuries require not only immediate action for survival, but also prolonged recovery and rehabilitation to accomplish a functional outcome. There are over 1.4 million head injuries each year in the United States. Of these injuries, 50,000 individuals die and over 235,000 arrive at the hospital for treatment. The majority of mechanisms resulting in head injury are falls (28%), followed by motor vehicle collisions (MVC) and other blunt and penetrating mechanisms. Rapid management of injury prevents further secondary brain injury. The Brain Trauma Foundation provides a resource for management of the brain-injured patient, *Guidelines for the Management of Severe Traumatic Brain Injury*. The guidelines were developed through extensive review of the literature and evaluation by leading neurosurgeons in the United States. The monitoring and management suggested in this text reflects the recommendations of these guidelines as well as of the trauma experts'. Adoption of the guidelines can result in a 50% reduction in mortality from head injury (Brain Trauma Foundation 2007).

ASSESSMENT

Neurologic assessment is part of the initial management of the trauma patient. The assessment of airway, breathing, and circulation (ABCs) takes priority and results in reduction of secondary brain injury. Secondary injury occurs from hypoxia, hypercapnia, hypotension/hypovolemia, hypothermia, coagulopathy, and increased intracranial pressure (IICP) (Henzler et al. 2007). Any decrease in mean arterial pressure within the first 4 hours after admission can result in death of the head-injured patient.

The majority of head injuries are mild (80%) (ATLS 2004). In the process of assessing the ABCs, the clinician has begun the neurologic assessment of response to verbal stimuli, orientation, and motor activity. A formal neurologic examination follows the ABCs. As noted in Chapter 2, necessary interventions occur while the assessment is undertaken to prevent delay in management.

History

Collect the initial history of mechanism of injury, any blow or direct impact to the head, or in penetrating injury, type of weapon and range from the victim. The history includes

- Estimated time of length of loss of consciousness (LOC) is usually provided by bystanders and is unreliable, but is a piece of initial assessment that should be documented. In the case of bystanders, especially family, the gravity of the situation often leads to exaggeration of the length of time that the patient was unresponsive. More accurate documentation of LOC can be collected from prehospital providers.
- Initial Glasgow coma scale (GCS) score obtained by prehospital providers is essential
- Any preexisting alteration in consciousness, such as confusion or dementia, or neurologic disorder such as seizures, should be documented in the history
- Headache, nausea, vomiting, prearrival seizure activity
- Personality changes, attention deficits, amnesia for event, memory loss, repetition or perseveration
- Alcohol or drug use

Trauma Assessment

Glasgow coma scale (GCS)

Immediately upon meeting the patient, the responsiveness of the patient is assessed through natural behavior, greeting the patient, and a quick observation of movement and eye opening. These are the initial components of the GCS (Table 4-1). The GCS

Table 4-1   Glasgow Coma Scale Score

Eye opening	
• Spontaneous	4
• To speech	3
• To pain	2
• None	1
Verbal response	
• Oriented	5
• Confused	4
• Inappropriate words	3
• Incomprehensible sounds	2
• None	1
Motor response	
• Obeys commands	6
• Localize to pain	5
• Withdraw from pain	4
• Abnormal flexion (decorticate posturing)	3
• Extension (decerebrate posturing)	2
• None	1
TOTAL	3 to 15

With permission from Teasdale G, Jennett B. Assessment of coma and impaired consciousness: a practical scale. *Lancet.* 1974;2:81-84.

is a measurement of the level of consciousness of the patient (Teasdale and Jennet 1974). It is not an evaluation of the spine or spine-controlled activity. It is a simple tool to provide consistent evaluation of the patient over time and across examiners. The GCS should be repeated at a minimum of every hour and more frequently if the patient's behavior is changing. The motor score of the GCS is the most accurate predictor of outcome (ATLS, 2004). Specific guidelines for GCS assessment are as follows.

GCS Guidelines

- **Assesses brain injury NOT spinal cord injury:** ask spinal-cord-injured patient to move body parts that are above the level of injury, (eg, stick out your tongue, blink your eyes)
- Obtain and document a GCS prior to sedation, neuromuscular blockade, or intubation
- If the patient is not spontaneous, verbal commands are next before inflicting pain to determine response; speak the primary language of the patient when giving commands
- If pain must be inflicted, use central areas such as pinching the supraclavicular area between the thumb and forefinger or pressing into the supraorbital notch with the thumb. DO NOT pinch the nipples. Applying pressure to nailbeds may obtain a response from the patient, but this can be a spinal reflex and not necessarily controlled by the brain
- **Localization:** the attempt to stop or prevent the source of pain
- **Withdrawal:** the movement away from the source of pain
- **Decorticate (abnormal flexion) posturing**—the hands curl inward and the arms will raise to the nipple line but not beyond; toes point downward (Figure 4-1)
- **Decerebrate (extensor) posturing**—the hands and feet extend, extremities are rigid

- **Intubated** patients receive a score of 1 for verbal response with a "T" added to indicate the intubation; if the patient is communicating by writing, the appropriate verbal score should be given
- **Eyes-swollen-shut** patients receive a score of 1 for eye opening with a note to indicate the swelling
- If **paralytics** are given, enter a motor score of 1 with a note regarding the presence of paralytics affecting the motor score
- GCS <8 indicates coma; GCS 9 to 13 indicates moderate head injury; TOTAL GCS = 3 to 15; there is no score <3 or >15!
- GCS is affected by hypovolemia, hypothermia, and the presence of alcohol and drugs; there may or may not be head injury if these are the source of the altered GCS
- Indicate the "best" score for each section; if the body responds differently on each side or changes, document the better of the responses

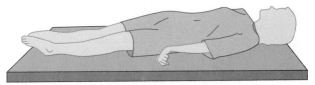

Decerebrate (extensor posturing)

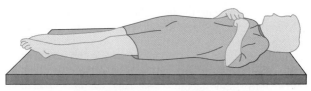

Decorticate (abnormal flexion posturing)

Figure 4-1   Abnormal posturing. (Illustration by Maggie Reynard.)

Table 4-2   Spanish Neurologic Examination

Question/Command	Spanish
Open your eyes	Abre sus ojos
Open your mouth	Abre su boca
Stick out your tongue	Saca su lengua
Squeeze my hand	Apreta mi mano
Release my hand	Solta mi mano
Show me two fingers	Enseña dos dedos
What is your name?	¿Cómo te llamas?
Where are you?	¿Donde estas?
What day is it? What year?	¿Qué dia es hoy? ¿Qué año es hoy?

Specific brain injuries display different responses determined by the role of the part of the brain affected. Individual descriptors of the responses are discussed under management. The GCS provides a global evaluation of head injury. Specific behaviors should also be described, especially as the patient lightens and becomes more interactive with the environment. Table 4-2 provides the Spanish for the basic neurologic examination that will allow the nurse to complete the GCS.

Inspection

As with all assessment, the head should be inspected and palpated for wounds. A scalp laceration can bleed profusely, especially in children. Immediate measures to reduce blood loss should be taken by application of pressure or clips to the edges of the wound until definitive closure later. Palpation of the skull may identify skull fractures especially within a laceration. Depressions in the skull from fracture are also palpable. During inspection of the head, observe for drainage from the ears or nose, which may reveal a basilar skull fracture. The most rapid way to determine if fluid from the nose or ear is cerebrospinal fluid (CSF) is to check for glucose. A drop of the drainage on filter paper will demonstrate separation of blood from CSF, a clear pale yellow liquid.

Motor strength

If the patient is able to cooperate with the examination, motor strength is assessed on a 5-point scale. A rapid assessment of upper and lower extremities involves having the patient lift the arms and legs from the bed. Notation is made if the patient can lift against gravity and against resistance. Motor strength is graded as follows.

Motor Strength Grading

5/5—Full range of motion (ROM) against both normal resistance and gravity
4/5—Full ROM against moderate resistance and gravity
3/5—Full ROM against gravity only
2/5—Full ROM but not against gravity
1/5—Muscle flicker in an attempt at movement but no movement
0/5—No muscle contraction or movement either visible or palpable

If the patient is alert and cooperative, pronator drift can be evaluated. The patient is asked to hold the arms out in front as if holding a tray, palms up, and close the eyes. If the motor strip is compressed, the palm will pronate and drop.

Extraocular movements—pupils

The eye examination is as essential as the GCS. In the case of pharmacologic paralysis, the pupils are the one motor activity that remains intact. Pupils are controlled by cranial nerve (CN) III, which results in constriction. Extraocular movements (requires a cooperative patient) are controlled by CN III, CN IV, and CN VI. Abnormal pupil responses signify early compression of CN III, which passes through the tentorium. When assessing pupils, nonreactivity or unequal pupils may be the result of head injury or intracranial pressure (ICP), direct injury to the globe, or the presence of a glass eye. It has occurred that nurses documented a nonreactive pupil for multiple assessments until the glass eye was recognized!

Pupil size is normally between 2 and 5 mm. Up to a 1-mm discrepancy between the pupils is considered acceptable (anisocoria). Figure 4-2 shows the sizes of pupils for comparison when documenting the size. Documentation should be made regarding pupil shape:

- Round pupil—normal
- Irregular pupil—evidence of eye surgery, cataracts, lens implantation
- Oval pupil—early CN III compression; will progress to dilation and nonreactivity

Pupil reactivity is another component of pupil documentation. Reactivity is a reflex response to light. The light should be shined from the outer canthus of the eye (not directly in front of the pupil). A normal response is constriction. The opposite pupil will also normally constrict in response to the light, consensual response. Pupil responses include:

- Brisk response—normal
- Sluggish response—IICP
- Nonreactive response—severe IICP

   Pupil abnormalities include:

- One fixed and dilated pupil—CN III compression on the side of the pupil

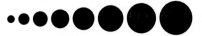

Figure 4-2   Pupil size gauge.

- Bilateral fixed and dilated pupils—CN III compression bilaterally, anoxia
- Pinpoint nonreactive pupils—pons compression
- Bilateral small, equal, reactive pupils—bilateral sympathetic injury at the hypothalamus
- Bilateral midline, nonreactive pupils—midbrain compression
- Bilateral pinpoint reactive pupils—effect of opiates

Frequently nurses document pupils equal, round, and reactive to light and accommodation (PERRLA). Examination of accommodation requires a conscious patient who must focus on an object held within 4 to 6 in from the face. As the object moves closer, the pupils constrict (accommodation). If the patient is not cooperative with the examination, make certain that documentation does not include "A" (accommodation)

Factors affecting pupillary response include

- Constriction—pontine hemorrhage, narcotics, pilocarpine, acetylcholine
- Dilation—drugs such as anticholinergics, dopamine, barbiturates, hallucinogens, antihistamines, amphetamines; instillation of mydriatics for ophthalmologic examinations, atropine, scopolamine

Extraocular movements are assessed with a conscious patient. Ask the patient to follow your finger from center to up, out, down, and in. Using a compass, the directions include north, northeast, east, southeast, south, southwest, west, northwest. (Figure 4-3)

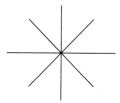

Figure 4-3   Extraocular movements.

- CN III palsy—outward gaze, dilated pupil, ptosis
- CN IV palsy—contralateral eye unable to move downward and in
- CN VI palsy—unable to look laterally

Cranial nerves

Cranial nerves control many sensory and motor activities. Several nerves cross from the head to other body regions, including the diaphragm and abdomen. Table 4-3 describes the 12 cranial nerves, their types, and functions. CN I is usually not assessed initially and requires a conscious patient, but injury may be apparent later when the patient cannot enjoy foods, especially favorites or food from home. Because the sense of taste is related directly to smell, a loss of the sense of smell alters the ability to taste foods. CN I can be injured when the brain slides across the sharp thin bones of the basilar skull.

Respiratory patterns

The pattern of respiration is determined by the midbrain and brainstem. Pressure on the brainstem or direct injury affects respiration. If the patient has been managed rapidly as expected, there may not be the opportunity to observe the respiratory pattern. Intubation and bag-valve-mask ventilation assist the patient but obscure the respiratory pattern. However, head-injured patients can appear alert and then deteriorate rapidly. The clinician should be able to recognize an alteration in respiration. Changes in the respiratory pattern, pupils, and GCS indicate alterations in ICP. Any of these respiratory patterns indicate severe IICP that requires immediate response. Table 4-4 describes the respiratory patterns associated with IICP.

Brain stem reflexes

The functions of the brainstem are usually the last reflexes to be lost when IICP is occurring. In the evaluation of brain death after herniation, the loss of brainstem reflexes is a confirmatory sign. Brainstem reflexes include

- **Cough**—stimulate by suctioning the patient
- **Gag**—stimulate by touching the posterior pharynx; movement of the orogastric tube

- **Corneal**—stimulate by lightly touching the cornea with a wisp of cotton or gauze
  - Long-time contact lens wearers have a decreased response to stimulus of the cornea
- **Pupils**—check reactivity, shape, and size as noted previously
- **Cold calorics**—instillation of 50 mL cold water into the external auditory canals, causing the eyes to deviate toward the stimulus
  - Test CN VII
  - Do not perform this test if there is a question of tympanic membrane rupture or evidence of basilar skull fracture with otorrhea
- **Oculocephalic**—eyes lag behind with a brisk turn of the head, then move back to center; the abnormal response is the eyes remaining midline when the head is turned (like a doll's eyes)
  - Do not perform this test if there is any question of cervical spine injury
- **Babinski reflex**—stroke the bottom of the foot; toes should curl downward >2.5 years; upgoing toes are abnormal unless <2 to 2.5 years
  - Not a brainstem reflex rather controlled by the corticospinal/pyramidal tract
  - Demonstrative of impending herniation

Cerebral monitoring—ICP bolt, ventriculostomy

In addition to close monitoring and management of blood pressure (BP), pulse, oxygenation, the brain can be monitored in various ways. Cerebral oxygenation and pressure are a means of directly observing the brain and its response to injury and edema. The brain attempts to provide itself with adequate oxygen (20% of total cardiac output, 25% of total glucose and oxygen) and nutrition. It is unable to store oxygen on its own. A hematocrit >30% to 33% provides optimal oxygen delivery. Cerebral autoregulation maintains the amount through adequate cerebral blood flow. Normal cerebral blood flow is ~50 to 55 mL/100 g brain tissue per minute.

Table 4-3 Cranial Nerve Function and Assessment

Cranial Nerve	Type	Function/Assessment
I Olfactory	Sensory	Smell: Test each nostril separately.
II Optic	Sensory	Vision: Read with each eye separately.
III Oculomotor	Motor	Extraocular eye movement, eye opening, pupil response, accommodation: Evaluate pupil for reactivity and accommodation.
IV Trochlear	Motor	Extraocular eye movement—superior oblique: Evaluate extraocular movements.
V Trigeminal	Sensory, Motor	Chewing, sensory—forehead, sensory-corneal: Clench teeth, corneal reflex; sharp-dull, pain, light touch, temperature sensory of face.
VI Abducens	Motor	Extraocular eye movement—lateral rectus: Evaluate extraocular movements.
VII Facial	Sensory, Motor	Facial expression, anterior two-thirds tongue taste, salivation, tears: Check smile, show teeth, raise eyebrows, close eyes; taste for sweet, sour, bitter, salt.
VIII Auditory	Sensory	Hearing, equilibrium: Cold caloric reflex, tuning fork vibration check.
IX Glossopharyngeal	Sensory, Motor	Posterior one-third tongue taste, salivation, swallowing: Swallow test, gag reflex.

Table 4-3 Cranial Nerve Function and Assessment (*Continued*)

Cranial Nerve	Type	Function/Assessment
X Vagus	Sensory, Motor	Pharynx and larynx sensory and motor activity; thoracic and abdominal viscera: Raise the soft palate (say "ah"), swallow, voice quality (hoarseness?), check cardiac rhythm for dysrhythmias.
XI Spinal accessory	Motor	Turn head, lift shoulders: Turn head and lift shoulders against resistance.
XII Hypoglossal	Motor	Moves tongue: Push tongue against cheek, move tongue side to side, stick out tongue.

Table 4-4 Respiratory Patterns

Respiratory Pattern	Source	Observations
Cheyne-Stokes	Bilateral cerebral hemispheres Diencephalon	Regular oscillations between periods of hyperpnea and apnea.
Central neurogenic hyperventilation	Low midbrain Upper pons	Sustained rapid respirations.
Apneustic	Midbrain Pons	Pauses at full inspiration.
Cluster	Low pons Upper medulla	Clusters of irregular respirations with apneic periods.
Ataxic	Medulla	Unpredictable, irregular respirations with apnea.

The brain, CSF, and blood are housed within the skull in equilibrium. According to the Monro-Kellie hypothesis, if one of these components increases in volume, the others must decrease. Cerebral edema and space-occupying lesions such as subdural or epidural hematomas, compete for space within the skull. The brain alters blood flow and CSF production to accommodate the extra volume. When it can no longer accomplish equilibrium, ICP increases and the brain will herniate through the foramen magnum, resulting in brain death.

ICP monitoring allows the clinician to observe the brain's response to injury. ICP monitoring should be initiated for the following patients: a patient in coma (GCS ≤8) with an abnormal head computed tomography (CT) scan for injury; a patient in coma with a normal head CT scan with either >40 years and unilateral or bilateral posturing, and/or any episode of hypotension. Cerebral perfusion pressure is calculated by subtracting the ICP from the mean arterial pressure (MAP). Cerebral perfusion pressure (CPP) indicates the degree to which blood flow to the brain exceeds the pressure within the skull providing adequate flow and oxygenation, global blood delivery. To maintain a CPP >60 mm Hg, a MAP of 80 mm Hg is required. It becomes evident that any hypotensive episode leads to secondary brain injury.

There are several methods to monitor cerebral blood flow. The most common is an ICP bolt/monitor and the ventriculostomy. The ICP bolt is the least accurate of the devices currently available. These monitors are placed by the neurosurgeon through a simple burr hole and attached to an external strain gauge transducer. The ICP monitor (bolt) is usually within the epidural space and is then zeroed and the waveform observed. A fiberoptic tipped catheter may be used as well. This catheter needs slight repositioning after insertion to remove any tissue from the tip itself. The fiberoptic catheters are a closed system, do not have a flushing system, and can be disconnected/reconnected without requiring recalibration. These surface monitors may not reflect the deep tissue ICP.

The ventriculostomy is inserted into the anterior horn of the lateral ventricle and is leveled at the foramen of Monro, most easily identified at the external auditory meatus. The ventriculostomy allows for monitoring similar to the bolt with the additional benefit of CSF drainage to relieve IICP. The drainage device is placed at the height determined in the orders and may be set to drain intermittently or determined by ICP readings. CSF drainage is first-line therapy for IICP. IICP threshold for drainage is usually 20 to 25 mm Hg. At the time the ventriculostomy is placed, the catheter is tunneled under the skin to decrease potential for infection. Infection rates without tunneling are 5.6% to 20% whereas the tunneled catheters show a rate of 0% to 4% (March 2005). Infection rates are also affected by positioning >5 days and where it was placed (ICU vs ED). Coagulopathies need correction prior to placement of the ventriculostomy to prevent hemorrhage.

Do not flush either the bolt or ventriculostomy system unless specifically trained to do so! When flushing is performed, preservative-free solution must be used. Be particularly careful that the correct transducer (external strain gauge) has been chosen to prevent error.

Cerebral monitoring—oxygen monitoring

A method of monitoring cerebral oxygenation is through the jugular bulb venous oxygenation saturation ($S_{jb}O_2$). Blood exiting the brain passes though the jugular bulb. A measurement of oxygen here reflects the oxygen uptake by the brain. This method does detect hypoxia but significant desaturation may occur prior to identification. To measure the jugular bulb saturation, a catheter is threaded into the jugular vein in a retrograde fashion into the jugular bulb.

Brain tissue oxygen monitoring measures the oxygen at the level of the white matter and is more sensitive than $S_{jb}O_2$. Hypoxia frequently occurs within the first 24 hours and its early identification prevents secondary brain injury. This triple lumen catheter measures brain oxygen, temperature, and ICP (LICOX). Approximately 1 to 1.5 hours after placement, the brain tissue has recovered from any microtrauma during insertion of the probe. This accurate method of determining cerebral oxygenation provides rapid information regarding hypoxia or worse, ischemia to the brain.

Cerebral Monitoring Measurement Norms

- Normal ICP = 0 to 15 mm Hg; maintain <20-25 mm Hg
- CPP = MAP − ICP
- CPP should be maintained >60 mm Hg
- Jugular venous oxygenation ($S_{jb}O_2$) = 60-75%
  - Cerebral extraction of oxygen (CEO_2) = $SaO_2 − S_{jb}O_2$ (normal 24-40%)
  - Oligemic cerebral hypoxia <50-54% (CEO_2 >40%)
  - Hyperemic >80-90% (CEO_2 <24%)
- Brain tissue oxygen ($PbrO_2$) = 30 to 35 mm Hg (range 25-50 mm Hg)
  - Hypoxia <20-25 mm Hg (critical)
  - Ischemia <15 mm Hg

Sedation monitoring

A component of management of the brain injured patient is sedation. Shivering, agitation, seizures, and many bedside procedures increase oxygen demand by the brain. Sedation is a method of decreasing that demand. Neuromuscular blockade provides a means of paralysis however does not manage awareness and pain. If neuromuscular blockade is used to synchronize ventilation and decrease activity, a neuromuscular transmission monitor (Train of Four) can be used to monitor an evoked response to peripheral nerve stimulation or level of paralysis.

For sedation, however, the bispectral index (BIS) monitor provides continuous evaluation of the degree of sedation. In this way, minimal drug usage can provide optimal sedation by maintaining an adequate hypnotic state. It also provides monitoring of periods of arousal or activities that cause arousal, return to consciousness, and the "waking up" of the sedated patient. A level of burst suppression is necessary if using barbiturate coma to manage IICP. The BIS monitor provides this assessment without oversedating the patient.

BIS Sedation Monitoring	
Awake	100
Responsive to commands	80
Unresponsive to verbal commands	<60
Hypnosis	40
Burst suppression	<20

DOCUMENTATION

Documentation includes all observations of the patient's verbal and motor activity as well as the reflexes noted above. The initial GCS should be documented before sedation or intubation has occurred so that at least one baseline GCS is available. GCS should be monitored no less than every hour for severe brain injury and approximately every 4 hours in minor concussions. Pupil checks should accompany the GCS and document size, reactivity, and equality. As the patient awakens, changes in behavior indicate the progress toward baseline preinjury status. Because of the importance of oxygenation, normothermia, and normovolemia, vital sign documentation is as essential as the GCS.

MANAGEMENT

Initial Resuscitation

Head injury can be prevented only through injury prevention efforts directed at protecting the head, such as helmet use. After the initial head injury, all efforts are focused on preventing secondary injury to the brain. The efforts begin immediately and are the same as the management of all trauma patients. Prevent any episode of hypoxia, hypotension, and hypothermia

- Secure the airway. If the GCS is ≤8, even if the patient appears to have a patent airway, intubation should be conducted.

  — Anticipate oral intubation to avoid possible facial fractures and intubation of the cranium through these fractures

  — An orogastric tube should be placed to prevent aspiration

  — During rapid sequence intubation (RSI), succinylcholine may increase ICP Use etomidate and vecuronium for RSI

- Prevent hypoxia! Apply 100% FiO_2 and maintain the PO_2 >100 mm Hg with oxygen saturations (SaO_2) >95%

  — Maintain PCO_2 = 35 to 38 mm Hg, low normal. Avoid hyperventilation in early management, especially if hand-bagging the patient.

  — Immediately manage any breathing complication, such as pneumothoraces

  — Consider continuing neuromuscular blockade and sedation after initial neurologic examination and to maintain synchronous ventilation without agitation

  — Activities that increase oxygen demand and should be minimized are

    ▪ Hypoxia

    ▪ Hypotension, hypovolemia, anemia

    ▪ Pain

    ▪ Shivering

    ▪ Agitation

    ▪ Seizures

    ▪ Fever

- Prevent hypotension by placing two large-bore IV using isotonic fluids (NSS or LR) and blood products. Avoid hypotonic solutions such as D5W that increase cerebral edema by decreasing osmolarity. Hyperglycemia leads to a poor outcome;

therefore glucose-containing solutions should be avoided during resuscitation.

— Control bleeding sources especially from the scalp

— Maintain MAP between 70 and 90 mm Hg with CPP >60 mm Hg

— To provide optimal oxygenation, Hgb should be ≥10 (Hct ≥30). Monitor coagulation.

— One incidence of hypotension (BP <90 mm Hg) can result in poor outcome for severe head injury

• Warm the patient to maintain normothermia

— Every 1°C change in temperature causes a 5% to 10% change in metabolism

— Brain temperature is approximately 1° to 2°C higher than the core

• After the secondary trauma survey and management as outlined in Chapter 2, a CT scan of the head is the gold standard for defining the head injury present. The remaining head injury management is dependent upon the ICP, presence of surgical lesions, or any evidence of transtentorial herniation, and is managed along with other life-threatening injury such as abdominal or thoracic hemorrhage which must be addressed rapidly to prevent hypotension. Head CT should precede a CT that will require contrast. Contrast will obscure findings on the head CT.

Scalp Injury

The scalp has five layers to provide protection to the underlying skull:

• S skin
• C connective tissue
• A aponeurosis (galea)
• L loose areolar tissue
• P periosteum

The scalp is vascular and therefore prone to bleeding especially in children. This blood loss can also occur as a subgaleal hematoma which is less obvious than a laceration. A "scalping" can also occur that results in blood loss and threatens the survival of the scalp tissue as is has been pulled free of its attachment to the skull.

Management

Scalp lacerations may be controlled with simple pressure or, in a large bleeding wound, surgical clips can be attached to the edges to control the bleed. A whipstitch suture can be placed rapidly to temporarily tamponade the wound edges. The wounds need eventual suture or staple closure and/or debridement as necessary. In the case of a scalping, plastic surgery should be involved to manage the injury.

Skull Fracture

The vault of the skull consists of the frontal, parietal bones, and the upper occipital and temporal bones. The names of the bones correspond to the lobes of the brain that they protect. The skull is made up of two layers of bone with a spongy layer in between to absorb impact. Vault skull fractures can be linear (70% incidence), usually requiring no specific management, or depressed skull fractures (Hoyt and Selfridge-Thomas 2007). Depressed fractures usually require elevation in surgery. These fractures involving both the inner and outer table of the skull can then impinge upon brain tissue causing laceration or contusion, tear the dura, or cause bleeding. Under 2 years of age, skull fractures are the best predictor of intracranial injury (Avarello and Cantor 2007). Skull fractures can result in

- Infection, especially if the bony sinuses are involved or the fracture is open
- Cerebral hematoma
- Seizures
- Pneumocephaly if the bony sinuses are involved or the fracture is open

The base of the skull consists of the lower temporal and occipital bones, and the sphenoid, ethmoid, and cribriform plate bones. The basilar skull is particularly thin at the temporal skull and vulnerable to injury. The major arteries and veins traverse the skull through the base. Because of the structure of the base of the skull, its thin sharp bones may cause injury to the brain and CN I (anosmia) during acceleration as the brain moves across the basilar skull. The posterior cranial fossa contains the brainstem and cerebellum and is housed at the posterior basilar skull. The most severe basilar skull fracture (BSF) is a hinge fracture, which crosses the base of the skull from one side to the other and usually disrupts the major arteries in the process (Figure 4-4). It can be caused by penetrating or blunt trauma. BSF can result in meningitis, encephalitis, and/or abscess. Epidural hematoma can occur from injury to the middle meningeal artery that crosses at the temporal skull.

Fractures that cross the carotid canals should be evaluated for carotid injury (transection, dissection, pseudoaneurysm, or

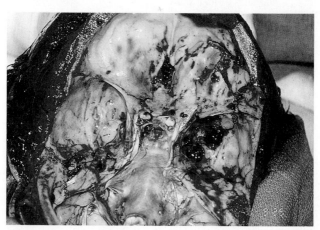

Figure 4-4   Hinge fracture.

thrombosis). Injuries can be identified prior to stroke if evaluated early and by using CT-angiogram. Management of the carotid injury can then occur prior to complication.

Signs and Symptoms of Injuries to the Anterior Basilar Skull

- Periorbital contusions (raccoon eyes) within 24 hours of injury
  — Can also be nasal or orbital fractures without BSF
- CSF leak from the nose (rhinorrhea)
  — Postnasal drip that tastes salty or sweet
- Conjunctival hemorrhage
- May include facial fractures and nasal tubes should be avoided

Signs and Symptoms of Injuries to the Middle Cranial Basilar Skull

- Posterior scalp contusion behind the ear (Battle sign), within 24 hours of injury
- CSF leak from the ear (otorrhea)
- Decreased hearing, vertigo
- Functional alteration in CN V
- Hemotympanum

Management

Management of skull fractures include

- Avoid blowing nose or sneezing
- Monitor CSF leak; if it continues, a lumbar drain can be placed to offload the pressure and assist the leak to seal

- Do not block the ear or nose
- Administer antibiotics for BSF, open-skull fractures, fractures through the sinuses
- Administer vaccines for *haemophilus influenza*, pneumococcus, and meningococcus for basilar skull fractures especially those involving sinuses
- Avoid nasal tubes to prevent intubation of the cranium
- Surgical repair of depressed and open skull fractures for elevation and debridement with possible dural repair
- Monitor for seizures

Fractures of the sinuses can result in pneumocephalus, air within the cranial cavity. Usually this will resorb on its own, however on rare occasion, the opening into the sinus cavity can suddenly "suck" air into the cranium resulting in severe pneumocephalus that acts in the same way as a hematoma. The clinician needs to be aware of this possibility while monitoring the neurologic examination. The pneumocephalus requires decompression as well as the skull fracture requiring sealing, usually with Teflon to prevent further pneumocephalus. Frontal sinus fractures may be obliterated with tissue to seal the fracture.

Carotid Cavernous Sinus

Injuries to the carotid cavernous sinus and the sagittal sinus are rare, approximately 1% to 2% (Ruffolo 2000). However when the injury occurs, the results can be devastating if not identified immediately. It is caused by shear forces or direct blow to the internal carotid artery (ICA) which tears the artery from its dural attachments resulting in injury. Associated injuries include subdural and epidural hematomas, depressed skull fractures, CN injuries, and pseudoaneurysm of the ICA.

Carotid cavernous sinus injury forms an abnormal arteriovenous anastomosis between the carotid and the cavernous sinus causing a high-flow shunt. It is the resulting venous congestion that results in symptoms. The changes can occur days to weeks after injury making the clinician ever-vigilant to the subtle signs and symptoms. Blindness is the most common and most serious change. Unnoticed and untreated, the injury can result in subarachnoid hemorrhage, intracranial hemorrhage, infarct, and death. At the least, blindness can be permanent from the hypoxic injury to the eye. Emergent treatment is necessary in the presence of epistaxis, blindness, sphenoid sinus aneurysm, and coma.

Signs and Symptoms of Carotid Cavernous Sinus Fistula

Visual disturbances including blindness, diplopia from an orbital mass or compression of CN III, CN IV, CN VI
Epistaxis
Pulsatile exophthalmos, pulsatile tinnitus—alert complaining of a pulse in the eye or face
Temporal bruit, orbital bruit
Chemosis, proptosis
Oculomotor palsies
Headache

Management

Angiography confirms the presence of the carotid cavernous fistula (CCF). They are classified according to the Barrow system (Barrow et al. 1985).

- A—direct, single ICA to cavernous sinus fistula, high flow
- B—indirect, meningeal branch of the ICA to cavernous sinus
- C—indirect, meningeal branch of the external carotid artery (ECA) to cavernous sinus
- D—indirect, meningeal branch of ICA and ECA to cavernous sinus

Indirect fistulas are described as such because they are low flow and will spontaneously resolve. The high-flow direct CCF requires treatment. During the angiogram, direct occlusion of the CCF is the optimal management. Coil embolization of the CCF occludes the fistula but maintains the integrity of the ICA. Complete occlusion will occur within days as a result of coagulation around the coils causing a fibrin plug. However clots from this plug can result in stroke. So in addition to coiling the CCF, administration of heparin and daily aspirin 325 mg is added to the therapy. The patient's associated head injuries must be able to tolerate the anticoagulation prior to initiating this therapy.

Diffuse Injury

Diffuse head injury occurs when the entire brain has undergone acceleration or blast effects. In some patients there is no clear evidence of the injury on CT scan of the head, yet there are clear neurologic deficits or effects after the event. In these patients the diagnosis of traumatic brain injury or concussion may be assigned. Most of these are minor head injuries and will resolve over the coming months. Approximately 3% will deteriorate, thus serial neurologic examinations are necessary to identify subtle changes (ATLS 2008).

Consciousness is the awareness of self and the surroundings with an ability to respond to the environment. Coma can occur (GCS <8) which results in the LOC and an unarousable state. An altered level of consciousness can occur when the patient is aware of the environment but may have altered or unexpected responses to it. This is not LOC, but only altered consciousness. Clinicians should be careful regarding the documentation of LOC versus altered consciousness. The GCS is a standard guide for this. Concussion involves a transient cessation of the reticular activating system, which is responsible for the normal sleep-wake cycle.

Signs and Symptoms of Concussion

- Transient loss of consciousness (<6 hours) with the following symptoms
  — Headache
  — Confusion, disorientation
  — Dizziness
  — Nausea, vomiting
  — Memory, concentration difficulties
  — Irritability
  — Fatigue
- Simple—brief loss of consciousness (~1-2 minutes), usually associated with resolution of symptoms within 7 to 10 days; GCS 13 to 15
- Complex—longer loss of consciousness, cognitive impairments can last >7 to 10 days; GCS 9 to 13, amnesia, focal deficits, confusion

There are other injuries which appear to have a negative CT scan, but have a deeper LOC and have a resultant positive magnetic resonance scan (MRI) for diffuse axonal injury (DAI), shear hemorrhages, or petechial hemorrhages. Some of the

Signs and Symptoms of DAI

- Prolonged LOC
- IICP
- Hypertension, hyperthermia
- Abnormal posturing
- Memory deficits

newer 64-slice CT scanners are capable of identifying these petechial hemorrhages. This injury occurs as the white and grey matter "slide" across each other during acceleration, resulting in tearing of the small vessels and axons crossing between the two. DAI may present as a minor injury or more commonly can be severe, even devastating.

Management

All patients with a documented LOC of >5 minutes and associated with amnesia of event, headache, and GCS <15 should receive a CT scan to identify injury (ATLS 2004). Minor traumatic brain injury management includes

- Asymptomatic—observe, then home with neurologic checks for 24 hours
    - Return to ED for any persistent or worsening headache, changes in level of consciousness, local deficits
    - Admit if there is no caregiver to perform neurologic checks
- GCS 9 to 13—repeat CT, monitor in ICU for 12 to 24 hours

Explain to the patient and caregivers that there are common signs and symptoms that involve thinking, communication, and the physical body following minor head injury, and can occur for approximately 3 months after the initial injury. If these symptoms worsen immediately after injury, the patient should return to the ED. If symptoms persist (>6 weeks), consultation with the primary care MD, neuropsychology, occupational therapy, and/or speech therapy is helpful (Cushman et al. 2001). For children and students, neuropsychology is very helpful with return to school. The "postconcussive" syndrome includes

- Headache
- Dizziness
- Nausea and vomiting
- Drowsiness and fatigue
- Blurry vision
- Concentration problems or thinking slowly
- Memory difficulties

- Building things or putting things together
- Solving problems, organization of daily activities
- Problems with sleep, not feeling rested
- Relationship problems, irritability, sadness, discouragement, tense
- Difficulty with word-finding
- Slow, hesitant, slurred speech
- Difficulty understanding complicated issues
- Difficulty expressing thoughts verbally or in writing
- Slow writing, spelling errors, math errors

Concussions which occur in sports or persons after nonsport concussions who participate in sports need special consideration regarding return to activity after injury. Second-impact syndrome has been described in which a second head injury occurs with relative proximity (before the symptoms of the first have cleared) to the first resulting in life threatening hemorrhages and sometimes death (Saunders and Harbaugh 1984, Cantu 1998). There should be no return to play or practice of sports until all symptoms have resolved. Unfortunately, some children hide the symptoms in order to return to play resulting in devastating second-impact injury. The guidelines intend to identify potential severe injury as well as protect the player from repeated head injury. Repeated injuries do not need to be severe to have a poor outcome. Per the EAST Mild TBI Guidelines (Cushman 2001), the set of suggested return to play guidelines briefly are described as follows.

Postconcussive Return to Play Guidelines

I Confusion without amnesia or LOC clearing within 20 to
   30 minutes
- Return to play; clearing >30 minutes, return to play in 1 week
- Second similar injury same season, return to play in 2 weeks
  with 1 asymptomatic week and a normal CT scan

- Third similar injury same season, no return to play; perhaps next season if asymptomatic

II Confusion with amnesia, no LOC
- Return to play after evaluation and asymptomatic for 1 week
- Second similar injury same season, return to play in 1 month if asymptomatic, normal CT scan
- Third similar injury same season, no return to play; may terminate play indefinitely

III LOC
- Hospital transport, CT scan
- Return to play if asymptomatic 2 weeks, LOC <1 minute, CT scan normal
- LOC >1 minute, return to play in 1 month if asymptomatic for at least 2 weeks
- Second similar injury same season no return to play; may terminate play indefinitely

Diffuse axonal injury patients are usually admitted as a result of the LOC and monitored for associated injuries as well as neurologic deterioration from IICP. IICP management is discussed later in this chapter.

Intracerebral Contusions, Subdural Hematoma (SDH), Epidural Hematoma (EDH), Subarachnoid Hemorrhage (SAH)

The brain is affected by direct injury in a profound way. Direct injuries can occur ranging from contusions or bruising of the brain parenchymal tissue to hematomas that are space-occupying lesions competing with the brain for space within the skull. Intracerebral contusions are exactly as described and affect the region of the brain in which they occur. They are like a bruise anywhere else on the body, developing from impact, increasing in size, and associated with swelling, then healing and being resorbed by the body. In the brain, however tissue can recover from the contusion or suffer permanent damage. The long-term damage is related to the degree of edema, IICP, and any episode of hypoxia or hypotension. Most contusions do not require surgery but may require ICP management.

Signs and Symptoms of Intracerebral Contusions

Prolonged LOC, focal neurologic signs dependent upon the
　　lobe involved or the lobe affected by edema
Personality, behavioral, speech deficits

The lobes of the brain perform different roles as defined below. The injuries will demonstrate changes within these areas as well as during the healing process.

Functions of the Brain

Frontal—personality/ behavior, inhibition, judgment, voluntary
　　motor functions, emotion and expression
Parietal—sensory, spatial orientation, motor strip along the falx cerebri
Temporal—speech reception and integration, memory; left-sided
　　speech in 100% of right handed people and 85% of
　　left-handed people
Occipital—vision
Diencephalon (thalamus, hypothalamus)—temperature,
　　hormone regulation, emotion, autonomic responses, peristalsis
Cerebellum—fine motor coordination, movement, balance, posture
Brainstem:
Midbrain and upper pons—reticular activating system
Medulla—heart rate, respirations, BP

Hematomas are epidural (EDH) or subdural (SDH). Their names identify their position in relationship to the three layers of dura. Epidurals are usually arterial in nature and are frequently associated with a temporal basilar skull fracture with subsequent middle meningeal artery laceration (Figure 4-5). In children, however these may be venous. They are positioned outside of the dura mater below the skull. When arterial, they grow rapidly requiring surgical intervention to evacuate the hematoma and control the bleeding.

Signs and Symptoms of EDH

Rapid deterioration to altered level of consciousness or LOC
   with lucid interval—hemiparesis, posturing
Rapid IICP—ipsilateral fixed and dilated pupil
Headache, nausea, vomiting
Dizziness
Sleepiness
Symptoms usually within 6 hours
Mortality up to 20%

Subdural hematomas (SDH) are located between the dura mater and pia mater and are usually venous in nature caused by injury to the bridging veins located here. They grow more slowly because of their venous nature, resulting in more severe brain injury as they may go unnoticed initially and can be asymptomatic until they are large enough to cause pressure on the brain and shift of the midline structures. They are frequent in the elderly, especially those on anticoagulants. A simple fall in these patients can result in the beginning of the bleed. Because of cerebral atrophy, symptoms can be delayed until the subdural is sizeable, up to 2 weeks or more. Alcohol abuse also results in coagulopathies, which can encourage a SDH after a simple low-energy impact as well. In children, the presence of a SDH is frequently a sign of abuse especially without an intensive mechanism such as an MVC. Figure 4-6 shows the CT scan of a SDH.

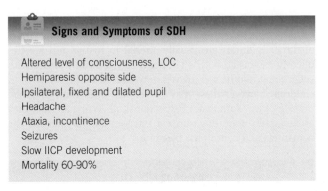

Signs and Symptoms of SDH

Altered level of consciousness, LOC
Hemiparesis opposite side
Ipsilateral, fixed and dilated pupil
Headache
Ataxia, incontinence
Seizures
Slow IICP development
Mortality 60-90%

Subarachnoid hemorrhages (SAH) occur within the sub-arachnoid layer, where the CSF flows through the ventricles, spine, and across the brain surface. Because of its closeness to the brain tissue, the presence of blood within the subarachnoid space is irritating to the brain. The brain responds to a trauma SAH in much the same way as a stroke SAH.

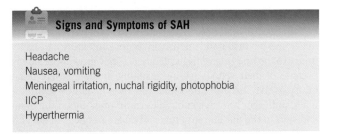

Signs and Symptoms of SAH

Headache
Nausea, vomiting
Meningeal irritation, nuchal rigidity, photophobia
IICP
Hyperthermia

Management

Maximal edema for contusions is usually at 18 to 36 hours after injury. This "blossoming" of the contusion can result in IICP during that time and needs neurologic and hemodynamic monitoring as well as secondary brain injury prevention. Most

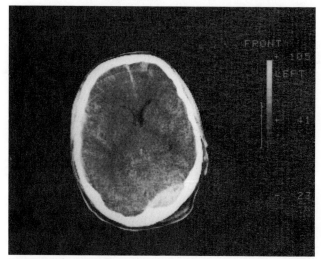

Figure 4-5   Epidural hematoma.

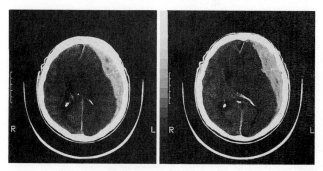

Figure 4-6   Subdural hematoma.

contusions are frontal and temporal caused by acceleration-sudden deceleration injuries. Some will evolve into an actual intracerebral hematoma that may require evacuation. Repeat CT scan is essential to monitor these lesions.

EDH and SDH may require surgical removal if they are of a considerable size that result in midline shift, neurologic deficits, IICP, and/or herniation of the brainstem. Rapid transport to surgery for decompression can save the patient's life as well as immediately decrease IICP. At times, only the hematoma needs to be removed. On occasion the skull flap is left off when there is significant edema of the brain tissue, allowing further space for the brain to swell without the restriction of the skull box. This is a decompressive craniectomy. The skull flap is protected in a special freezer in the OR or is placed in a fat layer flap of the abdomen. A football-like helmet is used to protect the brain in the ensuing period. A decompressive craniectomy may be done in the absence of a hematoma. It is also an effective means of managing IICP from edema as well. Later, the flap is returned to the skull.

The elderly patient with a slowly developing SDH but with neurologic deficit, may be managed with simple burr holes and drains to decompress the acute/subacute bleed. The drains are managed as any surgical drain with careful attention to prevent any air from entering the drain itself.

The only specific management of SAH beyond monitoring for vasospasm and managing IICP is to maintain a quiet environment to decrease stimulation of an already irritable brain. For all brain injuries, the potential for IICP is high. Constant vigilance is the key to identification of IICP, signs of ineffective management with the need to escalate therapy, and prevent herniation.

Penetrating Injury

Penetrating head injuries can result from various sources such as gunshots, stabbing with knives or other implements, impalement, arrows or any other possible implement. Low-velocity penetrating injuries usually affect the direct track of the implement.

High-velocity injuries are usually from gunshots in which the bullet creates a track and the pressure wave traveling in front of the bullet damages surrounding tissue as well from the blast effect. Not all penetrating injuries cross the skull and others both enter and exit the skull. Both symptoms and recovery are dependent upon the structures injured, time to resuscitation, depth of penetration as well as the blast effect. Figure 4-7 demonstrates the CT scan of a GSW to the head, with bullet and bone along the track of the bullet. Mortality from penetrating brain injury is approximately 60% (Hoyt and Selfridge-Thomas 2007).

Management

Wounds from penetrating trauma require debridement to prevent infection. Management focuses on prevention of IICP and

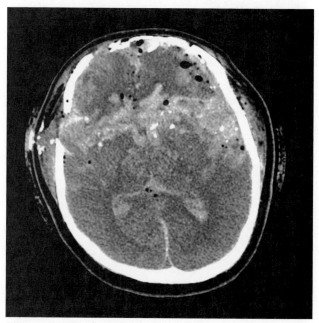

Figure 4-7   Gunshot wound to the head.

secondary brain injury as with all head injuries. The wounds may become a means for brain swelling herniation in severe injuries. Figure 4-8 shows the simplicity of the external wound in some GSW to the head as well as the forensic evidence of the muzzle marking, soot, and gunpowder. This is a fatal self-inflicted wound. Do not assume the injury is benign because the wound is small. Skull films may be used to determine the presence and position of the bullet or implement. CT scan will demonstrate the

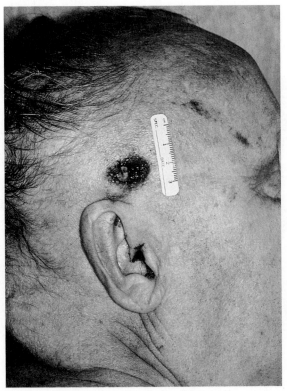

Figure 4-8   Gunshot wound to the head (external).

degree of intracranial injury. If the implement, such as knife or pliers, is still in place, removal occurs in the OR only.

IICP

ICP is affected by the contents of the skull—brain, blood, CSF, and in the case of trauma, edema and/or hemorrhage. The brain attempts to maintain control of the ICP by decreasing blood flow through vasoconstriction or decreasing CSF production. Vessels respond to PCO_2 levels. Increased PCO_2 results in vasodilation whereas decreased PCO_2 causes vasoconstriction. The patient may hyperventilate in an attempt to regulate ICP.

Actions should be taken to prevent IICP, however the following are the early signs and symptoms which indicate a need for immediate management.

Early Signs and Symptoms of IICP

Headache
Nausea, vomiting
Amnesia for event, LOC
Restlessness, drowsiness
Speech and judgment deficits

Late signs of IICP indicate impending herniation. Uncal herniation into the posterior fossa is the most common. Central transtentorial herniation places pressure directly on the brainstem and diencephalon. Pupillary changes are directly related to the presence of CN III passing along the edge of the tentorium. The pressure of IICP and herniation result in the pupillary changes. Treatment of IICP should be initiated or if already in place, then escalated prior to late signs or herniation. Herniation results in brain death if allowed to proceed.

Late Signs and Symptoms of IICP

Dilated nonreactive pupil(s)
Unresponsive
Posturing or no motor response
Cushing syndrome—widened pulse pressure, hypertension,
    bradycardia, altered respiratory pattern/rate

Signs and Symptoms of Uncal Herniation

Ipsilateral pupil dilation
Asymmetric pupil reactivity
Contralateral hemiparesis
Posturing

Signs and Symptoms of Transtentorial Herniation

Early—small and reactive to midline, unreactive pupils; upward
    gaze, agitated, negative Babinski reflex, contralateral
    hemiparesis to posturing, Cheyne-Stokes or central
    neurogenic hyperventilation, diabetes insipidus, hypertension
Late—fixed and dilated pupils; dysconjugate gaze; unrespon-
    sive, flaccid; positive Babinski reflex; ataxia, apnea; hyper-
    thermia; hypotension

IICP Management

The management of ICP, including simple nursing measures
that have a great impact on the overall prevention of IICP, is
outlined in Table 4-5. The management of IICP that is refractory to the standard management techniques is outlined in
Table 4-6. There is no substitute for vigilance in hemodynamic

Table 4-5   IICP Management

Therapy	Management
CSF Drainage	Requires ventriculostomy placement. First-line therapy ICP >20 mm Hg.
Osmotic Diuretics Mannitol 20%	Use with signs of herniation or progressive neurologic deterioration (dilated pupil, decreased LOC). Avoid hypovolemia, hypotension; assure adequate resuscitation before administration. Administer as intermittent boluses, 0.25-1 g/kg body weight over 5 minutes. Maintain serum osmolarity <320 mOsm to prevent renal failure.
Sedation/pain management Narcotics	Morphine inexpensive but has histaminergic properties and long half-life. Fentanyl shorter half life, more expensive. Naloxone reversal agent.
Benzodiazepines	Longer acting agents. Flumazenil reversal agent.
Propofol	Expensive but rapid emergence. Monitor lipids, especially with nutrition. Hypotension with rapid administration; ensure hemodynamic stability. Decreases cerebral metabolic rate.
Neuromuscular blockade	Use for ventilator asynchrony, which increases intrathoracic pressure, decreases venous return, results in IICP. Add sedation and analgesia. Prolonged use results in myopathy and postparalytic quadriparesis.
Steroids	There is no valid use for steroid therapy in severe head injury

(Continued)

Table 4-5   IICP Management (*Continued*)

Therapy	Management
Nutrition	Nutrition is essential for all critical patients to provide the energy needed for the hypermetabolic state, immunity, wound healing. Chemically paralyzed head-injured patient—replace 100% resting metabolic needs. Nonparalyzed head-injured patient—replace 140% resting metabolic needs. Ensure minimum 15% of calories are from protein. Use enteral (preferred) or parenteral feeds. Initiate no later than 7 days postinjury.
Antiseizure prophylaxis	Prophylaxis of late posttraumatic seizures is not recommended. Prophylaxis of early seizures (within first week) is effective for high-risk patients (cerebral hematoma, depressed skull fracture, penetrating head injury). Phenytoin, fosphenytoin, or carbamazepine are effective. Does not show improved outcome with prophylaxis. If seizures occur for a prolonged period, secondary brain injury will occur.
Nursing specific interventions	Elevate head of bed 30 degrees; avoid hip flexion to prevent impeding venous outflow; ensure hemodynamic stability first. Avoid hyperflexion of the neck; maintain midline. Minimize stimulation of cough or gag reflex. Plan activities to provide rest periods, quiet environment. Provide orientation, talk with patient, family photos in room. Separate stressful procedures—turning, suctioning. Suction <10 seconds with oxygenation between suctioning. Monitor ICP throughout all procedures. Provide sedation and analgesia for pain and stress relief. Antipyretics to avoid hyperthermia; Temperature >38.5°C within first 48 hours increases disability and length of stay. (Mcilvoy 2005)

Table 4-6   Management for Refractory IICP

Therapy	Management
Hyperventilation	Recommended only for brief periods if IICP is refractory to sedation, osmotic diuretics, paralysis, or ventriculostomy drainage.
	Should not be used prophylactically within the first 24 hours after injury when cerebral blood flow is reduced caused by the acute injury.
	If used, keep PCO_2 30 to 35 mm Hg, not lower.
	Suggest monitoring $S_{jb}O_2$, brain tissue oxygen levels to identify early ischemia.
	Be careful with hand-bagging for hyperventilation as PCO_2 can drop precipitously causing harm.
	Severe vasoconstriction can occur resulting in ischemia.
Barbiturate coma Pentobarbital	Use for IICP refractory to therapy or surgery.
	Reversible
	Must be hemodynamically stable.
	Decreases metabolic activity, recruits cerebral blood flow.
	Complications—increased ventilator days, pneumonia, hyperglycemia, thrombocytopenia, myocardial and respiratory depression, decreased GI motility, immunosuppression.
	Loading dose 10 mg/kg over 30 minutes pentobarbital; then 5 mg/kg/hour over 1 hour for 3 doses; maintain 1-3 mg/kg/hour to achieve EEG burst suppression (305 bursts/minute) or as demonstrated on BIS monitor.
	Serum pentobarbital level 30-40 mcg/mL
	Higher levels result in pupil dilation.
	Maintain 24-48 hours and begin withdrawal at 50% per day increasing analgesia and sedation; monitoring ICP and sedation level (BIS).
	Pentobarbital rapid onset within 10-60 seconds, half-life of 20 hours.

(Continued)

Table 4-6   Management for Refractory IICP (*Continued*)

Therapy	Management
Hypothermia	If used, initiate within 6 hours of injury in patients with GCS 3-5.
	Cool to 32°-34°C within 8 hours of injury and maintain for 48 hours.
	Prevent shivering during cooling and re-warming (increases ICP) with neuromuscular blockade or sedation.
	Rewarming can result in rebound IICP.
	Complications—increased risk of infection, pneumonia 40-45% (Mcilvoy 2005), cold-thermal burn from the device used; skin breakdown.
	Contraindicated for patients with coagulopathy.
	Monitor potassium, decreases with hypothermia but can rebound to hyperkalemia with rewarming.
	No definite improvement in outcome but increased complications and length of stay (Clifton et al. 2001).
Decompressive craniectomy	If performed, cranial flap is either frozen or placed in a subcutaneous adipose pocket in patient's lower abdominal wall.
	Surgery may be accompanied by evacuation of a space occupying lesion, lobectomy, debridement of injured tissue; durotomy is also performed to allow the brain room for swelling.
	Until cranioplasty, place a helmet as the patient awakens to protect the soft spot of the skull.
	Cranioplasty may occur during the hospital stay or rehabilitation.
Hypernatremia • Hypertonic saline	No definitive recommendations regarding hypertonic saline benefits.
	Consider use of 7.5% saline solution.
	Several small studies suggest there is some benefit (White et al. 2006); overall survival has not shown improvement with use.

(Continued)

Table 4-6   Management for Refractory IICP (*Continued*)

Therapy	Management
	Complications—central pontine myelinolysis not demonstrated in studies (not specifically monitored) but is associated with rapid increases in serum sodium in chronic hyponatremic patients.
	Maintain serum sodium 145-155 mMol/L in all head injured patients.
	White et al. 2006 suggest 250 mL of 3% saline; repeat until sodium level 155 mMol/L.
	If ICP remains increased after 3-4 days, administer furosemide to mobilize interstitial sodium.
	Monitor serum sodium and potassium every 4 hours.
	Use central line to prevent peripheral thrombophlebitis.

and ICP monitoring. There is no room for hypoxia or hypotension. If a therapy fails to control ICP, escalate treatment to that for refractory IICP. Uncontrolled IICP will result in herniation and brain death.

Traumatic Brain Injury

Management begins with routine care of trauma patients. Any episode of hypotension or hypoxia results in secondary brain injury and can lead to IICP. It is essential to manage airway, breathing, and circulation, manage the premise of trauma resuscitation and manage the head injury as well (Brain Trauma Foundation 2007). ATLS (2008) provides admission and discharge recommendations for asymptomatic patients that include:

- Discharge home after observation if neurologic checks can be provided for 24 hours after discharge with return to ED for headache, focal neurologic deficit, or LOC
- Admission if there is an abnormal CT scan, decreased level of conscious or LOC, moderate or severe headache, altered GCS

<15, skull fracture, CSF leak, a focal neurologic deficit, presence of alcohol or drugs of abuse, an associated injury, or the lack of a companion at home to assist with neurologic checks in the asymptomatic patient

If the facility that receives a severely head-injured patient (GCS <9) is not a trauma center, or a trauma center without immediate neurosurgical availability, arrangement for transfer to a level I or level II trauma center should begin immediately. There should be no diagnostic delay. The higher level trauma center should encourage immediate management of airway and prevention of hypoxia and hypotension. The nontrauma center can monitor hypoxia by maintaining SaO_2 >98% on 100% FiO_2. For the trauma center, head CT is delayed for immediate abdominal or thoracic surgery to control bleeding. During the procedure, of course, hypotension and hypoxia are avoided. An ICP monitor may be placed to assist with management through the trauma surgical procedure. If the initial BP is stable and >100 mm Hg, head CT may be obtained prior to surgery (ATLS 2004). Head CT is not recommended for nontrauma center facilities or trauma centers without available neurosurgeons. Transfer is the first priority in these patients. The basics of severe TBI management include:

- Secure airway; intubate if GCS ≤8, hypoxia with supplemental oxygen
- Administer 100% FiO_2
- Maintain Hct >33
- Ventilate; prevent hypoxia (SaO_2 >90%, $S_{jb}O_2$ >55%, $PbtO_2$ ≥20, PCO_2 35-40)
- Stop external bleeding—apply pressure, staples, scalp surgical clips
- Identify internal bleeding
  — Perform procedures necessary to stop internal bleeding including surgery, blood product administration
- Maintain MAP >90 mm Hg
- Maintain CPP >60 mm Hg; maintaining CPP >70 mm Hg can result in acute respiratory distress syndrome (ARDS)

- Monitor GCS, pupils
- Maintain normothermia

SPECIAL SITUATIONS

Diabetes Insipidus (DI)—Syndrome of Inappropriate Secretion of Antidiuretic Hormone (SIADH)

Antidiuretic hormone (ADH) is synthesized and released from the hypothalamus. Its purpose is to maintain fluid balance by increasing resorption of water by the distal tubules and collecting ducts of the kidney. The cause of altered ADH can be direct trauma to the hypothalamus or cerebral edema that creates pressure on the hypothalamus, resulting in dysfunction. DI is the result of insufficient ADH, either synthesis or release. The result is excess fluid loss. SIADH is caused by an excess of ADH, resulting in retention of water and increased thirst. Table 4-7 demonstrates the difference between DI and SIADH. SIADH can result quickly in hyponatremia, and may be the reason for diagnosis.

Signs and Symptoms of Hyponatremia

Headache
Decreased level of consciousness
Confusion, disorientation, irritability
Muscle weakness
Seizures
Cerebral edema
Nausea, vomiting
Impaired taste, anorexia, decreased bowel sounds

Management

DI Management focuses on control of fluid losses.

- Fluid replacement should be 1:1 or urine output + 10% with D5W or 0.5 NSS

Table 4-7   DI versus SIADH

Factor	DI	SIADH
ADH	Deficient	Excess
Urine output	↑; >200 mL over 2 hours	↓
Serum osmolality	↑	↓
Serum sodium	>145 mMol/L	<130-134 mMol/L
Urine osmolality	↓	↑
Urine specific gravity	1 to 1.005	>1.020
Fluids	Output > Intake	Intake > Output
Other	Poor skin turgor Dry mucous membranes Associated with herniation syndromes	Neurologic changes Restlessness Seizures

- If the patient is alert, encourage fluids by mouth as he or she begins to feel thirst
- Medications can be used and in the case of herniation or after brain death medications are necessary to control fluid loss
- Pitressin aqueous IV, IM, subcutaneous every 2 to 8 hours (short duration 1-2 hours) or desmopressin (DDAVP) IV, intranasal insufflations, or subcutaneous
    — Daily or twice daily (long duration 8-24 hours)
    — IV given via a central line

SIADH management begins with fluid restriction. This is usually the most difficult component for the patient who is intensely thirsty. The fluids should be measured and given to the patient. Restriction of patient access to other fluids is essential and includes family participation to maintain the restrictions.

- Fluid restriction 500 to 1000 mL/day
- IV D5NSS, NSS, or 3% hypertonic saline (stimulates ADH release)
- Offer high-sodium fluids, add salt to food or tube feedings
- Medications that may be used include
  — Demeclcycline
  — Diuretics
  — Phenytoin decreases ADH secretion
- Correct hyponatremia at a rate of no more than 1 to 2 mEq/L/hour

  For both situations, the clinician must carefully monitor
- Intake and output
- Electrolytes, specifically sodium and potassium
- Urine sodium and osmolality
- Daily weight
- Monitor volume status, vital signs

Cerebral Salt Wasting

Cerebral salt wasting (CSW) may be confused with SIADH and indeed appears much the same except for the loss of fluids. CSW results in hyponatremia with hypovolemia. There is a decrease in ADH with and elevated level of atrial natriuretic factor. CSW is often associated with a subarachnoid hemorrhage. Atrial natriuretic factor is released in response to atrial stretch and results in vasodilation, decreased ADH release, diuresis and natriuresis (excessive secretion of sodium). Thus the patient loses both sodium and water. The fluid shift can result in cerebral edema in a patient where edema is already occurring from injury. The fluid loss can also result in critical hypotension and possibly irreversible shock.

Management

When the decision is made to manage CSW versus SIADH, it is essential that the clinician is certain which is occurring.

Restriction of fluid in the CSW patient would result in severe hypovolemia. Differences in management include

* Hemodynamic monitoring, especially volume management
* Urine sodium and potassium > serum sodium and potassium
* Replace sodium without replacing volume; evaluate if patient is losing more sodium than is being replaced
* Administer hypertonic (3%) saline

Seizures

Seizures have been associated with cerebral hematoma, depressed skull fx, and penetrating head injury. If seizures occur, the clinician should note the type, duration, and expression of the seizure described.

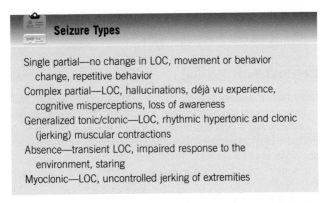

Seizure Types

Single partial—no change in LOC, movement or behavior change, repetitive behavior
Complex partial—LOC, hallucinations, déjà vu experience, cognitive misperceptions, loss of awareness
Generalized tonic/clonic—LOC, rhythmic hypertonic and clonic (jerking) muscular contractions
Absence—transient LOC, impaired response to the environment, staring
Myoclonic—LOC, uncontrolled jerking of extremities

Precautions to take in the event of a seizure and preferably before seizures occur include

* Padding side rails of the bed; keep side rails up
* Have suction readily available; turn patient to the right to decrease aspiration risk
* Monitor airway; check tongue for bite

- Note time of seizure and duration
- Note bowel or bladder incontinence
- Neurologic examination during and after the seizure
- Do not restrain or insert a padded tongue blade!
- Monitor vital signs and oxygen saturations
- Prophylaxis for a brief period with phenytoin or fosphenytoin may be ordered

Autonomic Hyperexcitability/Dysfunction Syndrome (AHS)

Autonomic hyperexcitability or dysfunction syndrome (AHS) has had different names, including diencephalic seizures, hypothalamic storms, and autonomic or sympathetic storms. It however, has a consistent description and management. AHS is the result of dysfunction of the hypothalamus and/or thalamus caused by pressure or direct injury. The symptoms are the result of a release phenomenon from the hypothalamus/thalamus. AHS occurs most commonly with diffuse injuries such as diffuse axonal injury (DAI) and cerebral contusions, as well as SDH and EDH (Nayduch and Reed 1996). It occurs most frequently in patients <50 years, who have a high injury severity score (>25), and in this study had a 98% survival. In a series of 42 traumatic AHS cases, AHS duration lasted less than 20 days and stopped when the patient began to have verbal communication, Rancho scale IV

Signs and Symptoms of Autonomic Hyperexcitability

Hyperthermia (40°–40.6°C)
Hypertension
Tachycardia
Profuse diaphoresis above the nipple line
Hypertonia, rigid posture

and V (Nayduch and Reed 1996). Of these patients, 65% left the hospital to rehabilitation without any AHS and a Rancho scale III through VI.

Signs and symptoms of AHS are directly related to the loss of autonomic control demonstrated by exaggerated autonomic response.

AHS results in severe increase in metabolic rate, even doubling caloric expenditure, during the event. AHS is not associated with IICP; however IICP can occur after the event. Efforts to control the episodes of AHS are essential to prevent the metabolic surge and the cerebral stress associated with it.

Management

Management of AHS includes:

- Morphine IV breaks the episode and is also useful for breakthrough events
- Bromocriptine can be administered routinely to continuously manage AHS and prevent recurrence; stops hyperthermia and diaphoresis (Nayduch and Reed 1996, Rossitch and Bullard 1988, Bullard 1987)
- Monitor hemodynamics especially with excess diaphoresis and fluid loss
- Assess for other signs of infection causing the hyperthermia
  — Perform routine cultures to rule out infection
  — Administer antipyretic in anticipation of infection until proven negative
- Assess for other causes of hypertension including IICP, underlying essential hypertension

Brain Death

When IICP becomes out of control or when no intervention impacts IICP, the outcome is herniation and thus brain death. The late signs and symptoms of IICP have occurred. Once herniation is complete, the body's response is opposite of the herniation. There is a rapid drop in BP due to the loss of sympathetic output from the brain. It is essential now to determine clinically that the patient has experienced brain death. Each facility has standards for brain death determination but in general, most require two separate physician examinations, one of whom must be a neurosurgeon or neurologist. The examination includes the following:

Brain Death Determination

- Documented absence of alcohol or drugs affecting response, especially if barbiturate coma has been used, benzodiazepines, opiates, neuromuscular blocking agents
- GCS = 3
- Nonreactive pupils
- Loss of other brainstem reflexes—cough, gag, corneals, oculo-cephalic, cold calorics
- Apnea
- Normothermia
- Flat electroencephalogram (isoelectric EEG)
- No cerebral blood flow

The apnea test is performed by respiratory therapy. After preoxygenation, the ventilator is removed and the patient is given the opportunity to breathe on his or her own. Hemodynamics are monitored and the test stopped if there is any sign of deterioration. A positive test is a PCO_2 >60 mm Hg and no evidence of attempt at respiration. The high PCO_2 should stimulate a living brain to breathe.

There are medications and situations that may alter the examination for brain death evaluation and could lead to an incorrect diagnosis (Table 4-8). Make certain that none of these agents is on board that can affect the diagnosis.

Table 4-8 Medications Affecting Neurologic Examination

Examination	Affecting Agent
Fixed or dilated pupils	Anticholinergic agents
	Dopamine
	Barbiturates
	Hallucinogens
	Antihistamines
	Amphetamines
	Instillation of mydriatics for ophthalmologic examinations
	Atropine
	Scopolamine
	Preexisting disease, false eye (glass)
	Eye injury
Lack of oculovestibular response	Ototoxic agents
	Vestibular suppressants
	Preexisting disease
Apnea	Posthyperventilation apnea
	Neuromuscular blockade
Lack of motor response	Neuromuscular blockade
	"Locked-in" neurologic state
	Spinal cord injury
	Sedation
Isoelectric EEG	Sedation
	Anoxia
	Hypothermia
	Encephalitis

Organ donation

After brain death diagnosis, the issue of organ donation becomes the focus. In anticipation of brain death, the staff should work closely with the family so that they are aware of the situation, understand the diagnosis, and the impact of the diagnosis. This is not something that can be accomplished in one meeting and should never be dealt with at the time of actual diagnosis and declaration to the family. Many trauma centers have specific staff assigned to begin the discussions with families regarding brain death and organ donation. The designated liaisons to the family have demonstrated successful outcomes for a family in understanding and accepting brain death as well as organ donation (Bair et al. 2006).

When the family visits with the patient after brain death diagnosis, be aware of spinal cord reflexes that may imply to the family that the patient is not dead. The hope that the diagnosis is not true is so strong, that any sign of possible awareness is grasped. Be certain the family has sufficient time with the patient. Be certain to reinforce that brain death and death are equivalent.

To be a potential organ donor, the patient must meet the following criteria:

• Declared brain dead

• Maintained on the ventilator

• Heart-beating donor (although some facilities can accommodate the nonheart-beating donor)

• Absence of infectious disease and cancer/metastasis

After these general criteria are met, organ specific criteria are applied to determine usability of each organ. There are at any given time 99,273 or more organs needed (http://optn.transplant.hrsa.gov/). It is essential that organ donation become the focus after brain death declaration with the hopes that the family will agree. While the organ procurement agency is evaluating the patient for possible organ donation, the family is making a decision and the patient is now unstable without the brain to control and monitor the body. The greatest loss of donors is from family refusal, unrecognized brain death until cardiac death follows, or instability after herniation (Arbour 2005).

The following common events after herniation must be anticipated, managed, and prevented when possible:

• Hemodynamic instability—after tachycardia, hypertension, increased oxygen consumption of herniation, the heart suffers autonomic collapse with loss of peripheral vascular resistance decreasing cardiac output

— Anticipate the instability and be prepared with fluids and vasopressors

— Rapid administration of crystalloid and colloid to replace fluid volume deficit

— Manage with vasopressors

▪ Dopamine <10 mcg/kg/minute for heart donors

▪ Norepinephrine 0.5 to 5 mcg/kg/minute

— Maintain CVP 8 to 10 mm Hg, BP >100 mm Hg

• Volume status—with the likely presence of DI, up to 1 to 2000 mL/hour volume loss in urine

— Manage DI as described above

• Bradycardia—caused by denervation of the heart

— Resistant to atropine

— Use small doses of epinephrine

• Neurogenic pulmonary edema—alterations in pulmonary capillary permeability cause acute lung injury

— Inflammatory mediators—cause vasodilation, further hemodynamic instability, and lung injury

— Pulmonary toilet, oral care to decrease infection, PEEP <7.5 cm H_2O

— Maintain peak inspiratory pressures ≤30 cm H_2O protective ventilation

— If the lungs continue to be refractory to these changes, inverse ratio ventilation is an option

• Hyperthermia during herniation very quickly becomes hypothermia

— Causes additional cold dierusis and fluid loss

— Provide warming blankets, fluids

• Hormonal loss results in decreased cortisol, T_3, T_4, vasopressin, insulin

— Inotropic agents assist with loss of cortisol

— Methylprednisolone 15 mg/kg every 24 hours also assists with loss of cortisol

— Decreased insulin and insulin resistance

  ▪ Monitor glucose that can result in an osmotic dieresis

  ▪ Maintain glucose at 120 to 180 mg/dL

  ▪ Administer insulin drip

• Coagulopathy is usually consumptive

— May require replacement with fresh frozen plasma, cryo-precipitate, platelets

The goal of therapy is to maintain the potential organ donor in a hemodynamically stable state to preserve the organs for retrieval. The donor team works as quickly as possible to organize the retrieval team to minimize the time between diagnosis, approval by family, and surgery. This salvages the organs as well as decreases the time the family is waiting for something to happen. The donor process for the family can provide tangible closure.

POSTRESUSCITATION MANAGEMENT AND REHABILITATION

The obvious goal of all head injury management, minor and severe injury, is optimal outcome with return to normal function. To achieve this goal, early therapy is initiated to provide gentle stimulation and escalate activities as the patient lightens. Cognitive rehabilitation assists the alert patient with improved memory and an understanding of the changes he or she is experiencing, ultimately decreasing anxiety and stress (Carney et al. 1999). Most cognitive rehabilitation programs assist the patient and families to understand the present deficits and how to deal with those deficits. Optimal outcome is the return to previous function if possible. If not possible, identify the optimal level that the patient can achieve and then alter home and occupation to meet the capabilities. Rehabilitation is physical, mental, and emotional. The attitude toward the outcome is as important as the outcome itself (Lefebvre et al. 2007).

Unfortunately, not all patients will achieve a functional outcome, nor will they progress to brain death. This vegetative state is like a wakeful unconsciousness. The patient often demonstrates the following signs and symptoms.

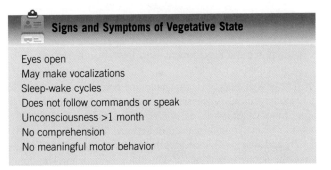

Signs and Symptoms of Vegetative State

Eyes open
May make vocalizations
Sleep-wake cycles
Does not follow commands or speak
Unconsciousness >1 month
No comprehension
No meaningful motor behavior

There are several scoring systems to identify the progress made by the head injured patient. A simplified scale is the Glasgow outcome score (GOS) (www.trauma.org/archive/scores/gos.html accesses 7-23-08)

- Good—normal or minor deficits
- Moderate—able to participate in most social and occupational activities, but has limitations; may work in sheltered setting
- Severe—severely limited communication, behavior, and emotional skills; partially or totally dependent upon assistance
- Vegetative—as described above
- Death

The Rancho Los Amigos Cognitive Scale (1974) developed at the Rancho los Amigos National Rehabilitation Center in Downey CA, is much better defined to provide a base from which rehabilitation activities can be planned. It provides the family with a guide to the awakening patient. Usually a multitude of rehabilitation personnel assist with this process, including occupational,

Table 4-9 Rancho Los Amigos Scale

Level	Response	Activities
I	None, unresponsive	*Nursing:* Prevent secondary brain injury; assist family *PT:* ROM, positioning, splinting, coma stimulation, maintain posture, teach family participation *OT:* Coma stimulation (touch, vision, sound), upper extremity splinting and ROM
II	Generalized—inconsistent reaction; nonpurposeful; may be the same response no matter the stimuli; delayed	
III	Localized—more specific reaction but inconsistent yet directly related to the stimulus; may follow commands, delayed; response to discomfort; may respond to family and friends	*Family:* Talk to patient, orientation, bring photos and music, provide periods of rest (no yelling at patient, remain calm)
IV	Confused, agitated—increased activity but decreased ability to process input; bizarre, nonpurposeful; incoherent or inappropriate verbalization; euphoric or hostile; short attention span	*Nursing:* Patient safety, privacy, prevent skin breakdown, quiet environment to prevent overstimulation *PT:* Short sessions, maintain flexibility, sitting, gait training. *OT:* Channel excess energy, goal purposeful response, retrains ADL, increase attention and memory *Speech:* Swallow study, feeding program, speech, assess communication *Family:* Limit visitors to control stimulation, allow sleep, be available

(Continued)

Table 4-9 Rancho Los Amigos Scale *(Continued)*

Level	Response	Activities
V	Confused, inappropriate, nonagitated—alert, responds to commands somewhat consistently; distractible but attentive to environment; inappropriate verbalization; severe memory impairment; lacks initiation for functional tasks; unable to learn new tasks; self-care with assistance; frustration; wanders!	*Nursing:* Self-care, reinforce rehabilitation plans, orientation, safety, encourage expression, monitor wandering *PT:* Modified exercise, increase strength and endurance, coordination and balance *OT:* Retrain ADL, problem-solving, memory, and judgment skills, upper extremity strength and coordination, self feeding *Speech:* Test attention, memory, learning potential, reading and writing, communication, compensation for memory and language problems *Family:* Tactful correction, self-care, orientation
VI	Confused, appropriate—goal-directed but needs cues; consistently follows commands; remembers relearned tasks; appropriate but may be incorrect caused by memory issues; functional in self-care; inconsistent orientation; increased awareness of family and friends, self	*Nursing:* Assist ADL, realistic self-care, discharge plan *PT:* Increase endurance, strength, coordination, balance, mobility with ambulation and/or assistive devices *OT:* Community reentry skills (telephone, money, safety), independent self-care, ADL skills for home, compensation for ADL limitations

VII	Automatic, appropriate—appears appropriate and oriented in structured setting; shallow recall; increased self-awareness; lacks insight into condition; decreased judgment and problem-solving skills; carryover of new learning but slow; minimal supervision for safety	*Speech:* Safe feeding, attention, memory, effective communication, compensation for memory and language issues, follow-up after discharge *Neuropsychology:* Test higher cognitive function, compensation for deficits, increase function at home, follow-up after discharge, tutoring for return to school *Family:* ADL reorganization at home, allow patient decision-making within safety margin, encourage visitation, encourage return to previous hobbies and activities *Vocational rehabilitation:* explore job opportunities based upon level of function
VIII	Purposeful, appropriate—alert, oriented, appropriate recall; no supervision once activity learned; physically independent at home and community (driving); decreased abstract reasoning, stress tolerance, judgment in emergencies; decreased but functional social and emotional capacity	

physical, speech, music therapy, neuropsychology, nursing, physical medicine and rehabilitation physicians, and families. Table 4-9 provides a brief description of the Rancho Los Amigos Scale levels and appropriate therapy activities for each.

Families should be encouraged to rest in the early phases of the patient's recovery. Their involvement increases rapidly as the patient lightens and needs their presence and assistance with memory and safety. It is difficult for families to go home and rest during the critical phase. Explain to the families the need for their energy as the patient recovers later and when the patient returns home. The patient who returns home may not be the same person they knew prior to the event. This requires patience, energy, and a positive attitude.

There are no guarantees in head injury or rehabilitation. The achievement of a functional outcome, discharge to rehabilitation, and return to home is a multidisciplinary activity from the moment the patient is found at the scene until the day they enter rehabilitation.

Critical Lifesavers

- GCS is a measurement of the level of consciousness of the patient. It is not an evaluation of the spine or spine controlled activity
- One incidence of hypotension (BP < 90 mm Hg) can result in poor outcome for severe head injury
- Emergent treatment of carotid cavernous fistula is necessary in the presence of epistaxis, blindness, sphenoid sinus aneurysm, and coma
- Constant vigilance is the key to identify increasing ICP and signs of ineffective management with the need to escalate therapy, and prevent herniation
- Ventriculostomy is leveled at the foramen of Monro, most easily identified at the external auditory meatus
- Correct hyponatremia at a rate of no more than 1-2 mEq/L/hour

REFERENCES

American College of Surgeons. *Advanced Trauma Life Support* (ATLS). 7th ed. Chicago, IL: American College of Surgeons; 2004.

American College of Surgeons. *Advanced Trauma Life Support* (ATLS). 8th ed. Chicago, IL: American College of Surgeons; 2008.

Arbour R. Clinical management of the organ donor. *AACN Clin Issues.* 2005.16(4):551-580.

Avarello JT, Cantor RM. Pediatric major trauma: an approach to evaluation and management. 2007. *Emerg Med Clin North Am.* 2007;25(3):803-836.

Bair HA, Sills P, Schumacher K, et al. Improved organ procurement through implementation of evidence-based practice. *J Trauma Nurs.* 2006;13(4):183-185.

Barrow DL, Spector R, Braun IF, et al. Classification and treatment of spontaneous cavernous fistulas. *J Neurosurg.* 1985;62:248-256.

Brain Trauma Foundation. Management of severe traumatic brain injury. *J Neurotrauma.* 2007;24(S1). http://www.cdc.gov/ncipc/tbi/TBI.htm. Accessed July 18, 2008.

Bullard DE. Diencephalic seizures: responsiveness to bromocriptine and morphine. *Ann Neurol.* 1987;21(6):609-611.

Cantu RC. Second impact syndrome. *Clin Sports Med.* 1998;17(1):37-44.

Carney N, Chesnut R, Maynard H, et al. Effect of cognitive rehabilitation on outcomes for persons with traumatic brain injury: a systemic review. *J Head Trauma Rehabil.* 1999;14(3):277-307.

Clifton G, Miller E, Choi S, et al. Lack of effect of induction of hypothermia after acuter brain injury. *N Engl J Med.* 2001;344(8): 556-563.

Cushman JG, Agarwal N, Fabian TC, et al. Practice management guidelines for the management of mild traumatic brain injury. *J Trauma.* 2001;52(5):1016-1026.

Henzler D, Cooper J, Tremayner AB, et al. Early modifiable factors associated with fatal outcome in patients with severe traumatic brain injury: a case control study. *Crit Care Med.* 2007;35(4): 1027-1031.

Hoyt KS, Selfridge-Thomas J. *Emergency Nursing Core Curriculum.* 6th ed. St Louis, MO: Saunders Elsevier; 2007.

Lefebvre H, Pelchat D, Levert MJ. Interdisciplinary family intervention program: a partnership among health professionals, traumatic brain injury patients, and caregiving relatives. *J Trauma Nurs.* 2007; 14(2):100-113.

March K. Intracranial pressure monitoring: Why monitor? *AACN Clin Issues.* 2005;16(4):456-475.

Mcilvoy, L. The effect of hypothermia and hyperthermia on acute brain injury. *AACN Clin Issues.* 2005;16(4):488-500.

Nayduch D, Reed RL. Clinical characteristics of autonomic hyperexcitability syndrome. Paper presented at: Western Trauma Association; February, 1996; Grand Targhee, WY.

OPTN. Organ donor statistics. www.optn.org/latestdata/step2.asp. Accessed July 18, 2008.

Rancho los Amigos National Rehabilitation Center. Rancho los Amigos Scale. Downey, CA: Rancho los Amigos National Rehabilitation Center, 1974.

Rossitch E, Bullard DE. The autonomic dysfunction syndrome: etiology and treatment. *Br J Neurosurg.* 1988;2(4):471-478.

Ruffolo DC. Carotid-cavernous sinus fistula in penetrating facial trauma. *J Trauma Nurs.* 2000;7(2):48-51.

Saunders RL, Harbaugh RE. The second impact in catastrophic contact-sports head trauma. *JAMA.* 1984;252(4):538-539.

Teasdale G, Jennett B. Assessment of coma and impaired consciousness: a practical scale. *Lancet.* 1974;2(7872):81-84.

Trauma.Org. Glasgow Outcome Scale. www.trauma.org/archive/scores/gos.html. Accessed July 23, 2008.

White H, Cook D, Venkatesh B. The use of hypertonic saline for treating intracranial hypertension after traumatic brain injury. *Anesth Analg.* 2006;102(6):1836-1846.

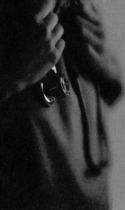

Chapter 5
SPINE AND SPINAL CORD INJURY

INTRODUCTION

Spinal cord injuries (SCI) are not the most frequent injury in the United States, however they are the injury associated with the highest cost. Approximately 12,000 SCI occur each year (NSCISC 2008). Motor vehicle collisions (MVC) are the most common cause (42%) followed by falls (27%) and disturbingly by violent acts (15%). The average age has increased from 28.7 to 39.5 years since 2005 (NSCISC 2008). As the population is aging and remaining active, SCI in individuals >60 years have increased from 4.7% to 11.5%. The most devastating injuries are in the cervical spine and are associated with the highest cost caused by care needs and loss of function. Quadriplegia above C4 average $775,000 for initial care and ongoing care $138,000 each subsequent year. Quadriplegia below C4 are less costly but not by much, $500,000 initially, with an additional $56,000 each year. From there, the costs are about $250,000 for incomplete injuries and paraplegia (NSCISC 2008).

In children, 60% to 80% of injury is to the cervical spine because of a large, heavy head, small neck muscles, and flat facets (Avarello and Cantor 2007). The increased flexibility of the neck results in ligamentous injury as well as spinal cord injury.

A significant percentage of SCI individuals die at the scene from loss of airway. However, those who survive need rapid emergent management and long-term care. In addition to SCI, fractures and dislocations of the spinal column occur. These patients may not have SCI but have the potential for the same. Thus management includes not only resuscitation and identification of other injuries, but also protection of the spinal cord and column.

ASSESSMENT

Because of the complexity of SCI, assessment includes the anatomy of the spine and spinal column. A complete understanding of the levels of function assists with rapid diagnosis and management. All injured patients are considered to have a spine injury until proven otherwise. The likelihood of a noncontiguous second spine injury is high. Only 5% of head injuries is associated with spine injuries. However, 25% of spine injuries is associated at a minimum with minor head injury (ATLS 2004).

History

As with all trauma, the history of the event is the most significant. Do not forget to include the patient's past medical and surgical histories as well. Life-threatening injuries are managed first. The presence of a spine injury may make diagnosis of other injuries difficult because of lack of pain sensation and neurogenic shock. The most common causes of spine injury include

- Rapid negative acceleration (deceleration) from motor vehicle crash (MVC)
- Axial load following a fall from a height
- Penetrating injury and/or blast injury
- Hyperextension during impact to the chin
- Hyperflexion occurring at fulcrum sites such as C5-C6, or T12-L1 with improper seatbelt use

In addition to the usual past medical history questions, include

- Any abnormal sensation after the event
  — Where
  — Description of the type of sensation—tingling, pins/needles, pain, numbness, burning

- Any abnormal motor activity after the event
  — Weakness
  — Loss of function, inability to move against gravity

Trauma Assessment

Begin all trauma assessments with airway, breathing, circulation, then neurologic assessment. Throughout the rapid initial exam, maintain spinal protection through use of the cervical collar and logroll maneuvers. When assessing, act on any life-threatening situations and proceed as outlined in Chapter 2. When assessing the neurologic system, knowledge of the anatomy of the spine is essential to document the injury correctly. Include palpation of the spine for tenderness or step-offs as a clue to spine injury.

There are 7 cervical vertebrae, 12 thoracic, 5 lumbar, and 5 sacral vertebrae which are fused (Figure 5-1). There are nerve roots associated with each level of vertebra. Of these, there are 8 cervical roots for the 7 vertebrae. Each vertebra from C3 down the spine is identical except for variations in size (Figure 5-2). The laminae form the ring around the spinal cord with the transverse and spinous processes. The pedicles complete the ring by attachment to the vertebral body. Fractures in these areas have the potential to impinge on the cord they protect. The facets are the articulating thumbprints and processes that align the vertebrae on top of each other. The vertebral bodies provide the structure with discs between for shock absorption. Injuries to the vertebral bodies are usually compression fractures or fractures that occur during subluxation. Nerve roots (31 pairs) exit between the vertebrae and the vascular supply runs the length of the spine through foramina. The brachial plexus consists of cervical roots 5 through 8 plus thoracic root 1. The plexus innervates the complex upper extremity.

The upper cervical spine has a unique anatomy that allows the body to turn the head. The articulations at the superior end start with the plain ring of C1 and the occipital condyles to protect the spinal cord (extension of the medulla oblongata) as it exits the skull. The ring of C1 then allows for the range of motion (ROM) of the neck as well as the head (Figure 5-3). C2 articulates with C1 via the dens (odontoid), a finger of bone

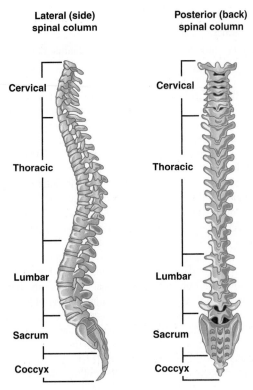

Figure 5-1   Spinal column. (Courtesy of http://www.spineuni-verse.com)

that stands upright from C2, allowing C1 to rotate. The elderly are particularly susceptible to fractures located here.

Motor assessment

As documented in Chapter 4, motor strength assessment is a 6-point scale with 0 = no movement and 5 = full motor strength with resistance. See Chapter 4 for further description. When assessing the spinal cord injury patient, note if there is a difference

Thoracic Vertebrae

Axial (Overhead) View   Lateral (Side) View

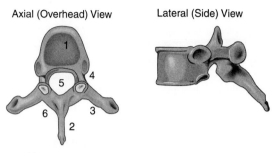

1 = Vertebral body   4 = Pedicle
2 = Spinous process   5 = Spinal canal
3 = Transverse process   6 = Lamina

Figure 5-2   Vertebra anatomy. (Courtesy of http://www.spineuniverse.com)

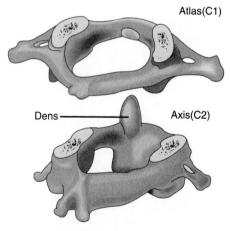

Atlas(C1)

Dens

Axis(C2)

Figure 5-3   C1-C2 vertebrae anatomy. (Courtesy of http://www.spineuniverse.com)

between right and left, upper and lower extremities. If there is loss of motor function, note at which level the loss initiates. The motor functions associated with the different levels of the spinal cord are described in Table 5-1. Any cord injury results in the loss of all functions below the level of injury.

Motor assessment is as follows. The anatomy of motor control includes the difference between upper and lower motor neurons and the spinal tracts that traverse the cord.

- Lateral corticospinal tract (pyramidal tract)
  — Posterolateral horns of the cord after crossing in the medulla
  — Lower extremity motor tracts are peripheral and upper extremity tracts are central
  — Ipsilateral motor control
  — Assess voluntary contractions
- Spinothalamic tract
  — Anterolateral horns of the cord
  — Contralateral pain and temperature sensation
  — Assess pinprick and light touch sensation
- Posterior spinal cord
  — Ipsilateral proprioception and vibration
  — Assess position sense of toes and fingers
- Upper motor neurons
  — Remain completely within the central nervous system
  — Present as paralysis, hypertonicity, and hyperreflexia
- Lower motor neurons
  — Begins in the central nervous system and exits to a muscle group
  — Final common pathway
  — Results in loss of motor tone (flaccidity), hyporeflexia or areflexia, fasciculations

Spinal reflexes are also assessed. Reflexes can remain intact despite loss of motor control as the reflex arc with the cord remains intact to the muscle group. In addition to assessment of reflexes, check for rectal tone, perianal sensation, and great

Table 5-1   Motor Assessment for SCI

Level	Motor Control
Cervical	
C3 through C4	Cervical plexus Diaphragm function (phrenic nerve) Respiratory arrest if injured above C4 Shrug shoulders
C5	Deltoid, bicep Flexion of elbows
C6	Extension of wrists
C7	Tricep Extension of elbows
C8	Hands Flexion of fingers (grip)
Thoracic	
T1	With C8—hands Spread fingers
T2 through T12	Intercostals, internal and external (T2 through T8) Ability to remain upright, cough, sigh, deep breathing Breathing
T8 through T12	Abdominal musculature
Lumbar	
L1 through L2	Flexion of hips
L3 begins cauda equina	Extension of knees
L4	Dorsiflexion of ankles
L5	Extension of great toe (#1)
Sacral	
S1	Plantarflexion of ankles
S2 through S5	Bowel and bladder control Sexual function

toe flexion to identify sacral sparing preferably after spinal shock has resolved. Reflexes are graded 0 to 3+ (2+ = normal). Reflex assessment includes

- Abdominal
  — Stroking of the upper abdomen results in umbilicus movement toward the stimulus
- Bulbocavernosus
  — Tug on Foley catheter results in anal sphincter contraction
- Superficial anal
  — Stroking the perianal area results in anal sphincter contraction
- Cremasteric
  — Males
  — Stroke inner thigh results in a pulling up of the scrotum
- Priapism
  — Males
  — Tug on Foley catheter results in an erection
  — An erection may be present on arrival in SCI due to the loss of connection with the upper motor neurons
- Babinski
  — Stroke bottom of foot, toes should curl
  — Toes are upgoing until 2 years of age or in the presence of upper motor neuron injury
- Deep tendon reflexes
  — Using a reflex hammer test
    ■ Achilles (S1, S2)
    ■ Quadricep (L3, L4)
    ■ Tricep (C7, C8)
    ■ Brachioradialis (C5, C6)
    ■ Bicep (C5)

Sensory assessment

The sensory assessment is one of the best means of describing the level of injury. The dermatomes (Figure 5-4) must be

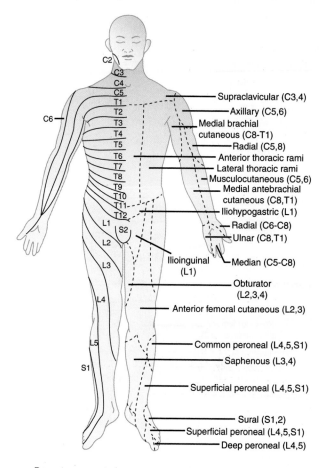

Dermatomes—anterior

Figure 5-4   Dermatomes. (With permission from Auerbach, PS. *Field Guide to Wilderness Medicine.* St Louis: CV Mosby; 2003.)

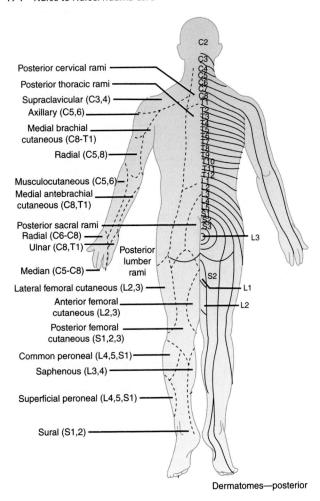

Posterior cervical rami

Posterior thoracic rami

Supraclavicular (C3,4)

Axillary (C5,6)

Medial brachial cutaneous (C8-T1)

Radial (C5,8)

Musculocutaneous (C5,6)

Medial antebrachial cutaneous (C8,T1)

Posterior sacral rami

Radial (C6-C8)

Ulnar (C8,T1)

Posterior lumber rami

Median (C5-C8)

Lateral femoral cutaneous (L2,3)

Anterior femoral cutaneous (L2,3)

Posterior femoral cutaneous (S1,2,3)

Common peroneal (L4,5,S1)

Saphenous (L3,4)

Superficial peroneal (L4,5,S1)

Sural (S1,2)

Dermatomes—posterior

Figure 5-4   (Continued)

described accurately. One of the most frequent mistakes is describing loss of sensation to the anterior upper chest as a T1-T2 level injury, yet the patient cannot move his or her arms. The cervical roots form a "shawl collar" effect on the anterior chest. Loss of sensation on the anterior upper chest identifies a C4-C5 injury, not T1. The dermatome diagram assists with understanding the distribution of the nerve roots, especially cervical and lumbar-sacral distributions. The lumbar-sacral roots form the cauda equina or plexus of roots leaving the end of the spinal cord (which concludes at L1-L2). The conus consist of the sacral segments at the immediate end of the spinal cord (L1).

ASIA impairment scale

The American Spinal Injury Association has developed a standard scale upon which spinal cord injury is graded. This allows for consistent description of spinal cord injury. The assessment includes motor and sensory evaluation to determine level of injury.

- Complete (A)—lack of motor or sensory function in the sacral roots S4-S5
- Incomplete (B)—sensory function is preserved but not motor function below the level of injury and includes the sacral roots S4-S5
- Incomplete (C)—motor function is preserved below the level of injury with more than half of the corresponding muscle groups with strength graded <3
- Incomplete (D)—motor function is preserved below the level of injury with at least 50% of the corresponding muscle groups with strength graded ≥3
- Normal (E)—all motor and sensory function normal
- Specific cord syndromes as described below are added to the above descriptors as needed

Cord injury

Spinal cord injury is described as complete or incomplete. Injuries may be with or without fracture, dislocation, or fracture-dislocation. Complete cord injuries are caused by transection of the cord or ischemia and death of a section of cord. Ischemia leads to necrosis, which then results in complete injury. Complete injuries are irreparable and are usually immediate. Injuries above T1 are considered quadriplegia. Complete injury presents as

Signs and Symptoms of Complete Cord Injury

Flaccidity
Loss of sensation, temperature, pain, pressure, vibration, proprioception
Loss of reflexes
Bilateral external rotation of hips
Loss of autonomic functions: hypotension, bradycardia, poikilothermia
Loss of bowel and bladder function
Ileus with distention
Priapism
Tachypnea, shallow respirations if cervical or high thoracic injury

Injuries below T1 result in paraplegia. Sacral sparing suggests an incomplete injury in which the sacral roots are intact. Sacral sparing is demonstrated by:

• Perirectal sensation
• Rectal tone
• Bulbocavernosus reflex

The incomplete cord syndromes are identified in Table 5-2. An incomplete injury has the potential for resolution or at least improvement over time except in the case of a Brown-Sequard injury. Brown-Sequard injuries result from a hemisection of the cord, usually from penetrating trauma, destroying a portion of the cord itself. The central nervous system is incapable of repairing itself. Peripheral nerves will usually regenerate and heal over time.

Diagnostic assessment

Facial and head injury suggests hyperextension mechanisms of injury, which can result in cervical spine injury as well

Table 5-2   Incomplete Cord Syndromes

Syndrome	Signs and Symptoms
Anterior cord	Loss of bilateral motor control, pain and temperature sensation below the lesion Proprioception, vibration intact If infarct of the anterior spinal artery, poor prognosis Associated with hyperflexion Recovery from lower extremities to bladder then upper extremities, finally hand
Posterior cord	Loss of proprioception Motor, pain, temperature intact Functional but with safety hazards Rare cord syndrome
Central cord	Impairment bilateral upper extremity motor control more than lower extremity Hyperextension of the anterior spinal artery Associated with hyperextension injury
Brown-Sequard	Loss of ipsilateral motor control and proprioception, vibration Loss of contralateral pain and temperature sensation Associated with penetrating trauma (hemisection of the cord)
Cauda equina	Injury to lumbar-sacral nerve roots (not cord injury) Areflexic bladder; saddle anesthesia Variable loss of lower extremity motor and sensory dependent upon injured root Areflexia of the affected limb Radicular pain in the affected extremity
Conus medullaris	S4-S5 spinal segment injury as they exit the cord (at L1) Areflexic bowel and bladder; flaccid anal sphincter Some degree of areflexia of the lower limbs Variable loss of lower extremity motor and sensory May have L1 fracture

(Hsu et al. 2007). It is important to note that if the patient is to be transferred to a higher level of trauma center, do not waste the time to identify spine injury. Maintain immobilization and protect the spine before and during transport. Even if a spine is "cleared," the transport crews will re-immobilize the patient for safety during transport. Protect the spine and arrange for rapid transport to the trauma center.

Plain films are usually the first diagnostics to be done to assess for spine injury. Fractures and dislocations can exist without cord injury and are evident on films or computed tomography (CT) scan. Three film views are usually obtained: anteroposterior (A-P) view (includes C2 through C7 spinous processes); lateral view (includes base of occiput to T1); open mouth odontoid view (entire dens and lateral masses of C1). If the C7-T1 junction cannot be seen, a swimmer's view may be of assistance.

CT scan of the neck is most frequently used to identify spine injury as the trauma patient is usually having scans of other body systems as well. An axial CT with 3-mm cuts is used. Helical spine CT identifies 99% of injuries especially if in addition to an A-P and lateral film. Identification of prevertebral swelling is an indication that cervical spine injury may be present (Hsu et al. 2007).

In addition to spinal fractures and distraction causing SCI, injury to the anterior vertebral artery can also result in SCI from ischemia to the cord. The anterior spinal artery feeds the anterior two-thirds of the cord where motor is controlled. Injury to the vertebral arteries can result in both cord ischemia as well as emboli to the cerebrum. Early identification and management can prevent progressive dissection, thrombosis, and embolization. There is approximately a 24% to 46% incidence of vertebral artery injury with vertebral fractures (Weller et al. 1999). The injury occurs as the artery enters the transverse foramina. Fractures involving the transverse foramina should have further workup to identify vertebral artery injury.

Magnetic resonance imaging (MRI) is particularly diagnostic of the presence of spinal epidural hematoma, disc injury, cord contusion, and/or ligamentous injury. It may also be used with CT scan in patients who are unable to participate in the exam to allow for cervical clearance and removal of the cervical collar.

Abnormalities on films that are normal variants include

- Pseudosubluxation of C2 on C3 in ~40% of children younger than adolescents
- Posterior fusion of C1 occurs at 4 years
- Anterior fusion of C1 occurs between 7 and 10 years
- Children also have flat facets until 7 to 10 years
- C2 epiphysis imitates an odontoid fracture in children <6 years

Types of fractures and dislocations

Hyperflexion can result in dislocation and jumped facets in which the upper vertebra no longer sits upon the "thumbprints" of the vertebra below.

- Jump-locked facets means the jump has occurred and the positioning of the facets prevents reduction. These injuries however are serious and unstable
- The posterior ligaments are frequently disrupted and there may be vertebral body compression or other fractures as well
- When the facets dislocate (sublux) there is often impingement or injury to the spinal cord as the canal is narrowed by the displacement of the vertebrae

Hyperextension results in central damage to the cord from compression.

- Intradural hemorrhage and edema result
- The anterior ligament ruptures

Flexion-rotation injuries can result in bilateral facet disruption when the vertebrae are displaced more than 50% of the width of the vertebral body.

- It can result in unilateral dislocation
- If the posterior ligament is disrupted, the injury is considered unstable.
- C5-C6 is the most common site for this injury.

Atlanto-occipital (A-O) dislocation is an avulsion of C1 from the occipital condyles.

- It usually results in immediate death from loss of airway
- Includes brainstem destruction
- This occurs more frequently in children because of underdeveloped ligaments
  — Can also be a sign of shaken-baby syndrome
- Cranial nerves IX, X, XI, XII exit at the A-O junction and can also be injured, demonstrating paralysis or severe weakness
- Classification is described as
  — Type I: anterior dislocation of the cranium from the atlas
  — Type II: longitudinal distraction without anterior or posterior displacement
  — Type III: posterior dislocation of the cranium from the atlas

C1 fractures are caused by axial load and can result in a blowout of the ring, a Jefferson fracture.

- The injury is unstable but rarely results in death.
- Open mouth odontoid plain film provides the best diagnosis
- If rotary subluxation occurs, results in torticollis
- Most common missed injury upper cervical spine C1-C2 (Powe 2006)

Atlanto-axial (A-A) dislocation (C1 and C2) is similar to A-O dislocation that results in stretching and tearing of the cord and immediate death from loss of airway (Figure 5-5).

Mechanical distraction of the posterior elements of C2 is called a hangman fracture. C2 can experience fractures as any other vertebra but includes fractures of the odontoid. If the patient survives, there is rarely cord injury.

- Odontoid fractures are usually caused by hyperextension
- Fractures of the odontoid are classified as
  — Type I: fracture above the base of the odontoid
  — Type II: fracture through the base of the odontoid
  — Type III: fracture extends into the vertebral body

C2 fractures are best identified with the lateral and open mouth odontoid plain films.

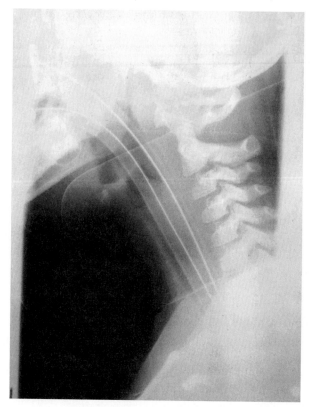

Figure 5-5   Atlanto-axial dislocation

C3 through C7 injuries with unilateral facet fractures have an incidence of SCI of 80%.

- If bilateral facet fractures occur, there is an 84% chance of complete cord injury (ATLS 2004)
- C5-C6 is the point of greatest flexion in the neck
- Most common missed injury of the lower cervical spine is C7-T1 (Powe 2006)

T1 through T10 fractures occur less frequently due to the stability provided by the ribs.

- Burst fractures of the vertebral body occur with axial load. The degree of compression determines the potential for further compression over time
- Fracture-dislocations result in SCI due to the narrow nature of the canal
- Chance fractures are a transverse fracture through the vertebral body
  — Frequently associated with abdominal or retroperitoneal injury
  — Caused by MVC where a lap-only belt is in place, particularly if worn too high on the abdomen or by children too small for an adult lap belt

T11 through L1 fractures are caused by hyperflexion or axial load. Conus and cauda equina injuries affect bowel and bladder as well as the lower extremities. These injuries are also due to hyperflexion or axial load.

DOCUMENTATION

Documentation of motor and sensory function should occur with the initial trauma assessment. Time of initial loss of function is necessary to determine treatment options as well as hypoxic or hypovolemic events that may have occurred since injury. As with head injury, secondary injury can occur to the spinal cord caused by any hypoxic or hypotensive event. Neurologic status should be reassessed frequently for changes or progression of neurologic symptoms. The SCI is then assessed throughout the patient's stay to monitor the progress of healing and to determine if an injury is incomplete rather than complete. It is possible for a SCI to appear complete on arrival and change over time.

Document any redness or pressure areas on arrival. These areas will need to be monitored continually to prevent decubiti. Continued skin assessment is necessary to identify any new pressure areas.

Temperature needs to be documented and monitored as well because a SCI patient above T6 is poikilothermic. They have the potential to lose enough heat to become the temperature of the surrounding environment. These patients cannot shiver to protect themselves.

MANAGEMENT

At the scene, spine protection is essential. Any mechanism where there is a significant transfer of energy requires immobilization of the spine in tandem with the airway, breathing, circulation (ABC) assessment on the scene. Penetrating injury to the cord also requires immobilization. When in doubt, immobilize at the scene with a backboard, cervical collar, head blocks, and straps. If the patient is under the effect of alcohol or drugs, has altered or loss of consciousness (LOC), a distracting injury, a neurologic deficit, and/or spinal pain, immobilization at the scene is required (ATLS 2008). If the patient is to be transferred from the local hospital to a trauma center, maintain the immobilization through transfer. When immobilizing children, place a towel roll or small pillow beneath the shoulder blades to align the body with the large occiput (Figure 5-6).

Resuscitation

Resuscitation for SCI and spine fracture patients is the same as all trauma patients with a few caveats specific to the spine, including the following:

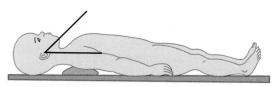

Figure 5-6   Pediatric spinal immobilization. (Illustration by Maggie Reynard)

Airway/breathing

Patients experiencing apnea at the scene may suddenly awaken once intubated. These are frequently the patients with A-O or A-A dislocations. Their need is an airway as their injury is above C4. However, they may now survive the insult as a profound quadriplegic, ventilator dependent. Nevertheless, airway, as always, is the first priority.

- Placing the airway requires cervical spine protection; maintain manual stabilization during intubation; DO NOT hyperextend the neck
- Cricoid pressure may assist with intubation
- Assess for shallow respirations, use of accessory muscles, paradoxical respirations, abdominal breathing as indicators that the patient is struggling to maintain respirations
  — Vital capacity <800 mL needs mechanical ventilation
  — Lesions above T10 have decreased cough
  — Quad cough maneuver assists with a more effective cough by placing the heel of the hand on the abdomen and pushing inward while the patient exhales
    ▪ Do not perform immediately after meals
    ▪ Possibility that the quad cough may affect the position of a vena cava filter
  — Chest physical therapy to move secretions and prevent atelectasis
  — Bronchoscopy can assist with persistent collapse to open the airways
  — Long-term ventilation requires a tracheostomy to ensure airway
- Initiate kinetic therapy early to enhance pulmonary toilet while immobilizing the patient
  — Use for patients that require logrolling
  — Can be used with cervical traction devices if necessary
  — Assure a snug fit but without pressure
  — Maintain constant rotation

- Vagus nerve exits above C1, which results in unopposed and uninterrupted flow, causing a vasovagal response to cough, suctioning, or position changes

Circulation

Circulation in the SCI patient is affected by both neurologic issues and associated injuries. If all potential sites for hemorrhage are ruled out, then treat the neurogenic and spinal shock.

Signs and Symptoms of Neurogenic Shock

Occurs with SCI above T6
Loss of sympathetic influence below the lesion—vasodilation, increased venous capitance, decreased venous return, decreased cardiac output, decreased perfusion
Hypotension
Bradycardia
Warm and dry skin
Lasts from 2 weeks to 2 years; average 3 months

Neurogenic shock should be managed as stated here (ATLS 2004)

- Administer fluids as per trauma resuscitation up to 2 L warm crystalloid
- Ensure there is no site of ongoing hemorrhage that requires management
- Continued fluid administration will result in pulmonary edema
- Administer vasopressors once fluid resuscitation is complete
  — Dopamine
  — Phenylephrine
  — Norepinephrine

Spinal shock is the response of the neurologic system to injury.

Signs and Symptoms of Spinal Shock

Flaccidity followed by hypertonicity/spasticity after resolution in
  cord injury
Areflexia
Loss of sensation
Atonic bladder
Return of function is heralded by bladder tone, sacral reflexes,
  and hyperreflexia
Reflexes usually return within 4-6 weeks

Maintain normothermia for the patient, especially quadriplegic
patients as they experience poikilothermia.

• Administer all fluids warmed
• Monitor core temperature continuously
• Warm the room
• Apply warm blankets or use a forced air warmer

Stabilization

Stabilization begins at the scene and continues until definitive
management. The backboard and cervical collar are placed prior
to arrival. Management includes

• Remove backboard as soon as possible after arrival to the
  definitive care facility to prevent decubiti
  — Remove backboard when logrolling the patient to assess
    the back
  — Logroll until cleared
  — Logrolling requires a minimum of 4 to 6 individuals: 1 to
    control the head and the roll itself, 2 with arms crossed across
    the patient's body, 1 to turn the legs; roll toward the staff

- Use the backboard for transport only
- After removal, logroll every 2 hours until injury is ruled out or definitive stabilization is accomplished (ATLS 2004)
- Philadelphia and extrication collars are acceptable for initial placement
- Long-term cervical collar is needed to provide stabilization and prevention of breakdown
  - Use Aspen or Miami-J collars for this purpose
  - Follow the guidelines for measurement and application or consult orthotics
  - Supply a set of pads so that they can be changed and cleaned daily
- C2 odontoid fractures usually fuse within 3 months of injury; stabilization is required during that time

  Specific management of various injuries includes

- Cervical strain—injury to muscle and ligaments only resulting in pain and stiffness usually 12 to 24 hours after injury
  - Apply soft cervical collar to remind patient to be gentle with their neck
  - Symptoms last ~2 to 4 weeks
- Fracture-dislocations requiring reduction
  - May be placed in Gardner-Wells tongs or halo tongs with traction to reduce especially if mechanical reduction is ineffective
    - Type II A-O dislocations should never be placed to traction (McElwee and Wargo 2006)
  - Once reduced, the patient may undergo surgery and/or halo placement
  - Frequently even with surgical fusion, the halo is placed in addition to maintain stabilization
  - Halo treatment includes cleansing pinsites daily with hydrogen peroxide and saline; application of betadine swab every 8 hours

— Tape halo wrenches to the vest itself in case of cardiac arrest where the anterior portion of the vest may need to be removed; some halo devices have breakaway vests
— Halo devices are also made of titanium and are MRI compatible
— Provide additional liner and wear t-shirt under the liner for hygiene
  ▪ Do not apply powder, lotion, or corn starch under the vest as these "gum up" and become skin irritants
  ▪ Monitor for skin breakdown
  ▪ Daily cleansing of the skin
— Provide instruction that the halo must remain in place at all times (usually 3 months) (yes, the author has had patients remove the device on their own or swim in it)
• Cervical-high thoracic injury
  — Use a somi or Minerva brace that essentially attaches a cervical collar device to a thoracic immobilizer
  — Fitted by orthotics
  — Use also when a halo cannot be placed such as pregnancy, obesity, or stable fractures
• Thoracolumbar fractures
  — Use a thoracolumbar orthotic device (TLSO or Jewett brace) fitted by orthotics for stable fractures or after surgical fusion
  — Logroll until placement of TLSO
  — A corset may be used for comfort in transverse process fractures; these do not require surgery but may indicate associated pelvic and abdominal injury
  — 50% of transverse process fractures are seen on CT but not on plain films (Homnick et al. 2007)
• Surgical fixation
  — Can be anterior or posterior or both at any length of the spine
  — Determined by the surgeon and the instability of the fracture and associated ligamentous injury

— Provides early decompression of epidural hematoma (EDH) or herniated discs to improve outcome (EAST 2000)

— Fusion allows for stability, early mobilization, early discharge to rehabilitation, and prevention of complications; early fixation allows the surgery to be done before any infectious complications start

— Usually performed within 1 to 4 days after injury

— If neurologically improving, surgery may be moved to 4 to 7 days

— Surgery may also include iliac crest bone graft (or vertebral) (ICBG) or cadaver bone to increase stability and calcification after surgery; laminectomy for decompression; reduction of dislocation

— Reduces hospital length of stay

• Methylprednisolone (steroid therapy)

— There remains considerable controversy regarding the use of steroids to reduce edema, act as an antioxidant, and prevent ischemia and cell death

  ▪ Initial studies demonstrate a possible benefit of return of 1 to 2 levels of function through the administration of high dose steroids (Bracken et al. 1990, 1998)

  ▪ Currently the American College of Surgeons has changed their instruction in the Advanced Trauma Life Support (ATLS) Course. They state that there is insufficient evidence for routine administration of high-dose steroids in acute spinal cord injury (Kortbeek et al. 2008)

  ▪ It is the decision of the treating physician to administer high-dose steroids

  ▪ See the box on page 190 for the guidelines for dosage

— Special considerations should be given to use in patients with the following as these were not included in the original studies

  ▪ Pregnancy

  ▪ Severe diabetes

  ▪ Age <13 years

- Human immunodeficiency virus (HIV) or fulminant infection, tuberculosis (TB)
- Penetrating trauma
— If used, the NASCIS II-III criteria must be followed (Bracken et al. 1990, 1998)

Methylprednisolone NASCIS II-III Criteria

Initiate ONLY if within 8 hours of initial onset of neurologic deficits
Administer bolus 30 mg/kg over 15 minutes
Prepare the long-term drip and begin by the end of the first hour
Administer long-term drip of 5.4 mg/kg/hour
If initiating within 3 hours of onset, use this drip for 23 hours
If initiating within 3-8 hours of onset, use this drip for a total of 48 hours from initiation of the bolus
Do not substitute other steroids
Do not add other steroids such as dexamethasone

Cervical Spine Clearance

There are various criteria for clearance of the cervical spine. The goal is removal of the collar as soon as possible but in a safe way to avoid missed injury.

- Alert, awake, and oriented patient (EAST 2000, Hoffman et al. 2000)
  — Without drugs or alcohol on board
  — Without distracting injuries (painful injuries)
  — Without midline posterior neck pain
  — Low probability of injury based upon symptoms and mechanism of injury
  — Without focal neurologic deficit
  — No films required to clear
  — Clearance should be performed by trauma surgery, orthopaedic spine surgery, neurosurgery, or emergency medicine

- Awake, alert, and oriented patient with neck pain (EAST 2000, ATLS 2004)
  — Perform a 3-view cervical spine film set—A-P, lateral, and open mouth odontoid views
  — Perform an axial cervical CT with 3-mm cuts
  — If C7-T1 junction is not visible on the plain films, add a swimmer's view and/or saggital reconstructions of the CT
  — If the films are normal, remove collar, then perform flexion-extension films
    ▪ These films are voluntary flexion and extension by the patient and must achieve ≥30 degrees without neck pain
    ▪ These films check for occult instability
    ▪ Preferably performed within 4 hours of injury
    ▪ If paraspinal muscle spasm limits films, maintain cervical collar for 2 to 3 weeks and reimage, achieving >30 degrees of flexion-extension
- Neurologic deficit—spine-related (EAST 2000)
  — Perform a 3-view cervical spine film set—A-P, lateral, and open mouth odontoid views
  — Perform spine MRI especially if plain films are normal
  — Preferably within 2 hours of arrival
- Altered level of consciousness that is expected to be prolonged >2 days
  — Perform a 3-view cervical spine film set—A-P, lateral, and open mouth odontoid views
  — Perform an axial cervical CT with 3-mm cuts and saggital reconstructions
  — Perform flexion-extension fluoroscopy with static images at the extremes of flexion and extension
    ▪ Excursion is performed by trauma surgery, neurosurgery, or orthopaedic spine surgery
    ▪ Preferably within 48 hours of injury to enable removal of the cervical collar and increased mobility

SPECIAL SITUATIONS

Spinal Cord Injury without Radiographic Abnormality (SCIWORA)

Spinal cord injury without radiographic abnormality (SCI-WORA) occurs in <10% of SCI and almost always in children. The children are usually <8 years of age. In children <8 years, hyperflexion is the cause, whereas in >8 years, hyperextension is the culprit (Koestner and Hoak 2001). Children have increased elasticity of the ligaments of the spine, maximum flexibility, and the flat facets that allow for dislocation and self-realignment after injury. Typical sites of injury include

- C2-C3 in infants
- C3-C4 in school age children
- C5-C6 in adolescents

In the lumbar spine, SCIWORA is caused by the improper use of a lap belt in an underage or underweight child, positioning the lap belt on the abdomen instead of the pelvis. A distraction injury occurs resulting in an ischemic cord.

Reasons for Delayed Diagnosis with SCIWORA

Transient paresthesias, numbness, and subjective paralysis are overlooked

Initial symptoms are followed by a latent period, then progressive paralysis for up to 4 days after initial injury

Recurrent impact because of improper immobilization or re-injury has a 50% chance of recurrence or worsening of the original injury

In the adolescent age group, football is often the cause of "stingers," which involve transient loss of function usually in the cervical spine. Stingers can be caused by mechanical injury or a congenitally narrow canal predisposing the cord to injury. As with SCIWORA, stingers can recur or worsen with subsequent impact.

Autonomic Dysreflexia

Autonomic dysreflexia (AD) occurs in SCI patients in whom the lesion is at or above T6. It does not occur until the spinal reflexes have returned. AD is the result of a noxious stimuli causing a sympathetic discharge below the level of the lesion that is uncontrolled by parasympathetic discharges. Vasoconstriction occurs below the injury. Baroreceptors in the carotid sinus and aorta respond by parasympathetic discharge that can only affect the body above the lesion causing vasodilation there.

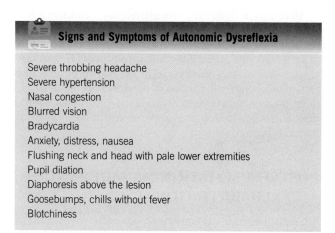

Signs and Symptoms of Autonomic Dysreflexia

Severe throbbing headache
Severe hypertension
Nasal congestion
Blurred vision
Bradycardia
Anxiety, distress, nausea
Flushing neck and head with pale lower extremities
Pupil dilation
Diaphoresis above the lesion
Goosebumps, chills without fever
Blotchiness

Management

Immediate recognition of the AD syndrome and actions to remove the noxious stimulus require emergent action. The syndrome may occur during the initial hospital stay, rehabilitation, or at home. Thus any area of the hospital may need to recognize AD.

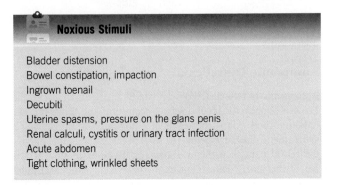

Noxious Stimuli

Bladder distension
Bowel constipation, impaction
Ingrown toenail
Decubiti
Uterine spasms, pressure on the glans penis
Renal calculi, cystitis or urinary tract infection
Acute abdomen
Tight clothing, wrinkled sheets

Management of AD requires identification and removal of the stimulus. Ganglionic blockers may be used to assist with managing the hypertension. If the syndrome is not controlled or prevented, myocardial infarction, subarachnoid hemorrhage, or stroke can occur. Prevention is the key. See the rehabilitation section following for discussion of preventive measures for SCI to be used on a daily basis. In addition, even minor surgical procedures require local anesthetic to prevent noxious stimuli from the incision, suturing, etc.

POSTRESUSCITATION MANAGEMENT AND REHABILITATION

Rehabilitation and prevention of complications begins on admission. Any complication has a serious impact on both the outcome and functional status of the SCI patient. Patients with spine structural injury only should be mobilized as soon as they are stabilized to prevent further complications. For the SCI patient, these are a lifetime commitment. Early discharge to rehabilitation removes the patient from sources of infection and further complications, and initiates all measures for future living. These measures include

- Physical therapy
  - Splinting of the extremities by physical therapist (PT) and occupational therapist (OT) to maintain functional position
  - Monitor splints for breakdown
  - Prevent foot-drop with foot splints
  - Provide ROM and activities of daily living (ADL)
  - Design adaptive devices for ADLs
  - Prism glasses to see people and TV from the supine position, especially during traction
- Orthostatic hypotension
  - Occurs in injuries above T6
  - Signs and symptoms include
    - Dizziness
    - Lightheadedness
    - Blurred vision
    - Loss of consciousness
  - Gradually increase the head of bed height to allow for changes in blood flow to the lower extremities
  - Place an abdominal binder and supportive stockings on the lower extremities
  - The addition of elastic wraps over the supportive stockings or the use of pneumatic compression booties also assists with prevention
  - Maintain hydration
- Speech therapy
  - Adapt communication devices for patient use, especially ventilator-dependent patients
  - Assess swallowing
- Nutrition
  - Initiate early enteral feedings to prevent ileus and provide wound healing
- Bowel and bladder program

— Bladder management

- Discontinue Foley catheter as soon as possible to prevent recurrent infection
- Some practices maintain the Foley, especially to enable thorough evaluation of fluid status and prevent dehydration and urinary retention
- Males—use an external device
- If flaccid, the bladder overfills but never completely empties
- Initiate intermittent catheterization every 4 hours once the Foley is removed
- With the return of reflex activity, lengthen intermittent catheterization to every 6 to 8 hours
- Use triggering maneuvers—stimulation in perineum, valsalva, crede (heel of hand to bladder) to initiate voiding and prevent involuntary voiding from a full bladder
- Urinary retention results in renal calculi and infection
- Maintain fluids at 2 to 2.5 L/day
- Annual urodynamic evaluation, antispasmotics

— Bowel evacuation programs are essential as ileus is likely

- Provide adequate fluids
- Daily laxatives or stool softeners
- Digital stimulation of the anal area can initiate evacuation if reflexes have returned

• Spasticity

— Use of muscle relaxants may assist with decreasing spasticity

- Intrathecal baclofen may be useful for chronic intractable spasticity
  ○ Administered through a surgically placed infusion pump
  ○ Continuous infusion

— Results in pain and contractures

— Use ROM, positioning, and splinting

- Psychosocial
  - Antidepressants may be helpful
  - Provide psychological and emotional support from admission
  - Counseling regarding the lifelong effects of the injury and the impact on home, family, and work
  - Vocational counseling Table 5-3 describes functional outcomes for the different levels of injury.
  - Sexuality counseling is essential for patients of a sexually active age
    - Note that pregnancy may precipitate AD in patients with injuries above T6
- Prevention of complications
  - SCI are at risk for
    - Deep vein thrombosis (DVT) and pulmonary embolism (PE)—use the usual methods of prevention (see Chapter 13); a permanent inferior vena cava filter may be the most effective method
    - Pneumonia—use quad cough; encourage incentive spirometry and as much mobility as possible for the patient; prevent aspiration while feeding
    - Decubiti—frequent position change; use of specialty cushions; massage, keep skin dry
      - Decubiti during the hospital stay can result in delayed fixation, increased immobility and length of stay
    - Contractures—lifetime splinting; monitor for breakdown; ROM
- Death commonly caused by pneumonia, sepsis, or pulmonary embolism

 Critical Lifesavers

- Loss of sensation on the anterior upper chest identifies a C4-C5 injury not T1
- If the patient is to be transferred from the local hospital to a trauma center, maintain the immobilization through transfer

Table 5-3   Functional Outcomes after SCI

Injury	Level	Functional Outcome
Quadriplegia	C1 through C4	Total dependency in ADL Ventilator dependence
	C5	Requires assistance with activities
	C6	Manual wheelchair mobility is possible if modified handrims ADLs possible with orthotic equipment
	C7 through T1	Self wheelchair transport Complete independence in ADLs Self-catheterization difficult at C7 level Bowel evacuation via suppository or rectal stimulation
Paraplegia	T2 through T6	Complete independence possible Self-catheterization Bowel evacuation via suppository or rectal stimulation
	T7 through T12	Complete independence includes driving (with adaptive car), dressing, and transfers out of wheelchair Bowel evacuation via suppository or rectal stimulation
	L1 through L3	Complete independence Bowel evacuation via suppository or rectal stimulation Bladder emptying by stimulation of sacral reflex Walking with long leg braces and crutches for short distances

(Continued)

Table 5-3   Functional Outcomes after SCI (*Continued*)

Injury	Level	Functional Outcome
	L4 through S1	All of the above with Independent walking with two canes or crutches Wheelchair unnecessary Bowel evacuation via strain or manual removal
	S2 through S4	As above with Bowel evacuation via strain or manual removal Bladder emptying via strain or crede Walking normal

REFERENCES

American College of Surgeons. *Advanced Trauma Life Support* (ATLS). 7th ed. Chicago, IL: American College of Surgeons; 2004.

American College of Surgeons. *Advanced Trauma Life Support* (ATLS). 8th ed. Chicago, IL: American College of Surgeons; 2008.

American Spinal Injury Association and International Medical Society of Paraplegia (ASIA/IMSOP). *International Standards for Neurological and Functional Classification of Spinal Cord Injury.* Atlanta, GA: American Spine Injury Association; 1996.

Avarello JT, Cantor RM. Pediatric major trauma: an approach to evaluation and management. *Emerg Med Clin North Am.* 2007; 25(3):803-836.

Bracken MB, Shepard MJ, Collins WEF, et al. A randomized, controlled trial of methylprednisolone or naloxone in the treatment of spinal cord injury (Results of the National Spinal Cord Injury Study). *N Engl J Med.* 1990;322:1405-1411.

Bracken MB, Shepard MJ, Holford TR, et al. Methylprednisolone or tielazad mesylate administration after acute spinal cord injury: 1-year follow up (Results of the third national Acute Spinal Cord Injury Randomized Controlled Trial). *J Neurosurg.* 1998;89:699-706.

Eastern Association for the Surgery of Trauma (EAST). Guideline for Determination of Cervical Spine Stability in Trauma Patients. 2000. Available at www.east.org

Hoffman JR, Mower WR, Wolfson AB, et al. Validity of a set of clinical criteria to rule out injury to the cervical spine in patients with blunt trauma. *N Engl J Med.* 2000;343(2):94-99.

Homnick A, Iavery R, Nicastro O, et al. Isolated thoracic-lumbar transverse process fractures: call physical therapy no spine. *J Trauma.* 2007;63(6):1292-1295.

Hsu KC, Tsai SH, Chang LW, et al. Prevertebral soft tissue swelling as a clue for spinal cord injury: case illustration. *J Trauma.* 2007; 63(6):1424.

Koestner AJ, Hoak SJ. Spinal cord injury without radiographic abnormality (SCIWORA) in children. *J Trauma Nurse.* 2001;8(4): 101-108.

Kortbeek JB, Al Turki SA, Ali J. Advanced trauma life support: the evidence for change. *J Trauma.* 2008;64(6):1638-1650.

McElwee K, Wargo CA. Traumatic atlanto-occipital dislocation: a pediatric case report. *J Trauma Nurse.* 2006;13(4):186-189.

National Spinal Cord Injury Statistical Center (NSCISC). Available at: http://www.spinalcord.uab.edu/show.asp?durki=19679. Accessed August 26, 2008.

Powe CB. Cervical spine clearance in the blunt trauma patient: overview of current management strategies. *J Trauma Nurse.* 2006;13(2):80-83.

Spineuniverse. Available at: http://ww.spineuniverse.com. Accessed August 28, 2008.

Weller SJ, Rossitch E, Malek AM. Detection of vertebral artery injury after cervical spine trauma using MRA. *J Trauma.* 1999; 46(4):660-666.

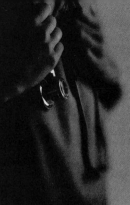

Chapter 6

FACE AND NECK INJURY

INTRODUCTION

The face plays many different roles in our lives, some of which we notice and some we do not. Obviously, the face is how we recognize each other. The face houses the five senses. In addition, the face is the first line of defense for the brain. It is designed to collapse on itself and deflect the kinetic energy load before the impact reaches the brain. Much like the steering column of a car collapses, so does the midface to protect the brain from the direct blow. There are multiple organs within the face that can sustain injury from both blunt and penetrating mechanisms.

ASSESSMENT

Assessment for facial injury begins, as all trauma assessment does, with airway, breathing, circulation and neurologic assessment. The face and brain assessments are intertwined, and a misinterpretation of data (eg. pupil dilation) could result in missing a brain injury or assuming there is one when it is simply a glass eye. Facial injury can very quickly result in airway loss; therefore airway is always the first priority. Facial injury can also be extensive, resulting in damages beyond recognition of the person. Long-term issues of reconstruction and self-image will be dealt with throughout the hospitalization and after discharge.

History

Understanding the mechanisms involved in injuries of the face is essential to anticipate airway issues and other potential problems. History should include

- Mechanism of injury
  - Impact to the face, such as assault, motor vehicle collision (MVC), steering wheel deformity, windshield starring
  - Use of safety devices, such as restraints, airbags, helmet
  - Penetrating injury may be self-inflicted unintentional or suicide attempt
- Scene and transport assessment
  - Airway issues, breathing difficulty or abnormality
  - Bleeding from nose, mouth
  - Intraoral or pharyngeal blood, secretions
  - Neurologic alteration
- Past medical and surgical history
  - Medications
  - Last meal

Trauma Assessment

Assessment follows the trauma standard of airway, breathing, circulation, and neurologic response. Focus initially on the essentials for patient survival. As with all trauma, action must be taken immediately if there are any issues with airway, breathing, circulation. The initial assessment must focus on stabilization and resuscitation as described in Chapter 2. Specific signs and symptoms related to individual injuries are listed below. Initial assessment with the focus on the face and neck includes

- Airway/breathing
  - Observe injury to the nose, mouth, oral cavity, pharynx, neck
    - Contusions, seatbelt sign across the neck
    - Lacerations

- ▪ Deformity
- ▪ Obstruction
- ▪ Bleeding
— Listen and observe respirations and manage the airway
  - ▪ Snoring, gurgling
  - ▪ Retractions
  - ▪ Obstruction nasal, oral, pharyngeal
  - ▪ Check position of the tongue
— Do not place airway or any tubes through the nose if facial injury is suspected; tubes can be placed directly into the cranium if cribriform plate fractures are present
- Circulation
  — Observe for bleeding and control
  — Check pulses in the neck for equality
  — Listen for bruit over the carotids
  — Note any oral or pharyngeal bleeding that may be coming from nasal or maxillary sources
    - ▪ Rapid control of nasopharyngeal bleeding is required
    - ▪ Assess for coagulopathy and manage
- Neurologic deficit
  — Evaluate neurologic status
  — Maintain airway
    - ▪ Prevent hypoxia
  — Maintain normovolemia
    - ▪ Prevent hypotension
  — Cranial nerve assessment (see Chapter 4)
- Facial assessment
  — Observe for deformity
    - ▪ Penetrating implements should be stabilized to prevent movement
    - ▪ Check for sensation and symmetrical movement

— Palpate the bones of the face for
  - Crepitus
  - Deformity
  - Movement of bony structures
— Maxilla
  - Hold the upper teeth and wiggle gently
  - Be careful as the patient may bite
  - Observe for movement at the alveolar ridge, antrum, and/or across the orbits
— Mandible
  - Check bite/occlusion
  - Crepitus
  - Check missing, loose, or fractured teeth
  - Palpate temporal-mandibular joint for alignment, tenderness
  - Assess oral cavity for lacerations, bleeding, swelling, tongue injury
— Eyes
  - Check pupils (see Section Extraocular movements—pupils, Chapter 4)
  - Visual acuity can be assessed by asking the patient to count examiner's fingers at a distance of three feet
  - Extraocular movements (see Chapter 4)
  - Enucleation or deformity of the globe
  - Ophthalmologic examination if there is question of injury to check lens, retina (funduscopic examination), vitreous, vessels, optic nerve, intraocular pressure
— Ears
  - External auricular injury, check for amputation/near-amputation
  - Blood or fluid from the external auditory canal; check for cerebrospinal fluid (CSF) leak (see section on Inspection, Chapter 4)

- Contusion behind the ear
- Check tympanic membranes for rupture or hemotympanum
- Check bilateral hearing

DOCUMENTATION

Documentation of facial injury must define any visible deformity, skin injuries, and injuries to the facial organs, such as the eyes, tongue, teeth and ears. Penetrating injury should be described, especially gunshot wound (GSW). The neurologic examination should be included as well as sensation and movement of the face.

MANAGEMENT

Some injuries to the face are managed immediately. These are injuries that affect airway, breathing, and circulation. Organ-threatening injuries such as enucleation or globe rupture are also managed early. Tongue lacerations can bleed profusely and will require rapid control for both the bleeding and to maintain the airway.

Penetrating facial injuries require immediate airway management caused by edema, hemorrhage, hematoma, and other debris that can obstruct the airway.

Upper Third of Face

The upper third of the face includes the zygoma, orbit, and nasal bones, frontal skull/sinus and globes. Injury here can result in total craniofacial dysjunction as this is the means of connecting the face to the cranium. Multiple cranial nerves and vessels are also present in this part of the face. All vessels within the face are under pressure due to the proximity to the aorta and carotids.

Ear injury/management

Because the ear is mostly external to the skull, it is easily injured with a blow to the head. Injuries to the auricle and external auditory canal (EAC) are visible. Blood from the EAC should be evaluated for CSF by use of the halo test on filter paper or a glucose dipstick testing positive. If negative, blood from the EAC is likely an external laceration or may be from a ruptured tympanic membrane. Blood from the face may also run toward the EAC caused by gravity in the supine position. Evaluate for the source of bleeding. Internally, a basilar skull fracture may also affect the ossicles causing disruption and decreased hearing. Other causes of decreased hearing include hemotympanum, ruptured tympanic membrane, and cranial nerve injury.

Hemotympanum and ruptured tympanic membranes heal on their own. Antibiotics may be given to prevent infection if basilar skull fracture is involved. Ossicular disruption is managed nonoperatively. Hearing evaluations will be necessary to monitor hearing function over time.

Amputations and near-amputations of the ear are treated as any amputation and require urgent surgery for reattachment. In the case of a severely mangled ear, reconstructive surgery will be needed to rebuild the structure. After repair, a bolster is usually attached to the ear for stabilization and protection. Amputations are discussed in Chapter 9.

Orbital fractures/management

There are multiple bones within the orbit, including the sphenoid, ethmoid, lamina papyracea. The fractures of the orbit thus also include the basilar skull. These bones are fragile and thin and easily fractured during a direct blow from increased pressure. The orbits are the bones that connect the face to the cranium, as well as the cup holding the globes and cranial nerves controlling the eyes. A fracture across the orbits, nasal bones and zygoma-maxillary complex becomes a Le Fort III maxilla fracture known as craniofacial dysjunction (Figure 6-1).

Signs and Symptoms of Orbital Fractures

Periorbital ecchymosis with swelling, inability to open eyes
Asymmetry of the eyes/orbits
Extraocular movements may be affected if muscle entrapment
Vision loss
Crepitus, subcutaneous air
Infraorbital paresthesias
Subconjunctival hemorrhage
Proptosis, check globes
Cranial nerve entrapment

Surgical management of the orbital fractures may be delayed unless the globe is injured and needs repair or entrapment is evident. A "blowout" orbital fracture involves the orbital floor without an orbital rim fracture (Lelli et al. 2007). If enopthalmos is present, immediate surgical repair is usually undertaken. Management includes

- Assess for neurologic injury in addition to facial injury
- Computed tomography (CT) scan to determine degree of fracture, impingement, enopthalmos or exophthalmos
- Ice packs to decrease swelling and pain management
- Increase head of bed to decrease swelling
- Do not blow the nose (basilar skull fracture may be involved and increases intraocular pressure)
- Operative management may involve otorhinolaryngologists, oral-maxillofacial surgeons, ophthalmology
  — Can be delayed if there is no entrapment or signs of cranial nerve involvement
  — Surgery should be within 2 weeks if symptomatic diplopia or soft tissue entrapment (Burnstine 2003)
  — Lateral and medial wall fractures, supraorbital fracture and nasoethmoid fracture respond best to repair within

2 weeks to avoid difficulties due to the healing process (Burnstine 2003)

- Antibiotics may be necessary if basilar skull fracture is present with cerebrospinal fluid leak

Eye injuries/management

Eye injuries can include injury to the internal globe as well as to the external surface and eyelids/lacrimal ducts. Signs and symptoms of eye injuries are listed below. Globe rupture and enucleation require emergent management.

Signs and Symptoms of Eye Injuries

Globe rupture
Decreased or lost vision, penetrating object present
Pain
Extrusion of aqueous/vitreous humor, prolapse
Teardrop-shaped pupil
Examination—shallow anterior chamber, decreased intraocular pressure

Hyphema
Blurred vision, decreased visual acuity
Pain
Blood-tinged vision
Increased intraocular pressure

Lens dislocation
Unilateral diplopia

Retinal detachment
Unilateral loss of vision, cloudy, veil
Flashing lights and/or floaters, shower of black dots
Painless, gradual or sudden onset

Corneal Abrasion
Sensitivity to light, tearing
Redness, sharp pain
Excessive blinking

Management of eye injuries include

- Nonsalvageable eye must be enucleated
  — If the eye remains, an antigenic response causes blindness in the uninjured eye
- Traumatic enucleation
  — Cover with sterile saline-soaked gauze and protect from injury
  — Surgery for replacement or removal determined by the degree of destruction to the globe. If removed, a conformer may be placed in the orbit to retain shape until a prosthetic eye is placed
- Globe rupture (sclera injury)
  — If a penetrating object is present, secure to prevent movement and further injury
  — Do not open the eyelids until ophthalmologic examination
  — Abnormal pupils may indicate globe injury or neurologic injury
  — CT scan to evaluate damage
  — Place a shield on both eyes (ou) to decrease consensual movement
  — Pain management
  — Antibiotics IV; antiemetics as needed
  — Increase head of bed and promote rest
  — Surgical repair
- Hyphema
  — Accumulated blood within the anterior chamber; injury and bleeding from the iris and can be associated with severe intraocular injury
  — Graded by the amount of blood accumulating in the anterior chamber
  — Secondary bleeding can occur up to 3 to 5 days after initial injury (Hoyt and Selfridge-Thomas 2007, ATLS 2004)
  — Shield the eye for protection
  — Increase head of bed and promote rest

— Do not administer nonsteroidal anti-inflammatory drugs (NSAIDs), aspirin, anticoagulants because of the potential for further bleeding

— Administer cycloplegic agents; steroids to decrease intraocular pressure

— Glaucoma may develop over the long term after hyphema in ~7% of patients (ATLS 2004)

• Retinal detachment

— Vision threatening; requires rapid identification to prevent blindness from loss of blood supply

— Shield both eyes to prevent consensual movement

— Promote rest

— Surgical repair

— Of note, in child abuse, retinal hemorrhages result from severe shaking or severe blunt trauma; funduscopic examination identifies the hemorrhages

• Retrobulbar hematoma

— Caused by hemorrhage from the infraorbital artery

— Can be the result of acute orbital compartment syndrome

— Ischemic optic neuropathy occurs and results in blindness; increased intraocular pressure

— Increase head of bed

— Avoid any pressure on the eye

— CT scan may assist in diagnosis

— Management includes

▪ Lateral canthotomy to decompress the orbit; can be done in the emergency department (ED)

▪ If visual acuity does not return or intraocular pressure remains increased, surgical decompression of the orbit with hematoma evacuation is necessary

• Corneal abrasions

— Can be caused by any foreign body, especially contact lenses; be sure to assess for lenses and remove to prevent iatrogenic abrasions

— Fluorescein stain uptake in the cornea will demonstrate the defect
— Apply topical anesthetics and cycloplegics to decrease pain
— Apply topical antibiotics to prevent infection
— Promote eye rest, wear sunglasses to decrease light sensitivity

• Extraocular foreign body
— Stabilize the foreign body to prevent movement
— Metal objects if left on the eye can result in rust on the cornea which then invades
— Large objects require removal in surgery and repair of the globe if ruptured
— Small or microscopic objects can be removed with a moist cotton swab usually by the ophthalmologist
— If rust is present, surgery is required for removal
— Apply topical anesthetics for discomfort; topical antibiotics if there is also a corneal abrasion
— Assess for contact lenses and remove
— Pain management
— Tetanus

• Eyelid lacerations
— Evaluate for involvement of the lacrimal duct, which would require ophthalmologic repair
— Laceration repair can occur in the ED
— For lacerations requiring ophthalmology evaluation, cover with saline gauze to keep the wound moist
— Ptosis will be present if there is cranial nerve injury or levator muscle injury
— If the canthus is involved, ophthalmology is needed to assess the injury and determine appropriate repair

Zygoma fracture/management

The zygoma (cheekbone) is the malar eminence and part of what makes the face distinctive. In a Le Fort III fracture, the zygoma is part of the fracture complex. Of its own, a zygoma may not need repair; however, because of self-concept issues related to the face, repair prevents permanent deformity and asymmetry. A tripod fracture involves the lateral zygoma, orbit, and maxilla.

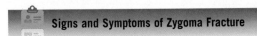

Signs and Symptoms of Zygoma Fracture

Deformity of the "cheekbone," flattened
Facial ecchymosis
Pain
Cheek, nose, upper lip paresthesias
Subcutaneous emphysema resulting from sinus involvement
May effect lower jaw movement

Zygoma fracture management is dependent upon deformity and effect on facial nerves. Other management includes

- Pain management, apply ice packs to decrease swelling
- Increase head of bed to decrease swelling
- May need antibiotics if sinuses are involved
- Surgical repair with open reduction and internal fixation (ORIF) or reduction with external fixation

Frontal sinus fracture/management

The frontal bone forming the forehead is part of the vault of the skull. Within the frontal bone, the sinus is large and if fractured can result in pneumocephalus as well as infection. Unless there is forehead deformity or palpable fracture, the diagnosis is usually made by CT scan. Repair is dependent upon deformity and communication with the cranium. Repair may include obliteration of the sinus by filling the space with soft/fatty tissue and sealing the posterior defect with Teflon or other plate.

Fractures involving the anterior and posterior walls may also be associated with dural tear and brain injury. If the cranium is involved and not just the anterior table of the skull, antibiotics are usually administered to prevent infection, and the patient should not sneeze or blow the nose to prevent increased pressure in the sinuses. CT monitoring of pneumocephalus should occur until repair. Sudden increase in pneumocephalus behaves as any extracerebral hematoma and can result in enough increased intracranial pressure (IICP) to alter level of consciousness or cause herniation.

Nasal fracture/epistaxis/management

As with most of the facial bones, the nose also contains numerous thin, small bones that communicate with the basilar skull via the cribriform plate. Nasal fractures are the most common isolated facial fracture (Alvi et al. 2003). The nose is also divided by the septum and has a very rich blood supply under pressure from the aorta which can result in severe hemorrhage. Epistaxis can be associated with fracture or simply laceration. Increased pressure to the head can also cause epistaxis in patients with hypertension or the presence of antiplatelet medications.

Signs and Symptoms of Nasal Fracture

Periorbital ecchymosis, swelling
Deformity
Pain
Epistaxis
Septal hematoma
Airway loss, inability to breathe through the nose

Nasal fracture management begins with protection of the airway and the avoidance of any tubes through the nose. Hemorrhage must be controlled as a significant amount of blood loss can occur.

• Apply ice to the face and to the back of the neck to decrease bleeding and swelling

- Direct pressure to stop hemorrhage by compressing the nostrils
- Direct pressure will not affect a posterior hemorrhage
  — Nasal tampons or packing may be inserted and gently pulled forward into position to tamponade the bleed
    ▪ Be aware that if there is a cribriform plate fracture, the packing can be passed into the cranium
  — A 14-g Foley catheter can also be used to tamponade epistaxis (Harrahill 2005)
    ▪ Partially inflate the balloon after insertion, then gently pull forward into position
  — Silver nitrate may be used to cauterize the bleeder directly; endoscopic cautery can also be used
  — An otorhinolaryngologist may also choose to suture the bleeder directly
  — Cocaine may be "snorted" or cocaine/lidocaine-soaked gauze/pledgets can be inserted into the nose to vasoconstrict the vessels
  — A nonallergenic hydrophilic polymer/potassium salt product (Quick Relief) is a powder applied directly to the bleeding site and is particularly useful for epistaxis in patients on anticoagulation
  — Packing should be removed within 24 to 48 hours to reassess bleeding and prevent infection
- Evacuate the septal hematoma to open the nasal passages and prevent septal necrosis
- Administer
  — Antibiotics because of the proximity of sinuses and the basilar skull
  — Antihistamines to decrease nasal swelling
  — Topical anesthetic
- Pain management but avoid aspirin, NSAIDs, antiplatelets until bleeding is controlled
- Nasal fractures are most often reduced and an external splint placed; ORIF may be necessary

Midface

The midface is formed by the maxilla and the associated upper alveolar ridge and teeth. The maxilla is also formed by several small bones including the pterygoid, which forms part of the articulation of the face to the mandible/lower jaw. The midface is where the protective mechanisms of the structure of the face belong. It is here that the bones begin to collapse until the impact involves the nasal, orbital and zygomatic bones of the upper third of the face.

Maxilla fractures/management

The maxilla shapes the rest of the face and houses sinuses that drain to/from the nose into the nasopharynx. Air-fluid levels are frequently seen on CT scan of the maxilla and are usually caused by chronic inflammation of the sinuses or in the case of trauma may represent blood from fracture. Le Fort fractures may involve only one side of the face, or may be of two different types on each side of the face (Figure 6-1).

The pattern of maxilla fractures are described as

- Le Fort I: transverse fracture across the lower maxilla (upper jaw) and may involve the alveolar ridge along with teeth fractures, pterygoid, and can include the hard palate
- Le Fort II: pyramidal fracture upward from the maxilla and across the nasal bones, pterygoid, medial orbits

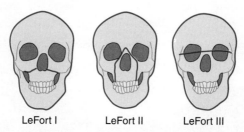

LeFort I   LeFort II   LeFort III

Figure 6-1   Le Fort fracture patterns. (Illustration by Maggie Reynard.)

Signs and Symptoms of Maxilla Fracture

Airway compromise (Figure 6-2)
Paresthesias primarily cranial nerves II-III
Deformity, asymmetry
Pain
Facial ecchymosis, swelling, epistaxis
Visual changes
Malocclusion, lip swelling/contusion (Le Fort I-II)
Cerebrospinal fluid leak (Le Fort II-III)
Flattening zygoma, cheek paresthsias, diplopia (Le Fort III)

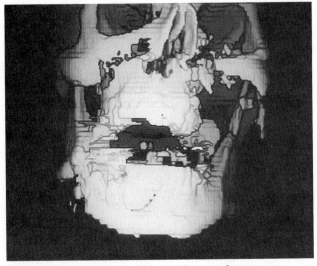

Figure 6-2 Gunshot wound face with severe fracture.

- Le Fort III: craniofacial dysjunction crosses the orbits, zygoma, maxilla, pterygoid, nasal bones

    Maxilla and Le Fort fracture management begins with airway and hemorrhage control.

- Control airway, rapid sequence oral intubation
- Apply ice to decrease swelling
- Increase head of bed if other injuries permit
- Pain management
- CT scan to identify degree of fracture involvement
- Surgical repair may be delayed depending on severity and the involvement of the sinuses
- ORIF is usually required to stabilize and maintain the integrity of the face
- Le Fort I fractures are often stabilized through maxillo-mandibular fixation (MMF), discussed below.

Lower Third of Face

The lower face includes the mandible and the temporomandibular joint (TMJ) as well as the oral structures of the teeth, tongue, pharynx, and parotid/salivary glands. The lower face provides for mastication and swallowing, clearance of secretions, airway and its relationship to the trachea/larynx, and the beginning of the gastrointestinal tract involving the mouth, pharynx and esophagus.

Mandible fracture/management

The mandible (Figure 6-3) provides the power for mastication and the attached tongue is the strongest muscle of the body, which provides taste as well as swallowing. The alveolar ridge of the mandible attaches the teeth. The parotid gland and duct are the source for saliva, which lubricates and initiates digestion. The TMJ is the attachment of the mandible to the skull. The mandible forms a partial ring and because of its structure is frequently fractured in more than one place. If one fracture is identified, the patient should be evaluated for a second.

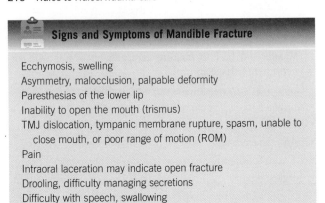

Signs and Symptoms of Mandible Fracture

Ecchymosis, swelling
Asymmetry, malocclusion, palpable deformity
Paresthesias of the lower lip
Inability to open the mouth (trismus)
TMJ dislocation, tympanic membrane rupture, spasm, unable to
    close mouth, or poor range of motion (ROM)
Pain
Intraoral laceration may indicate open fracture
Drooling, difficulty managing secretions
Difficulty with speech, swallowing

Mandible fracture management begins with airway and may preclude intubation, forcing an emergent surgical airway if the mouth cannot be opened sufficiently for visualization of the vocal cords.

- Maintain airway—intubation or surgical cricothyrotomy
- Apply ice pack to decrease swelling

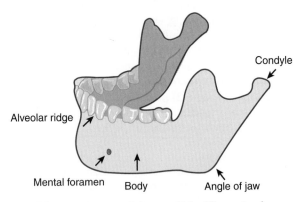

Figure 6-3   Components of the mandible. (Illustration by Maggie Reynard.)

- When assessing for mandible fracture, check malocclusion
  — May place tongue blade between the teeth and twist; blade breaking with pain is 100% diagnostic for mandible fracture and ~50% diagnostic for maxillary sinus or Le Fort fractures (Haydel et al. 2005)
- Raise head of bed
- Provide suction to clear secretions especially when a definitive airway is not present
- Pain management
- Surgical repair includes ORIF/closed reduction (CR)/CR with internal fixation (CRIF) and frequently includes MMF; external fixation may be necessary for comminuted and extensive fractures
  — Dental wiring requires that wire cutters be kept with the patient at all times
  — Repair includes realignment of the mandible to approach normal occlusion as possible
  — In the case of vomiting or loss of airway, the wires must be cut immediately
  — Nutrition consult is necessary to provide meal plans with pureed foods and liquids
  — Oral hygiene is necessary to prevent infection and protect teeth from caries and the incisions from infection; swish with hydrogen peroxide/Cepacol, tooth-brushing
- TMJ closed reduction
- Requires a soft diet to decrease stress on the joint
- Reduction may be included in the mandible repair and MMF

Oral injury/management

Injuries to the oral cavity may not require treatment if they are minor. However, lacerations may indicate open fractures or parotid injury. Parotid injury requires surgical repair. Oral lacerations can be sutured unless open fracture is involved, and then require debridement and fracture repair.

- Teeth may be fractured, loosened, or avulsed from the socket

- Fractured teeth may involve only the enamel or through the tooth to the root and pulp
  — Dentin only: sensitive, painful; cover exposed area with gauze and calcium hydroxide or zinc oxide; consult dentist within 24 hours
  — Pulp: dentistry consult immediately because of potential for infection; cover with gauze and keep moist
- Loose tooth
  — Usually heals within 2 weeks if there is minimal mobility (Hoyt and Selfridge-Thomas 2007)
  — Soft diet
  — If primary teeth, not adult teeth, recommend allowing the tooth to fall out as the adult tooth will follow in time
- Tooth loss/avulsion
  — If the tooth is found at the scene, bring with the patient
  — If tooth not found, it may have been aspirated; check chest x-ray (CXR) for foreign bodies in the lungs or esophagus
  — Touch only the crown of the tooth
  — Transport and preserve in milk after rinsing off debris with saline
  — If the tooth can be cleansed with saline immediately, place back into the socket until repair (within 30 minutes to 6 hours maximum) (Hoyt and Selfridge-Thomas 2007)
  — Delayed repair, maintain the tooth in milk or Hanks solution
  — After repair/replacement, avoid temperature extremes of food; eat soft foods, and try to avoid chewing on the injured tooth
- Tongue laceration/contusion
  — Tongue is attached to the anterior mandible, thus any fracture to the anterior mandible can result in tongue injury and posterior displacement into the airway
  — The tongue may be bitten during the injury event and result in contusion and swelling or laceration

— Laceration usually needs repair and can bleed profusely
- Deep sutures can be placed to close the laceration (Ceallaigh et al. 2006)

— Contusion may result simply in swelling, however any swelling of the tongue can obstruct the airway

— Airway management is the first priority and if possible an oral airway should be placed even if an endotracheal tube is determined to not be necessary; the oral airway will keep the tongue in proper position while airway is continually reassessed

Neck Injury

The neck includes numerous structures that pass through the neck en route to their final destination and a few structures that reside solely within the neck itself. Transitory structures include the larynx/trachea, esophagus, cranial nerves, carotid arteries and jugular veins. The thyroid, parathyroid, and hyoid reside within the neck and have the potential for injury when there is a direct blow or penetrating injury there. The cervical spine resides in the posterior neck and is discussed in Chapter 5. Common mechanisms of injury include direct blow (assault, clothesline, steering wheel) or penetrating injury (GSW, stabbing).

 General Signs and Symptoms of Neck Injury

Tachypnea, loss of airway, dyspnea
Contusion, abrasion, subcutaneous emphysema
Hemoptysis, hematemesis
Pulsatile or expanding neck hematoma
Carotid bruit
Hemorrhage from external wound
Dysphagia, hoarseness
Stroke symptoms: aphasia, hemiparesis/hemiplegia
Cranial nerve deficits

Thyroid injury/management

The thyroid is a vascular organ with endocrine properties and is located in the anterior neck. It is rarely injured; however, it may be affected by penetrating injuries to the neck or an iatrogenic injury during cricothyrotomy or tracheostomy. The thyroid requires direct surgical repair or resection if lacerated (Heizman et al. 2006). Hormone levels should then be monitored to ensure proper function.

Hyoid fracture/management

The hyoid is the only bone other than the cervical spine that resides within the neck. The hyoid is located in the anterior neck and in males is known as the Adam's apple, the prominent bone at the point of the thyroid cartilage. Hyoid fracture may occur with impact to the steering wheel, for example, but is most commonly caused by strangulation and is in fact, a clue to potential homicide when no mechanism is known. There is no management necessary for hyoid fracture.

Larynx injury/management

Laryngeal injury can occur from a direct blow or a stabbing or laceration to the neck. The steering wheel is often the culprit of such a blow but may also be from hanging, strangulation, or a penetrating injury. In sports, this injury is not common but could be fatal if not identified (Paluska and Lansford 2008).

Signs and Symptoms of Laryngeal Injury

Airway compromise, stridor, tachypnea, respiratory distress
Hoarseness, altered voice, breathy quality
Cough, hemoptysis
Contusion, swelling
Subcutaneous emphysema
In males: loss of the thyroid cartilage prominence (Adam's apple)

Management must be immediate and airway control is essential.

- Maintain airway likely requiring surgical cricothyrotomy
- Diagnosis may require direct laryngoscopy, fiberoptic endoscopy
- Nasogastric/orogastric tube insertion to prevent vomiting
- Pain management
- Vocal cord paralysis
  — Resulting from injury to the recurrent laryngeal nerves
  — Protection of the airway during swallowing is compromised
- Surgical repair of anatomy and to restore voice quality and may include injection of Teflon or other substance to increase cord bulk into the paralyzed vocal cord

Vascular and neck injury/management

The large carotid arteries and jugular veins pass through the neck to and from the cranium. They are large high-pressure vessels in which injury can result in rapid exsanguination. Blunt injury may result in intimal injury and pseudoaneurysm formation. The most common blunt mechanism is a misplaced seatbelt across the neck. The intimal injury can result in clot formation and a resultant stroke from an embolism. Early identification of neck vessel injury is essential to provide management prior to stroke occurrence.

Vascular injury can be identified through CT-angiogram or actual angiogram. Auscultation over the carotids is >95% sensitive for diagnosis of vascular injury (Tisherman et al. 2008). Anticoagulation is typically the management of intimal tears. When anticoagulation is contraindicated, operative repair or endovascular stenting is beneficial in reducing the rate of stroke. Intimal tears can be coiled or gelfoam can be placed to seal a large pseudoaneurysm. The angiogram should assess all other vessels to ensure collateral circulation prior to occlusion of the vessel with coils or other management.

In a patient with penetrating neck injury, surgical exploration and repair of identified injuries must be undertaken. It is possible for penetrating trauma never to cross the platysma and therefore not injure any underlying structures. The neck is sectioned into three zones to assist with identification of possible injury and determine if exploration is necessary. Injuries through the platysma are typically taken for exploration as the risk of morbidity is low for the surgery itself and morbidity is high if an injury is missed (Tisherman et al. 2008).

- Zone I: horizontal area between the clavicle and the cricoid
  — Includes clavicles, lung, trachea, esophagus, subclavian arteries and veins, and the thoracic duct
  — Surgical exploration is difficult
- Zone II: cricoid to mandible angle
  — Includes jugular veins, carotid arteries, larynx, trachea, esophagus, and subclavian arteries and veins
  — Penetrating injury can be managed with selective exploration using helical CT angiogram to rule out injury (Tisherman 2008, Insull et al. 2007, Inaba et al. 2006, Brywczinski et al. 2008)
  — CT angiogram should be used for penetrating injuries near vascular structures
- Zone III: above the mandible angle to the base of the skull
  — Includes jugular veins, vertebral arteries, internal carotid arteries
  — Surgical exploration is difficult

Esophagus injury/management

Injuries to the esophagus are discussed in Chapter 7. For the purposes of neck evaluation, esophageal injuries are identified by contrast esophagoscopy and/or neck exploration (Tisherman et al. 2008). Subcutaneous emphysema and free air on cervical spine films or CT scan may indicate esophageal or tracheal injuries. An injury requires surgical management with postoperative nutrition management until the esophagus is healed. Mortality is increased for any delayed diagnosis of >24 hours for esophageal injury (Tisherman et al. 2008).

POSTRESUSCITATION MANAGEMENT AND REHABILITATION

As with any injury, face and neck injuries have the potential for infection. Because of the involvement of sinuses and the oropharyngeal cavity, wounds and incisions are contaminated by the natural environment. Common signs and symptoms of infection include the following:

Signs and Symptoms of Infection of the Face/Neck

Fever, increased white blood cells (WBC)
Purulent drainage from incisions or wound sites
Halitosis
Neurologic signs of infection/meningitis: altered level of consciousness, headache, photophobia, neck stiffness

Prevention of infection include

- Diligent wound care
- Oral hygiene
- Surgical irrigation and debridement of open fractures and removal of foreign bodies
- Avoid nasal tubes to prevent sinusitis
- Remove nasal packing as soon as hemorrhage is controlled to prevent bacterial growth on packing material
- Decongestants/antihistamines to maintain open nasal passages
- Avoid nose-blowing/sneezing to prevent intracranial infection with basilar skull fracture

Management of facial infections is the same as any infection, including administration of antibiotics and identification of the source. Antibiotics should be culture driven. The site of injury may include irrigation and debridement with or without the removal of hardware used to fixate the bony fracture. If neurologic infection is suspected, a lumbar puncture is done to identify the presence of the infection and assess opening pressure.

Psychosocial Impact

The psychosocial impact of facial trauma cannot be denied. It is by our face that we are recognized and introduced. It is through our eyes that we see the world, smell food through the nose, taste that food with the mouth, and hear the world with our ears. All of the senses are involved in the face and can be changed for life after injury. Simple scarring after a laceration on the face can affect self-confidence, let alone a devastating facial injury. In addition, a self-inflicted GSW, or worse, a shot-gun wound to the face can result in years of reconstructive surgery along with the preexisting psychological circumstances.

Management includes early acknowledgement of the injury to provide

- Opportunity for the patient to express feelings regarding his or her appearance
- Demonstrate acceptance of the patient's appearance
- Offer counseling, chaplain services for the patient to express grieving and loss
- Provide psychiatric or psychology consultation as needed and for the patient with a suicide attempt
- Prepare the patient for home
- Provide cosmetic consultation with plastic surgery for repair; cosmetics for scar coverage

Facial injuries can be simple with suture repair and delayed surgical fixation. However, facial injuries can also be devastating open fractures or crush-like injury in which there is loss of airway and hemorrhage. These injuries require immediate management of the airway, breathing, and circulation in addition to extensive repair. No facial or neck injury should be ignored or assumed to be minor until it is proven to be.

Critical Lifesavers

- Do not place airway or any tubes through the nose if facial injury is suspected; tubes can be placed directly into the cranium if cribriform plate fractures are present
- If a penetrating object [in the eye] is present, secure to prevent movement and further injury

REFERENCES

Alvi A, Doherty T, Lewen G. Facial fractures and concomitant injuries in trauma patients. *Laryngoscope.* 2003;113(1):102-106.

American College of Surgeons. *Advanced Trauma Life Support* (ATLS). 7th ed. Chicago, IL: American College of Surgeons; 2004.

Brywczynski J, Barrett T, Lyon J, et al. Management of penetrating neck injury in the emergency department: a structured literature review. *Emerg Med J.* 2008;25(11):711-715.

Burnstine M. Clinical recommendations for repair of orbital facial fractures. *Curr Opin Ophthalmol.* 2003;14(5):236-240.

Ceallaigh P, Ekanaykaee K, Beirne C, et al. Diagnosis and management of common maxillofacial injuries in the emergency department part I: advanced trauma life support. *Emerg Med J.* 2006; 23(10):796-797.

Harrahill M. Epistaxis following an assault: practical consideration in stopping the bleeding. *J Emerg Nurs.* 2005;31(6):597-599.

Haydel MJ, Meyers R, Mills L. Use of the tongue-blade test to identify patients with mandible and maxillary sinus fractures: *Ann Emerg Med.* 2005;46(3):S66.

Heizmann O, Schmid R, Oertli D. Blunt injury to the thyroid gland: proposed classification and treatment algorithm. *J Trauma.* 2006;61(4):1012-1015.

Hoyt, KS and Selfridge-Thomas, J. Emergency nursing core curriculum, 6th ed. St Louis: Saunders Elsevier; 2007.

Inaba K, Numera F, McKenney M, et al. Prospective evaluation of screening multislice helical computed tomographic angiography in the initial evaluation of penetrating neck injuries. *J Trauma.* 2006;61(1):144-149.

Insull P, Adams D, Segar A, et al. Civil, I. Is exploration mandatory in penetrating zone II neck injuries? *ANZ J Surg.* 2007; 77(4):261-264.

Lelli GJ, Milite JM, Maher E. Orbital floor fractures: evaluation, indications, approach, and pearls from an ophthalmologist's perspective. *Facial Plast Surg.* 2007;23(3):190-199.

Paluska SA, Lansford CD. Laryngeal trauma in sport. *Curr Sports Med Rep.* 2008;7(1):16-21.

Tisherman SA, Bokhari F, Collier B, et al. Clinical practice guidelines: penetrating zone II neck trauma. *J Trauma.* 2008;64(5): 1392-1405.

THORACIC INJURY

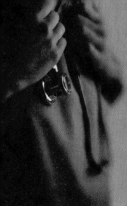

INTRODUCTION

Thoracic injury involves airway, breathing, and circulation. In the initial resuscitation of the patient, these issues are assessed and managed as they are recognized. In this way, the majority of chest injuries are identified immediately. Approximately 20% of trauma deaths are related to chest injuries (McQuillan et al. 2009). Most chest injuries occur from blunt trauma, primarily motor vehicle collisions (MVC) (Ziglar et al. 2004). The design of the chest itself protects major vessels and organs. When injuries are identified, a high index of suspicion must be present to identify common concomitant injuries. A small percentage of these injuries require surgery. Most are controlled by simple and immediate procedures and fast critical thinking.

ASSESSMENT

Airway is essential and breathing cannot be accomplished without one. Chapter 2 on resuscitation reviews the immediate actions necessary for assessment problems regarding airway. Breathing and cardiac circulation issues are discussed here.

History

The history of the patient provides clues about associated injuries, past problems, and primary problems. Fractures in the chest are important clues to underlying problems. Scapula fractures are associated with rib fractures, clavicle fractures, lung injury or pneumothorax, and spinal injury with a frequency of 80% to 95% (Baldwin 2008). Rib fractures are associated with pneumothorax even more than scapula fractures. The first and second ribs are well protected. Injury to these two ribs is frequently associated with aorta, brachial plexus, head, and spinal cord injuries (TNCC 2007). Sternal fractures have a 13% correspondence with spine fractures. If displaced, the sternum is associated with lung and cardiac injury (von Garrel et al. 2004). An assumption that chest injury has occurred should be evident with any mechanism implying impact to the sternum or scapula.

Collection of history includes

- Mechanism of injury with special attention to steering wheel deformity or impact with the steering wheel, side impact and depth of intrusion into the vehicle, use of restraints (proper use?), airbag deployment especially if without shoulder restraint, falls from a height
- Past medical history affects the patient's ability to tolerate thoracic injury and should include specific attention to
  — Recent upper or lower respiratory infection
  — Asthma or chronic obstructive pulmonary disease
  — Chronic sinus infections
  — Smoking history
  — Drug and alcohol history
  — Cardiac history
- Prehospital response and initial assessment
  — Administration of oxygen, airway adjuncts, suctioning needs, needle thoracostomy, intubation
  — Assessment of breath sounds, respirations, and any changes en route
  — Vocalization, level of alertness

Trauma Assessment

Thoracic injury assessment is essential to the initial resuscitation and management of the patient. Assessment begins with airway and progresses to breathing. All alterations from the normal require immediate management. Symptoms of impending hypoxia include altered level of consciousness, tachypnea, and an altered breathing pattern. The assessment of airway and breathing are discussed in Chapter 2. Brief assessment includes

- Observe
  - Color, cyanosis, or pallor
    - Cyanosis is a late sign of loss of airway, breathing
  - Position of comfort for the patient: upright, refusing to lie down
  - Work of breathing: use of accessory muscles, nasal flaring, struggling
  - Dyspnea
  - Respiratory rate, rhythm, depth, effort
  - Symmetrical chest movement versus paradoxical movement
    - Paradoxical movement is evident only in the spontaneously breathing patient
  - Chest pain: localized to the site or generalized
  - Jugular vein distention (may not be visible in the presence of hypovolemia)
  - Penetrating injuries: site, size, bubbling/sucking
    - Include observation of the back and neck
    - Lower chest injuries may include abdominal injury
    - High chest injury may include great vessels and neck structures
- Listen
  - Gurgling respirations or stridor
  - Vocalization normal, hoarse, none
  - Auscultate lungs
    - Breath sounds equal bilaterally
    - Adventitious sounds: rales, rhonchi

- Lack of breath sounds
  - With intubation—check tube placement (esophageal or mainstem?)
  - Without intubation—requires management (see section on Pneumothorax and Hemothorax)
- — Auscultate heart sounds
  - Rate, rhythm, murmur
  - Point of maximal impulse should reside at fourth to fifth intercostal space midclavicular line
    - Altered positioning may indicate tension pneumothorax with deviation of heart
- — Blood pressure (BP)
  - Auscultate manual BP initially after airway, breathing, circulation evaluation
  - Continue to monitor BP every 5 minutes throughout the resuscitation
- Palpate
  - — Crepitus (subcutaneous emphysema)
  - — Chest movement
    - Symmetrical
    - Paradoxical (a segment of ribs moving in opposition to the chest)
  - — Trachea midline
  - — Peripheral and central pulses: presence, rate, quality
- Percussion
  - — Dull sound represents fluid within the chest
  - — Hyperresonant sound represents air within the chest cavity outside the lung
- Diagnostics
  - — Pulse oximetry
    - Must manage and prevent hypoxia
    - Altered by hypothermia and hypovolemia where distal extremities are cold

— Chest x-ray (CXR)
  - Portable, supine
  - Anteroposterior (A-P) view
  - Place markers at sites of penetrating injury
  - If thoracic spine cleared, upright film decreases the incidence of false positive widened mediastinum; best visualization of vascular injury and volume of hemothorax
— Chest computed tomography (CT)
  - Helical multislice; if abdominal CT is expected, perform at the same time to decrease dye load
  - Strong negative predictive value for aortic injury
  - Sensitive to pneumothorax
  - More likely to identify pulmonary contusions earlier than CXR
  - Helical CT-angiography is the gold standard for vascular evaluation primarily aortic dissection
— Angiography
  - May be ordered for confirmatory evaluation of aortic injury and branch vessels or if helical multislice CT is not available
  - Invasive
— Arterial blood gas (ABG): normals (Table 7-1); acidosis versus alkalosis (Table 7-2)
  - Monitor for respiratory acidosis which demonstrates hypoperfusion
  - Increasing PCO_2 demonstrates inadequate ventilation
  - Ventilation: perfusion mismatch indicates pulmonary contusion and/or alveolar collapse
— Electrocardiogram (ECG)
  - 12-lead ECG for analysis of alterations indicating myocardial contusion is helpful but should not interrupt the primary survey
  - Observe for rhythm alterations and S-T changes

Table 7-1 Arterial Blood Gas Results

ABG Parameter	Normal	Abnormal
pH	7.35-7.45	Acidosis <7.35 Alkalosis >7.45
PCO_2	35-45 mm Hg	Low—hyperventilation High—hypoventilation
PO_2	80-100 mm Hg	Low—hypoxia
Bicarbonate (HCO_3)	22-26 mEq/L	Low or high—compensation for respiratory issues; metabolic issues
Base excess/ deficit	–2 to +2	Low—uncompensated shock
Oxygen saturation	96-100%	Low—hypoxia; saturations may appear normal when saturated with CO not O_2

DOCUMENTATION

The documentation of chest injury is straightforward and includes the full assessment of the chest and any activities surrounding management of alterations. Ongoing vital sign assessment including cardiac rhythm and pulse oximetry is essential. Changes over time may indicate subtle injury or decompensation. Penetrating injuries should be diagramed with all wounds labeled. Do not distinguish between "exit" and "entry" wounds.

Table 7-2 Acidosis versus Alkalosis

Abnormality	pH	PCO_2	Bicarbonate
Respiratory acidosis	↓	↑	↑
Metabolic acidosis	↓	↓	↓
Respiratory alkalosis	↑	↓	↓
Metabolic alkalosis	↑	↑	↑

MANAGEMENT

As stated, these injuries in general are managed as they are identified. Rapid identification is essential as most of these injuries are life-threatening and require immediate resolution. All trauma patients need

- Oxygen on arrival even if alert, oriented, and seemingly uninjured
- Pulmonary hygiene which includes incentive spirometry (IS) to prevent atelectasis and pneumonia
- Early mobilization to heal pulmonary injury and prevent pneumonia
- Pain management without oversedation to enable pulmonary hygiene and mobilization

Pneumothorax and Hemothorax

Pneumothorax and hemothorax can occur independently or in conjunction with each other. They occur when air or blood leak into the potential space between the parietal and visceral pleura and are usually caused by lung laceration or thoracic spine injury. A hemothorax is frequently the result of lung, intercostal or internal mammary artery laceration. Most hemothoraces are self-limiting. While the blood and/or air accumulates, pressure is applied to the lung restricting the space for lung ventilation and ultimately lung collapse.

A penetrating chest wound results in an "open" chest. Blunt chest trauma with impalement or large wound that enters the chest cavity can also result in an open chest wound. In the case of an open pneumothorax or hemothorax, air enters (is "sucked" into) the pleural space caused by the gradient of intrathoracic pressure to atmospheric pressure equilibrating the two. An opening in the chest wall that is two-thirds the size of the trachea is large enough to result in a sucking chest wound.

Both of these situations can rapidly result in a tension pneumothorax in which the internal organs of the chest are forced to the healthy side of the chest resulting in not only lung collapse but cardiac dysfunction as well (mediastinal shift with cardiac compression). Venous return is compromised resulting in hypotension, decreased cardiac output, and vascular collapse. A tension pneumothorax is a life-threatening situation that must be rapidly identified. It should be recognized by clinical assessment, however occasionally it is not seen until CXR. Figure 7-1 demonstrates a tension pneumothorax. The most

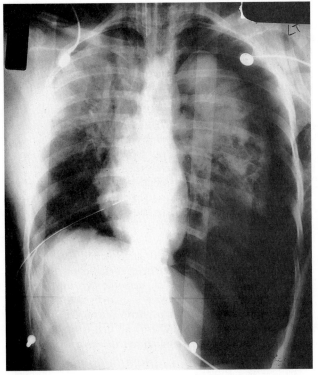

Figure 7-1 Tension pneumothorax.

common cause of tension pneumothorax is positive pressure ventilation in the presence of visceral injury or even a small pneumothorax.

More pneumothoraces are evident on the sensitive helical CT. Many are very small and may not be evident on a CXR. In some cases the physician may choose to monitor them without placement of an immediate tube thoracostomy (Kortbeek et al. 2008). They may also be asymptomatic because of their size. A pneumothorax seen on CT in a patient going to the OR or undergoing positive pressure ventilation requires treatment to prevent conversion to a tension pneumothorax.

Signs and Symptoms

Pneumothorax—Open Pneumothorax
Hypoxia
Labored respirations, dyspnea, tachypnea
Absent or decreased breath sounds on the side of injury
Asymmetrical chest expansion
Hyper-resonant to percussion
Restlessness, tachycardia, pain, discomfort
Open pneumothorax—"sucking" chest wound evident
Subcutaneous emphysema (crepitus)
Cyanosis (late sign)

Hemothorax
Hypoxia, cyanosis
Labored respirations, dyspnea, tachypnea
Absent or decreased breath sounds on the side of injury
Asymmetrical chest expansion
Dull to percussion
May require 200-300 mL of blood before evident on CXR

Signs and Symptoms of Tension Pneumothorax

Rapid deterioration of vital signs (hypotension, tachycardia, tachypnea)
Hypoxia, chest pain
Increased airway pressure, difficulty bagging
Labored respirations, feeling of impending doom, air hunger
Disorientation, confusion
Absent or decreased breath sounds on the side of injury
Distended neck veins (absent if hypovolemia exists)
Tracheal deviation away from the side of injury

Management

Management of pneumothoraces and hemothoraces is accomplished during primary survey of resuscitation. Both can have a delayed presentation. An increased awareness of this potential should be carried out throughout the patient's initial stay. In addition, a pneumothorax can convert to a tension pneumothorax, especially with positive pressure ventilation and altitude. Transport of the patient by air can result in this complication even with a chest tube in place. The provider should not become complacent because a chest tube has been inserted. Even with CXR confirmation of placement, a chest tube can be displaced or become obstructed. Diligence is essential.

- Open sucking chest wound
  — Stabilize any impaled object; do not remove
  — Cover immediately with an occlusive dressing that is sealed on three sides
  — The dressings act as a flutter valve to allow air exit during exhalation but not air entry during inhalation
  — The patient requires immediate chest tube placement
  — The defect in the chest wall is usually closed

- — Penetrating injury anterior and medial to the nipple or posterior and medial to the scapula may involve the mediastinum and require an evaluation for great vessel or tracheobronchial injury in addition to managing the pneumothorax and hemothorax
  - — Penetrating injury to the lower chest may involve the abdomen and diaphragm
- Needle thoracostomy
  - — Large-bore 14- to 16-g needle is placed on the midclavicular line, over the third rib into the second intercostal space; the catheter is left in place
  - — May be used in the prehospital setting to relieve a tension pneumothorax
  - — Placement requires chest tube placement as the catheter can now act as an open chest wound
  - — Upon release of the tension pneumothorax
    - Vital signs should return to normal if other causes for abnormal vital signs have also been corrected
    - A rush of air confirms the diagnosis of tension
- Tube thoracostomy
  - — To relieve both pneumothoraces and hemothoraces, a chest tube is placed in the fourth or fifth intercostal space just anterior to the midaxillary line
    - If the patient is ventilated, do not apply positive pressure ventilation until the chest tube is in place to prevent a tension pneumothorax
  - — Chest tube should be 32 to 40 Fr in size to allow for both air and blood to escape without obstruction
  - — Connect tube to a drainage device that provides a water seal environment to prevent "intake" of air into the chest
    - Tubes are taped lengthwise to prevent separation
    - Usually the setup is then attached to 20-cm wall suction to provide negative pressure and maintain an inflated lung

- Suction may be removed for transport but should be reconnected upon arrival to CT or the definitive destination
- Peri-insertion antibiotics have not been shown to decrease the risk of empyema or pneumonia (Maxwell et al. 2004, Luchette et al. 2000)

— Assessment after insertion
  - CXR is necessary after placement to confirm
  - Reassess breath sounds for inflation, symmetrical chest rise/fall
  - Recheck vital signs for stabilization
  - Check for fluctuation in the chamber, type of output, airleak
  - Monitor volume of output—initial output of 1500 mL on insertion or 200 mL/hour for 2 to 4 hours will likely require surgery to identify the cause (ATLS 2004)
  - Hemothorax may require blood replacement therapy as well

— Check insertion site to assure that all holes are within the chest and not exposed

— Cleanse the site and dress with Vaseline gauze and an occlusive dressing daily

— For large hemothoraces, an autotransfusion device may be attached to the chest tube setup. Autotransfusion is discussed in Chapter 2.

— Chest tubes remain in place until the lung remains inflated when placed on waterseal only
  - CXR evaluation on waterseal
  - NEVER clamp the chest tube as a tension pneumothorax could result

— Removal of the tube thoracostomy
  - Provide an occlusive dressing on removal with Vaseline gauze at the center over the site itself
  - CXR evaluation after removal

- If a small pneumothorax remains, a trial of 100% oxygen administration may assist in the resorption of any small pneumothorax through an increased nitrogen gradient
- If there is a large pneumothorax after removal, a chest tube will likely need to be reinserted
- Nonsurgical management
  - For pneumothoraces managed by observation, diligent monitoring of lung sounds, vital signs is essential
  - Any sign of respiratory compromise requires
    - Immediate assessment of vital signs and breath sounds
    - CXR to identify if the pneumothorax has increased in size

Pulmonary Contusion

Like any other organ or body part, the lung can bruise after impact. The contusion can range from minor to severe involving one or both lungs, one or more lobes of the lung. As with other contusions in the body, these also accumulate edema surrounding the bruised area within the interstitial tissue and alveoli. The injury most often associated with pulmonary contusion is a flail chest. The transfer of energy to result in a flail segment of ribs is significant and therefore injures both the ribs and underlying lung. Blast injuries also result in lung contusion. The onset of respiratory failure with pulmonary contusion can be insidious.

Signs and Symptoms of Pulmonary Contusion

Dyspnea
Ineffective cough, hemoptysis
Hypoxia, PO_2 <65 mm Hg, saturations <90% on room air
Chest contusion
Pain
Increased pulmonary vascular resistance (PVR), decreased compliance
Consolidation on CXR within 24 to 48 hours after injury

Management

Pulmonary contusions require recognition and then identification of the impact of the contusion. Some contusions are minor and do not require any management other than pulmonary hygiene. Some minor pulmonary contusions will resolve within 48 to 72 hours (McQuillan et al. 2009). The goal is adequate tissue perfusion. Severe pulmonary contusion can result in respiratory failure and acute respiratory distress syndrome (ARDS).

- Pulmonary hygiene
  - Incentive spirometry (IS)
  - Chest physiotherapy (chest PT)
  - Positioning and early ambulation
  - Goal is avoidance of respiratory failure and intubation if possible (Simon et al. 2006)
  - Kinetic therapy with continuous rotation especially if positioning is difficult because of other injuries
  - If able, prone positioning is effective in lung recruitment
- Oxygenation and ventilation
  - Supplemental oxygen
  - Use continuous positive airway pressure (CPAP) ventilation as an alternative to intubation if tolerated by the patient
  - Intubation with mechanical ventilation if unable to maintain airway, impending hypoxia (as above), altered level of consciousness, immobilization because of other injuries
  - Use positive end-expiratory pressure (PEEP) and wean early
  - Independent lung ventilation may be useful if there is severe unilateral pulmonary contusion when conventional ventilation does not reverse shunt (Simon et al. 2006)
  - In severe pulmonary contusion high-frequency oscillating ventilation is lung protective by providing a low tidal volume (Funk et al. 2008). Use when
    - Mean airway pressure >30 cm H_2O
    - FiO_2 >60%

— Other ventilator modes that are useful in managing pulmonary contusion include pressure control ventilation with reverse inspiratory:expiratory (i:e) ratio

— Avoid neuromuscular blockers if possible during ventilation because of the long-term postparalytic weakness that occurs with withdrawal of the medication. The patient will need strength to maintain pulmonary hygiene after extubation

• Provide initial resuscitation necessary but avoid unnecessary fluid administration

— Pulmonary-arterial catheter (Swan-Ganz) may be useful in determining fluid status

— Avoid pulmonary edema and maintain euvolemia

— Diuretics may be useful in the presence of increased pulmonary capillary wedge pressure (PCWP) with hemodynamic stability or current congestive heart failure (CHF)

— Do not administer steroids; benefits are anecdotal only

• Analgesia

— Manage pain associated with the flail segment

— Avoid oversedation

▪ Avoid intubation if possible

▪ Early extubation

Tracheobronchial Injury

Although rare, a tracheal or bronchial injury is a severe threat to patient survival. Many of these cause arrest at the scene and never present to the hospital. The trachea and bronchi are injured when there is a sudden increase in intrathoracic pressure against the closed glottis. Penetrating trauma can also result in a perforation of the main airways. Most of these injuries will require surgical management and patients need to be transferred rapidly to a trauma center. The injuries tend to occur within 2.5 cm (1 in) of the carina and occasionally involve the bronchi as well (ATLS 2004). They are often missed injuries and carry a high mortality. Small injuries or injuries in which the fascia maintains the integrity of the trachea may have delayed presentation of up to 3 to 4 days (Hoyt and Selfridge-Thomas 2007). Delayed presentation is usually a sudden onset of pneumothorax and subcutaneous emphysema. Persistent atelectasis may be a clue to evaluate for this injury.

Signs and Symptoms of Tracheobronchial Injury

Severe respiratory distress, combative, restless
Upper airway obstruction
Subcutaneous emphysema
Tension pneumothorax with a persistent air leak
Pneumothorax, pneumomediastinum, retro-esophageal air,
   peribronchial air
Rib fractures
Hoarseness, dysphagia
Stridor
Airway hemorrhage, hemoptysis
Pain
May be alert and conversant at the scene with sudden
   respiratory arrest upon supine positioning

Management

The management of tracheobronchial injury involves the usual airway and breathing assessment. Because airway is the first priority in the primary survey, the primary management of this injury is already being addressed.

- Provide an airway
  — May require a surgical airway if the patient cannot be intubated

— Intubation may be successful but tenuous if the trachea is a circumferential injury

   ▪ Especially with movement of the patient

— If total tracheal transection, a surgical airway will not be successful as the two components of the trachea will not be "connected" by the short tracheostomy tube

   ▪ Requires operative intervention

— Patient will need a mechanical airway and ventilation until edema resolves

— May require independent lung ventilation if severe

• Tube thoracostomy insertion

— As above, a chest tube must be inserted to manage the pneumothorax

— May require more than one chest tube to manage massive airleak

— Monitor airleak, increase in subcutaneous air, airway pressures

• Evaluation

— Bronchoscopy is the definitive means of evaluation unless the patient has gone directly to surgery

— Surgical repair is necessary in tears >33% of the circumference

— Long-term these patients have a decreased sensitivity to cough and airway clearance

• Rupture of bronchus can result in air embolism

— Signs and symptoms

   ▪ Sudden cardiovascular collapse or arrest without evidence of hemorrhage

   ▪ Focal neurologic signs that are not related to a head injury

— Management

   ▪ Immediate Trendelenburg position to prevent the air from moving out of the apex of the heart

   ▪ Thoracotomy with lung clamping at the hilum and cardiocentesis to remove the air

- Hyperbaric oxygen (HBO) chamber rapid decompression to 168 fsw on 100% oxygen to minimize the size of the embolus and promote resorption into the circulation
- For HBO the patient needs to be stable (not actively in arrest) and will require a long decompression from the depth of 168 fsw

Rib and Sternum Fractures

Rib fractures are the most common chest injury, yet they are also the key to associated injuries. High rib fractures (#1-2) are associated with great vessel injury, mid rib fractures (#3-9) involve the lungs, whereas low rib fractures (#9-12) may highlight an abdominal injury. Frequently hemothoraces and pneumothoraces are associated with ribs that have fractured and injured the lung. Both rib and sternum fractures require a large transfer of energy to fracture, so associated injuries should be expected and evaluated.

In children, rib fractures are a sign of significant force as their ribs are elastic and not prone to injury. In the elderly, it is just the opposite, as their ribs are fragile and prone to fracture. In addition, the elderly are less likely to tolerate the pain and decreased chest expansion associated with these fractures. Age is a predictor of mortality in the presence of rib fractures and/or multisystem injury (Brasel et al. 2006). Almost 30% of individuals >65 years with rib fractures will require mechanical ventilation and have five times the odds of dying in comparison with younger individuals with rib fractures (Bergeron et al. 2003).

A flail chest is a series of rib fractures (>2) that are consecutive and have more than one fracture per rib. This results in a free-floating segment of ribs that no longer moves with the rest of the chest wall. This "paradoxical motion" decreases effective ventilation. There is also a high association of significant pulmonary contusion with a flail segment.

Sternum fractures can be associated with great vessel or airway injury especially in the case of sternoclavicular dislocation.

Signs and Symptoms of Rib Fractures, Flail Chest, Sternum Fracture

Rib fractures
Inspiratory pain, tenderness to palpation, pain with movement
Hypoventilation to splint chest, atelectasis
Visible on CXR or CT
Chest contusion may be present

Flail chest
Paradoxical chest wall motion visible (with spontaneous respiration) or palpable over the flail segment
Hypoxemia caused by ineffective respiration and associated pulmonary contusion
Increased work of breathing, respiratory failure
Pain, crepitus
Low tidal volume, alveolar collapse
Visible on CXR or chest CT frequently with pulmonary contusion (may be delayed presentation)

Sternum fracture
Pain
Movement of sternum with respirations
Palpable defect
Hoarseness, stridor, voice quality changes indicative of airway injury

Management

Management of rib fractures focuses mainly on pain relief so that the patient may maintain effective ventilation. Rib fractures in and of themselves rarely require mechanical ventilation. A flail segment may require ventilation for management of the pulmonary contusion more so than the management of the flail.

Rib fractures are usually "sticky" within 3 weeks with healing evident at 6 weeks. The pain associated with the fractures unfortunately can last for weeks to months after the initial injury. Pain increases with the number of ribs fractured. Management includes

- Internal fixation
  — Sternum fractures do not usually require surgical fixation although if healing is delayed or severe movement is associated with respiration, the surgeons may choose to internally fixate the sternum
  — Rib fractures including flail segments, may also receive internal fixation if they do not show evidence of healing or are seriously affecting ventilation. Experimental use of bioresorbable plating systems reduce ribs early with the hope of more rapid healing and less need for mechanical ventilation (Vu et al. 2008)
- Sternoclavicular dislocation can be reduced by extension of the shoulder (ATLS 2004)
- Ventilation
  — Maintain ventilation and provide intubation if the patient cannot manage effective respirations or is at risk for respiratory failure
    - Maintain PO_2 >80 mm Hg
    - Positive pressure ventilation
    - Attempt trial of CPAP to avoid intubation if possible
  — IS and pulmonary hygiene are essential
  — Early ambulation or kinetic therapy if the patient cannot mobilize to prevent atelectasis and pneumonia
  — Ineffective ventilation results in retained secretions
  — Patients with flail segments are sensitive to fluid overload caused by the associated pulmonary contusion
- Pain management
  — Provide analgesia without over-sedation or respiratory depression

- — Pain management of chest injury is discussed in the next section of this chapter
- — Reduce pain to expand the lung
- — Long-term, patients with flail segments may have persistent residual pain (Ziglar et al. 2004)
- DO NOT splint the flail segment with tape, binders, or sand bags
  - — Results in restriction of ventilation and long term sequelae
  - — May result in pneumothorax

Cardiac Contusion-Rupture

As with the lung, the heart is also subject to injury from a direct blow to the chest or penetrating injury. The most common cardiac injury is contusion. Much like pulmonary contusion, the impact to the chest can result in a bruising of the heart. Myocardial contusions range in depth from subepicardial petechiae to full transmural contusions. The majority of myocardial injuries are caused by MVC particularly in individuals >65 years. Falls from significant heights are also associated with cardiac injury. The majority of cardiac contusions is undiagnosed or has no symptoms or residual effects. In some cases the contusion results in serious conduction abnormalities, wall motion abnormalities, or death from cardiac rupture or infarction. An ECG has a 96% sensitivity of predicting myocardial injury. Transesophageal echocardiography (TEE) may be used to evaluate the myocardium. Most significant cardiac injuries demonstrate symptoms within the first 24 hours after injury, primarily an abnormal ECG (Salim et al. 2001).

Rupture is caused by compression or direct impact with increased venous return and over-distention of the heart itself. Shear forces may also result in rupture. Falls >18 feet have an incidence of >50% cardiac injury, particularly causing tears at the junction of the inferior vena cava and the right atrium. The higher the fall the more extensive and irregular the tears become (Turk et al. 2004). Sternal fractures occur in these falls in 76% of all patients with cardiac injury. The most common site is the right ventricle which is anterior in the chest and has a thinner myocardium. Cardiac rupture has up to an 85% mortality (Van Horn 2007). Likely survivors of rupture will demonstrate tamponade and vital signs. An atrial rupture results in a slow tamponade (ATLS 2004).

Signs and Symptoms of Myocardial Injury

Chest pain
ECG abnormalities: ST-T wave changes (most prevalent), PVCs, atrial fibrillation, bundle branch blocks (particularly right), supraventricular tachycardia
New CHF with holosystolic murmur may indicate interventricular septal rupture

Management

If a blunt cardiac injury is suspected

- 12-lead ECG should be obtained after primary and secondary surveys to identify any rhythm disturbances
  — ST-T wave changes
  — Evidence of ischemia
  — Bundle branch blocks
- Monitor for 24 to 48 hours if the ECG is positive primarily to manage rhythm disturbances
- Hemodynamically unstable patients may undergo an echocardiogram to determine degree of wall motion abnormality
- Nuclear medicine studies are not helpful in diagnosing blunt cardiac injury (Pasquale et al. 1998)
- Sternal fracture without evidence of altered ECG does not require cardiac monitoring in and of itself (Pasquale et al.1998)
- Manage cardiac rhythm disturbances
  — Conduction abnormalities are susceptible to sudden dysrhythmias

- Monitor for pericardial tamponade
- Measurement of cardiac troponin I and CPK-MB have not demonstrated usefulness in identifying cardiac injury
  - It is not recommended that enzymes or troponin levels be drawn
  - In the presence of a normal ECG and a negative cardiac troponin I, there is confidence that there is no cardiac injury and therefore monitoring is not required (Salim et al. 2001)

Pericardial Tamponade

Pericardial tamponade can result from blunt or penetrating trauma to the heart, although penetrating is more frequent. The pericardial sac normally contains only 20 to 30 mL of fluid in the potential space between the heart and the pericardium itself. Bleeding into the sac results in expansion of the sac to its limit and compression of the heart impeding contractility. Decreased diastolic filling results in decreased stroke volume and cardiac output.

Signs and Symptoms of Pericardial Tamponade

Pulsus paradoxus: drop in systolic BP >10 mm Hg during inspiration

Beck's triad (10-40% occurrence):
- Muffled heart tones
- Jugular venous distention (may not be evident with hypovolemia)
- Narrow pulse pressure: normal = 40 mm Hg; tamponade <30 mm Hg

Sense of impending doom, anxiety

Refuses to lay supine, dyspnea

Kussmaul sign—increased venous pressure with spontaneous inspiration

Pulseless electrical activity without tension pneumothorax or hypovolemia

Management

The management of pericardial tamponade requires a high index of suspicion and rapid identification. Further resolution of the tamponade follows along with definitive operative treatment.

- Echocardiogram has a 5 to 10% false negative rate for diagnosis
    — FAST exam is used increasingly during resuscitation to identify abdominal and cardiac injury and provides a reliable diagnosis of pericardial tamponade (McQuillan et al. 2009)
    — Pericardiocentesis provides relief of congestion
        ▪ It is preferable to perform a thoracotomy and definitive pericardial window and management of the cardiac injury itself (Kortbeek et al. 2008)
        ▪ If pericardiocentesis is necessary it should be performed with
            ○ Elevated head of the bed at 45 degrees
            ○ 14- to 16-g long needle with stopcock or syringe
            ○ Entry is ~1- to 2-cm subxiphoid at a 15-degree angle to the skin aiming at the left scapula
            ○ Aspirate upon entry into the pericardium; nonclotting blood should return
            ○ Leave catheter in place as the self-sealing pericardium will close over the site if removed and tamponade can recur
            ○ Pericardiocentesis is a temporizing procedure only; definitive management with a pericardial window and cardiac repair is required

Thoracic Aorta Injury

One of the most rapidly devastating thoracic injuries is a thoracic aorta tear. Up to 80% of these patients die at the scene and that statistic has not changed in more than 20 years. The remaining 20% arrive at the hospital and will either deteriorate or remain stable. Aortic injury is caused by, for example, MVC with lateral impact to the driver, unrestrained ejected driver, penetrating mediastinal wounds, and falls >10 feet.

Diagnosis and management of the aortic injury must occur rapidly. Those who survive suffer an incomplete laceration of the aorta with an intact adventitia (pseudoaneurysm) or a contained mediastinal hemorrhage. Any free rupture into the left chest whether at the scene or in the hospital is fatal unless immediate transfer into the operating suite occurs. Even with rapid transfer, survival is unlikely.

Most aortic injuries occur at the ligamentous arteriosum where the aorta is rigidly bound to the chest from birth. Other common sites are the bifurcation of the innominate artery from the aorta, the aorta's entry through the diaphragm, and the superior aortic valve annulus.

Signs and Symptoms of Thoracic Aorta Injury

Chest, mid-back, scapula pain
Hoarseness, stridor, dyspnea, dysphagia
Chest contusion
Upper extremity hypertension with lower extremity hypotension
Paraplegia
Hypovolemic shock
Systolic murmur parascapular
CXR abnormalities: widened mediastinum, obscured aortic knob, left apical cap, tracheal or gastric tube deviation to the right (most sensitive), depressed left mainstem bronchus, first or second rib fractures

Management

Rapid identification and management of the aorta are paramount to the survival of these patients. Diagnosis starts with the routine CXR.

- Upright CXR (preferably) can provide the first radiographic evidence of aortic injury as listed above in the signs and symptoms (Nagy et al. 2000)
  — Placement of a nasogastric or orogastric tube prior to CXR increases the visibility of deviation of the esophagus
  — Figure 7-2 shows the widened mediastinum with positive aortic pseudoaneurysm; Figure 7-3 shows the deviated trachea and esophagus with positive aortic pseudoaneurysm; Figure 7-4 shows the thoracic aorta pseudoaneurysm at the ligamentum arteriosum in a child with paraplegia and no spinal cord injury
- Helical multislice CT of the chest is accurate in diagnosing aortic injury

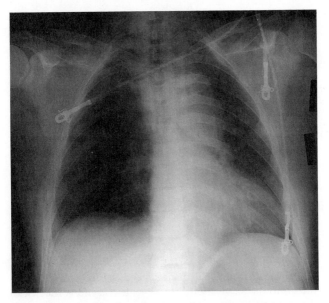

Figure 7-2   Widened mediastinum in positive aortic pseudoaneurysm patient.

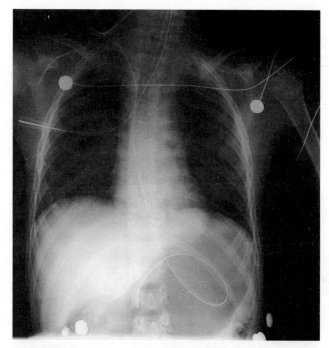

Figure 7-3 Deviated trachea and esophagus with positive aortic pseudoaneurysm.

— Surgeons may request an aortogram after CT to further define the injury

• BP (Nagy et al. 2000) and heart rate control is the first line therapy prior to surgery

— Beta-blockers and calcium channel blockers may be used to maintain systolic BP at 80 to 100 mm Hg until repair

■ Vasodilators such as nitrates and nitroprusside may also be used

■ This becomes a challenge in the presence of head injury where a minimum BP 90 mm Hg systolic is required to prevent secondary head injury; These patients may benefit

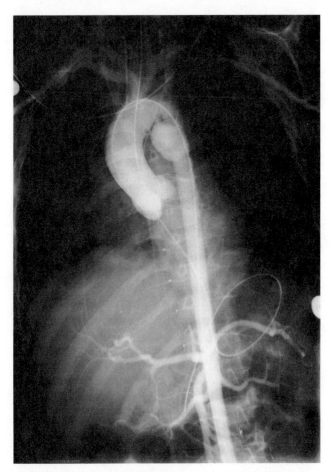

Figure 7-4   Thoracic aorta pseudoaneurysm in a child.

from early endovascular repair if acceptable to the neurosurgeon managing the head injury

— Heart rate is maintained at 60 to 80 bpm (McQuillan et al. 2009)

- Delayed management
  — May be necessary for emergent craniotomy or laparotomy
  — Poor operative candidates are patients with extensive past medical history and age
  — From 1997 to 2007 there is demonstrated increase in time to repair from 16.5 hours to 54.6 hours with a concomitant increase in the use of stents, decreased incidences of paraplegia and mortality (22-13%) (Demetriades et al. 2008); the same study demonstrated no difference in the complications of pneumonia and renal failure

- Direct repair
  — Repair may be performed in a delayed fashion if there is no evidence of impending rupture (Pacini et al. 2005)
    ▪ Manage other life-threatening injuries first
    ▪ Unstable injuries are those with uncontrolled BP, hemothoraces >1000 mL, circumferential lesions, extravasation on CT or angiography, enlarging pseudoaneurysm
  — Resection with interposition graft placement or direct suture repair
    ▪ Cardiopulmonary bypass requires full heparinization, which may result in hemorrhage in the abdomen or brain
    ▪ Left heart bypass with a centrifugal pump can be done without heparinization and is spine protective
    ▪ Direct clamping of the aorta is associated with neurologic complications; neurologic complications correlate directly with ischemia time >30 to 35 minutes (Nagy et al. 2000, Johnson 2007, Hunt et al. 1996)
  — Distal perfusion bypass or shunt is spine protective
  — Proximal injury and those extending into the transverse arch or crossing the subclavian/innominate roots require circulatory arrest and hypothermia for repair

- Endovascular repair
  - Negates the risk of rupture by placement of the stent spanning the pseudoaneurysm
    - Injuries distal to the subclavian artery with a proximal neck of the aorta ≥5 mm and the absence of thrombus
    - Peripheral vascular access must be obtainable
    - Complete exclusion of the pseudoaneurysm
  - Allows time to stabilize other life-threatening injuries while controlling the aorta
  - Can be done early or delayed
  - Allows increased systolic BP to manage head injury more appropriately
  - Deployment can take significant time dependent upon the skill of the interventional radiologist and the specific injury
  - Delayed placement allows scarring of the pseudoaneurysm first and management of coagulopathy but carries the risk of rupture
  - Complications associated with stent placement include endovascular leak, injury to the access vessel, carotid occlusion, stroke, paraplegia, infection, and partial collapse of the stent (Demetriades et al. 2008)
  - Long-term
    - Requires lifetime beta blockade
    - Monitor for migration or leak
    - Migration can result in subclavian artery obstruction
    - Strict BP management
- Complications of the management of thoracic aorta injury include
  - Pulmonary embolism
  - Paraplegia from the injury causing ischemia to the vertebral artery or after repair from cross-clamp time
  - Vocal cord paralysis
  - Renal failure
  - Rupture of the pseudoaneurysm or leak from the graft or stent

— Cerebral ischemia
— Ischemic bowel or infarction
— Critical care complications include pneumonia and ARDS

Diaphragm Injury

Increased intrathoracic and intra-abdominal pressure push on the only organ shared by both, the diaphragm. Although elastic, there is a limit to the degree of pressure it can tolerate without rupture. MVC are frequently the cause primarily frontal or near-side impact collisions at high speed (Reiff et al. 2002). Penetrating injuries that involve both the abdomen and chest include a diaphragm injury. Blunt trauma most often causes a large tear, and a penetrating injury is usually small.

The most common site of rupture is the left diaphragm, where the right diaphragm is relatively protected by the liver. The left diaphragm also experiences herniation more frequently as the hollow viscus stomach and small bowel slide up through the rupture into the chest. A missed diaphragm injury can result in strangulation of the herniated organs or with any increased abdominal pressure, the tear can enlarge. In addition, the presence of the abdominal organs in the thoracic cavity can also compress the lungs, decrease venous return, and cause ineffective ventilation.

Signs and Symptoms of Diaphragm Injury

Dyspnea, orthopnea, decreased breath sounds
Abdominal pain, sharp, epigastric
Kehr sign—pain referred to the shoulder (also reflects splenic injury)
Bowel sounds in the chest on auscultation
Chest tube drainage includes contents of the gut
Heart may shift to the right
CXR: gastric tube in the chest, elevated diaphragm on the injured side, gastric dilatation, loculated hemopneumothorax, mediastinal shift

Management

Diagnosis of diaphragm injury is often made after CXR or chest tube placement. The surgeon may also identify the injury during exploratory laparotomy. Even then, it can be missed if the tear is subtle. Management is straightforward. Diaphragm ruptures are repaired in surgery. The patient frequently has other serious injuries to the abdomen or extremities. Preparation for imminent laparotomy should be expected.

Transmediastinal and Esophageal Injury

Penetrating injury that crosses the mediastinum can result in injuries to the great vessels, trachea, bronchi, and esophagus. Mortality is ~40% (ATLS 2004). One should anticipate pericardial tamponade, hemorrhage, and tension pneumothorax. On CXR, mediastinal air implies tracheal, bronchial, and/or esophageal injury. If hemodynamically stable, a helical CT is useful to identify the structures involved. Esophagoscopy and bronchoscopy also identify injury and are usually performed in the operating suite to provide the opportunity for immediate management. In the unstable patient, prepare for bilateral chest tubes and/or bilateral thoracotomy. In patients with esophageal injury, repair must be undertaken quickly to decrease leak of gastrointestinal fluids into the chest. This leak results in mediastinitis and empyema. Mortality increases if the injury is missed or delayed in diagnosis (McQuillan et al. 2009).

Penetrating injury involving vessels or near to vessels can result in foreign body embolus. If the bullet has not resulted in serious injury, thoracotomy is not usually undertaken for simple bullet removal. However, awareness that a bullet near a vessel can enter that vessel is essential. In addition peripheral bullets can also embolize. The foreign body within the vessel results in turbulent blood flow and thrombosis. The presence of a foreign body in the esophagus can also result in an esophago-aortic fistula and movement of the bullet into the circulation.

SPECIAL SITUATIONS

Trauma Arrest

There remains the time when a decision must be made either to perform a thoracotomy or not. In the case of blunt trauma, death is death. There is no evidence that thoracotomy in the patient with CPR from the scene to the hospital and continued is of any benefit to the trauma patient in arrest. ATLS (2008, Kortbeek et al. 2008) provides guidelines for the use of thoracotomy. The recommendations include

- Penetrating injury with CPR in the field
  - Evaluate for signs of life including cardiac electrical activity
  - No signs of life or activity, resuscitation should cease
  - If pulseless electrical activity is present, thoracotomy may be beneficial
- Blunt trauma with CPR in the field
  - Even with pulseless electrical activity, thoracotomy is not valuable

If the resuscitating physician determines that a thoracotomy may assist the patient, prepare for

- Left anterior thoracotomy by opening the thoracotomy tray and ensuring that adequate airway and IV lines are in place
- Procedures that may occur during the thoracotomy, including
  - Initiating open cardiac massage and defibrillation
  - Opening the pericardium to relieve a pericardial tamponade
  - Controlling hemorrhage by cross clamping the aorta
    - Document the time of cross clamp
  - Provide direct hemorrhage control to the site of injury if evident
  - Rapid repair of the heart for cardiac laceration
    - Suture with Teflon pledgets or stapler should be available for cardiorrhaphy

Tracheoarterial and Tracheoesophageal Fistula

Fistula is a rare complication that can occur in both thoracic and abdominal injuries. Fistulas can occur from either blunt or penetrating trauma. Tracheoarterial fistulas can involve the innominate, right carotid, or lower thyroid arteries. Although injury itself can cause these fistulae, trauma from tube placement can cause them more frequently. Pressure from the tracheostomy or endotracheal tube on the retropharynx and trachea can lead to erosion and fistula formation. The usual cause is an overinflated cuff. Diligent cuff pressure (20-25 mm Hg) assessments are essential to critical care. The critical symptom is hemorrhage into the airways. Control may be temporarily obtained by inflating the tube cuff to maximal inflation. A finger compressing the artery against the sternum may also temporize blood loss while transitioning to surgery. Exsanguinating hemorrhage can be rapidly fatal.

Tracheoesophageal fistulas occur when the pressure causes necrosis between the trachea and the posterior esophagus. The gastric tube can also result in fistula formation. Monitor all tubes for necessity. A gastric tube may be able to be replaced with a percutaneous gastrostomy to relieve irritation to the esophagus. Again, cuff pressure of tracheal tubes must be diligently monitored. Observe for symptoms of cough with swallowing, suction of gastric fluids/contents from the lungs, and distention of the stomach. These fistulae are diagnosed with an esophagoscopy and/or bronchoscopy. Immediate management includes repositioning of the tracheal tube more distal in the airway, anticipate placement of a percutaneous gastrostomy or jejunostomy and surgical repair.

Empyema-Retained Hemothorax/Pneumothorax

Most hemothoraces are relieved with chest tube management. Any remaining blood is usually resorbed by the body. However on occasion, the hemothorax becomes loculated, cannot be removed by chest tube and restricts respiration. In addition, the retained blood provides the opportunity for infection resulting in empyema. Early video-assisted thoracoscopy (VATS) within 72 hours of presentation removes any residual hemothorax and prevents loculation and empyema. If the hemothorax is not resorbed, the surgeons may choose to perform a VATS with decortication to remove the loculation. A thoracotomy may be necessary if the collection cannot be removed thorascopically. In the case of recurrent pleural effusion, in addition to drainage, a formal pleurodesis may be performed. Pleurodesis involves the instillation of bleomycin, tetracycline, or more commonly talc to the surface of the lung. This irritant encourages the lung visceral and parietal pleura to adhere, decreasing the space available for effusion to collect.

If infection is present, the empyema requires appropriate antibiotic management (after cultures) and simple chest tube drainage. If the empyema is not amenable to chest tube drainage, a decortication is the next option for treatment.

Note: ARDS and ventilator management are addressed in Chapter 13.

POSTRESUSCITATION MANAGEMENT AND REHABILITATION

The optimal outcome for thoracic injuries is rapid progression to independent ventilation and return to activity. For the patient on mechanical ventilation, minimal sedation is encouraged to move the patient toward weaning and extubation. In the meantime, turning and pulmonary hygiene is essential to prevent atelectasis and pneumonia. Coordination of pulmonary management complements the other injuries experienced by the patient. If sedation and long-term ventilation are necessary to manage other injuries, it is the roles of nursing and adjunctive therapy to maintain pulmonary hygiene by turning every 2 hours, providing chest physical therapy, suctioning without saline instillation, and oral care. Pain management of rib fractures is discussed below.

Once the patient is extubated, pulmonary hygiene, including coughing and deep breathing and incentive spirometry hourly maintains open airways. Encouraging ambulation and activity with therapy also maintains open airways. Regaining previous strength and endurance is necessary to maintain pulmonary health and return to optimal function after discharge.

Pain Management

One of the key interventions after thoracic injury, especially rib fractures, is pain management. Specifically, the elderly patient with more than three rib fractures, requires pain control to enable effective ventilation. As noted under flail chest, taping, elastic bandages or binders, and sand bags are not acceptable means of splinting the chest to decrease pain. These methods are ineffective and result in poor ventilation and the associated complications of pneumonia, pneumothorax, and respiratory failure.

There are numerous methods of pain control. These include

- Epidural analgesia
  - Preferred method for severe blunt thoracic injury management (EAST 2005)
  - Preferred for patients >65 years with more than three ribs fractured and/or comorbidities of diabetes and chronic obstructive pulmonary disease (COPD)
  - Bilateral rib fractures are also managed best with epidural analgesia
  - Most effective combination is local bupivacaine with a narcotic, such as fentanyl
    - Uses low-dose medication
    - Fewer side effects
  - Does not require critical care monitoring when in place
    - Some hospital protocols may require cardiac monitoring and pulse oximetry
  - Improves perception of pain
  - Improves pulmonary function/ventilation
    - Effective during weaning

- — Less respiratory depression, sedation
- — Avoids constipation/ileus associated with narcotics
- — Contraindicated in spine injury (Karmakar and Ho 2003)
- Paravertebral and extrapleural infusion
  - — May improve pulmonary function
- Intrapleural and intercostal blocks
  - — May be useful for minimal trauma
  - — Regional analgesia
  - — Regional blocks are invasive but more effective than systemic narcotics
  - — Intercostal blocks must be placed both above and below the fractures
- IV narcotics
  - — Beneficial as initial management and in low-risk patients with hemodynamic stability
  - — Monitor hemodynamics
  - — Convert to oral medication if needed
    - If fewer than three ribs are involved, oral pain medication should be sufficient (Karmakar and Ho 2003)
- Use of complementary and nonnarcotic therapy is also essential to management of the whole patient
  - — Transcutaneous electrical nerve stimulation (TENS) is very effective
  - — Nonsteroidal anti-inflammatory drugs (NSAIDs) also reduce inflammation
  - — Imagery, meditation, acupuncture, reiki, massage, and other forms of complementary medicine can be effective adjuncts to pain management
    - The effectiveness of each method of alternative medicine is dependent upon the patient's ability to participate, willingness, individuality, perception of pain, and pain tolerance
    - Not all or necessarily any of these methods will be effective for each patient

— Positioning and activity also assist with pain management and prevention of complications of immobility

- When managing pain
  — Monitor and maintain airway and ventilation
    ▪ Avoid sedation or neuromuscular blockade without analgesia
    ▪ Patients with head injury also experience pain; analgesia should not be withheld
  — Assess pulmonary function, ABG
    ▪ Provide IS and coughing/deep-breathing exercises in addition to pain management
  — Use a numeric or visual pain scale appropriate for the patient's communication and understanding to assess the patient's experience with the pain and analgesics
  — Assess vital signs and behavior for signs of pain
    ▪ Tachycardia, tachypnea
    ▪ Restlessness
    ▪ Anxiety
    ▪ Verbalizations or lack of verbalization; individuals in different cultures express their experience of pain differently; do not assume a quiet patient is comfortable
    ▪ Assess sleep/rest
    ▪ Monitor nutrition as opiods can frequently cause nausea and constipation

Thoracic injuries, although managed nonoperatively most of the time, present serious challenges to the management of the trauma and especially multitrauma patient. Rapid identification of the injuries is essential to survival. Prompt management of the injuries is required. Throughout the patient's stay, airway, breathing, and circulation are monitored and managed to attain and maintain a hemodynamically stable state.

Critical Lifesavers

- A tension pneumothorax is a life-threatening situation that must be rapidly identified clinically.
- DO NOT splint the flail segment with tape, binders, or sand bags.
- Measurement of cardiac troponin I and CPK-MB have not demonstrated usefulness in identification of cardiac injury.
- Pericardiocentesis is a temporizing procedure only.

REFERENCES

American College of Surgeons. *Advanced Trauma Life Support* (ATLS). 7th ed. Chicago, IL: American College of Surgeons; 2004.

American College of Surgeons. *Advanced Trauma Life Support* (ATLS). 8th ed. Chicago, IL: American College of Surgeons; 2008.

Baldwin K, Ohman-Strickland P, et al. Scapula fractures: a marker for concomitant injury? A retrospective review of data in the national trauma database. *J Trauma.* 2008;65(2):430-435.

Bergeron E, Lavoie A, Clas D, et al. Elderly trauma patients with rib fractures are at greater risk of death and pneumonia. *J Trauma.* 2003;54(3):478-485.

Brasel KJ, Guse CE, Layde P, et al. Rib fractures: relationship with pneumonia and mortality. *Crit Care Med.* 2006;34(6):1642-1646.

Demetriades D, Velmahos GC, Scalea TM, et al. Diagnosis and treatment of blunt thoracic aortic injuries: changing perspectives. *J Trauma.* 2008;64(6):1415-1419.

Eastern Association for Surgery of Trauma (EAST) Guidelines Committee. Pain management in blunt thoracic trauma. *J Trauma.* 2005;59(5):1256-1267.

Emergency Nurses Association. *Trauma Nursing Core Curriculum* (TNCC). 6th ed. Des Plaines, IL: Emergency Nurses Association; 2007.

Funk D, Lujan E, Moretti E, et al. A brief report: the use of high frequency oscillatory ventilation for severe pulmonary contusion. 2008. *J Trauma.* 2008;65(2):390-395.

Hoyt KS, Selfridge-Thomas J. *Emergency Nursing Core Curriculum.* 6th ed. St Louis, MO: Saunders Elsevier; 2007.

Hunt J, Baker C, Lentz C, et al. Thoracic aorta injuries: management and outcome of 144 patients. *J Trauma.* 1996;40(4):547-556.

Johnson SB. Operative approaches for traumatic thoracic aortic injury: immediate versus delayed therapy. *J Trauma.* 2007;62(6): S24-S25.

Karmakar MK, Ho AM. Acute pain management of patients with multiple fractures ribs. *J Trauma* 2003;54(3):615-625.

Kortbeek JB, Al Turki SA, Ali J, et al. Advanced trauma life support: the evidence for change. *J Trauma.* 2008;64(6):1638-1650.

Luchette FA, Barie PS, Oswanski MF, et al. Practice management guidelines for prophylactic antibiotic use in tube thoracostomy for traumatic hemopneumothorax: EAST PMG work group. *J Trauma.* 2000;48(4):758-759.

Maxwell RA, Campbell DJ, Fabian TC, et al. Use of presumptive antibiotics following tube thoracostomy for traumatic hemopneumothorax in the prevention of empyema and pneumonia: a multi-center trial. *J Trauma.* 2004;57(4):742-749.

McQuillan KA, Flynn Makic MB, Whalen E. *Trauma Nursing From Resuscitation Through Rehabilitation.* 4th ed. St Louis, MO: Saunders Elsevier; 2009.

Nagy K, Fabian T, Rodman G, et al. Guidelines for the diagnosis and management of blunt aortic injury. *J Trauma.* 2000;48(6): 1128-1144.

Pacini D, Angeli E, Fattori R, et al. Traumatic rupture of the thoracic aorta: ten years of delayed management. *J Thorac Cardiovasc Surg.* 2005;129(4):880-884.

Pasquale MD, Nagy K, Clarke J. Practice management guidelines for screening for blunt cardiac injury. *J Trauma.* 1998;44(6):941-956.

Reiff D, McGwin G, Metzger J, et al. Identifying injuries and MVC characteristics that together are suggestive of diaphragmatic rupture. *J Trauma.* 2002;53(6):1139-1145.

Salim A, Velmahos GC, Jindal A, et al. Clinically significant blunt cardiac trauma: role of serum troponin levels combined with electrocardiographic findings. *J Trauma*. 2001;50(2):237-243.

Simon B, Ebert J, Bokhari F, et al. Management of pulmonary contusion and flail chest. Practice management guidelines. 2006. Available at: http://www.east.org. Accessed December 9, 2008.

Turk EE, Tsokos M. Blunt cardiac trauma caused by fatal falls from height: an autopsy-based assessment of the injury pattern. *J Trauma*. 2004;57(2):301-304.

Van Horn JM. A case study of right ventricular rupture in an elderly victim of MVC: incorporating end of life care into trauma nursing. *J Trauma Nurs*. 2007;14(3):136-143.

von Garrel T, Ince A, Junge A, et al. The sterna fracture: radiographic analysis of 200 fractures with special reference to concomitant injuries. *J Trauma*. 2004;57(4):837-844.

Vu KC, Skourtis ME, Gong X, et al. Reduction of rib fractures with a bioresorbable plating system:preliminary observations. *J Trauma*. 2008;64(5):1264-1269.

Ziglar M, Bennett V, Nayduch D, et al. *The Electronic Library of Trauma Lectures*. Chicago, IL: Society of Trauma Nurses; 2004.

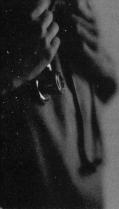

Chapter 8
ABDOMINAL INJURY

INTRODUCTION

The abdomen is protected by the pelvis and rib cage, nevertheless it is vulnerable to blunt and penetrating trauma. Tools meant to protect the body in motor vehicle collisions (MVC), such as seat belts and air bags, can harm the abdomen when used improperly. The lap belt worn above the pelvis can result in mesenteric avulsion, ruptured bowel, or vascular injury. The lumbar spine fracture or cord injury associated with the lapbelt occurs when it is worn without the shoulder harness. This is especially important in children who need a booster seat, but instead are harnessed into a lap belt. In the pregnant patient, these injuries can also include the uterus or fetus.

The abdomen is complex in its function as well as structure, consisting of both hollow and solid viscus. The hollow viscus, when ruptured or perforated, results in leakage of bacteria, fecal and food matter, enzymes, and stomach acid. The abdomen, consisting of both the peritoneum and retroperitoneum, is also the largest cavity into which blood loss can occur. The retroperitoneum itself can hold up to 4 L of blood. Injury here must be identified rapidly and decisions made regarding management to prevent uncontrolled hemorrhage and death. This chapter discusses only the internal organs of the abdomen. Management of the pelvis and vascular injuries associated with the pelvis are discussed in Chapter 9.

ASSESSMENT

Assessment of the abdomen is confounded by distracting injuries, spinal cord and head injury, and body habitus. Even diagnostic studies can be equivocal or miss injuries. An intense index of suspicion based upon mechanism of injury and diligent monitoring will identify injury.

The upper peritoneal cavity contains the ribs, diaphragm, liver, spleen, stomach, and transverse colon. The lower cavity holds the small bowel, sigmoid, ascending and descending colon. The pelvic cavity contains the bladder, rectum, and female reproductive organs. The retroperitoneum contains the duodenum, kidneys, pancreas, ureters, aorta, and inferior vena cava. Penetrating injury to these organs occurs most frequently to the liver followed by small bowel, and the diaphragm, whereas blunt trauma more frequently involves the spleen and liver.

Assessment begins with history and involves assessment of the mechanism of injury to assist with determination of potential injury.

History

As with all trauma, the history begins with the mechanism of injury. Knowledge of the transfer of energy to the body increases alertness to specific injuries. Questions specific to abdominal injury include

- Mechanism of injury: blunt
  — MVC: speed, intrusion into the passenger compartment, air bag deployment
  — Use of restraints? Proper positioning? Shoulder belt in place or behind the shoulder?
  — Impact with the steering wheel; damage to the steering wheel
  — Position of a child in the vehicle: front seat, booster seat/car seat, air bags
- Mechanism of injury: penetrating (stabbing and gunshot wound [GSW])

— Proximity of the weapon for penetrating injury

— Type of weapon: knife/ sharp object, gun type/ size

• Impact to the abdomen—handlebars, assault, fall onto an object; is the object still present? impaled

• Allergies, especially iodine (contrast), seafood, strawberries, medications, foods

• Medications—be aware of contrast issues with metformin

— Contrast has the potential to induce acute renal failure

— Acute renal failure in the presence of metformin can result in dangerously high levels of the drug and lactic acidosis

• Last meal

• Last menstrual period

• Vomiting, hematemesis

• Past medical and surgical history, particularly previous abdominal surgery

Trauma Assessment

Trauma assessment is the same for all trauma patients and begins with airway, breathing, and circulation. These areas must be assessed and issues managed as they are identified. The assessment of the abdomen is part of the secondary survey. The interventions that occur during the abdominal assessment are performed only after the primary issues are controlled and a full brief secondary survey is completed. Continued reevaluation is essential.

• Observe

— Inspect the size and shape of the abdomen; note distention

— Identify any contusions or abrasions across the pelvis (seat belt sign): bowel, lumbar spine injury

— Contusions around the umbilicus (Cullen sign): retroperitoneal injury

— Contusions in the flank (Grey Turner sign): renal injury, retroperitoneal injury

— Complaints of left shoulder pain while lying flat (Kehr sign): referred pain from spleen injury with blood below the diaphragm irritating the phrenic nerve
— Note any holes from GSW, stabbing, or impalement
  ▪ Identify position and place a marker for any radiographs of the abdomen
  ▪ Photograph if possible (follow hospital standards for permission)
  ▪ Count holes from GSW—even number MAY indicate through-and-through injury
  ▪ For penetrating injuries above the umbilicus, expect plain film of the abdomen and chest to identify any foreign bodies present (ATLS 2004)
— The diaphragm relaxes at the fourth intercostal-space on full expiration. Therefore any penetrating wound below the fourth intercostal-space should be considered thoracoabdominal until proven otherwise
— Observe for evisceration that can also occur in the flank or posterior
  ▪ Immediately cover the exposed gut with saline-soaked gauze to keep it moist until surgery
— Stabilize any impaled object to prevent further damage or hemorrhage
— Place an oral gastric tube (nasogastric if there is no facial or head injury) to decompress the stomach and prevent aspiration
  ▪ If the patient begins to vomit with or without a gastric tube, turn the patient to the right
  ▪ If the patient is still on the backboard, tilt the board to the right
— Observe the perineum for bleeding, open wounds
  ▪ If open wounds are present, open pelvic fracture should be considered
  ▪ Observe the urinary meatus for bleeding—indicates urethral injury; DO NOT place a Foley catheter

- Blood at the urinary meatus requires further evaluation with a retrograde urethrogram and likely suprapubic catheter placement
- Observe the scrotum and penis for external injury
- Identify perineal contusion, especially a butterfly pattern
- Observe for frank blood from the rectum
— Identify patient complaints of pain, note location, type, radiation, diffuse or localized

- Auscultate
— Listening to bowel sounds may be difficult during trauma resuscitation
— Absence of bowel sounds may be caused by ileus from multisystem injury or from abdominal injury (nonspecific sign)
— Auscultation of bowel sounds in the chest is a sign of diaphragmatic injury with herniation
— Listen for bruit over the abdominal aorta and renal arteries
— Auscultate over the stomach after placement of the gastric tube
  - Once position is confirmed, place to low intermittent wall suction
— Listen over the epigastric area after placement of the endotracheal tube as well to ensure placement is not in the esophagus

- Percuss
— Percussion is also difficult to hear in the trauma room
— Dullness indicates an underlying solid organ or hemo-peritoneum
— Resonance over the stomach indicates gastric dilatation; place a gastric tube to decompress if not done; check placement if resonant with the tube in place
— Other tympanic areas of percussion may indicate air within the abdomen from a ruptured hollow viscus
— Aggressive bag-valve-mask ventilation can result in gastric distention from air entering the stomach

— Do not perform an assessment that involves touching the abdomen prior to auscultation and inspection; once the abdomen is touched, if pain is present, further assessment may be impossible

  ▪ In children, do not touch the abdomen until the final assessment as any pain elicited will prevent future evaluation

• Palpate

— Palpation of the abdomen is intended to initiate guarding, rigidity, or rebound tenderness

— Light palpation may indicate areas of tenseness/rigidity from underlying organ injury

— Guarding: involuntary, indicates peritoneal irritation

— Rebound tenderness: deep compression of the abdomen with quick release results in pain and indicates peritonitis

— Digital rectal examination is also performed to identify

  ▪ Gross blood from rectal/sigmoid injury

  ▪ Prostate position—boggy, high riding prostate is indicative of urethral injury

— After the rectal examination, a Foley catheter can be placed if the prostate is normal

— All pulses should be palpated for rate and quality

  ▪ Diminished lower extremity pulses may indicate injury to abdominal or lower extremity vascular structures

Diagnostics are necessary in the case of blunt trauma and questionable penetrating injury. In a patient who is hypotensive, a trip to the computed tomography (CT) scanner is unacceptable. This patient needs to be in the surgical suite for exploration. The environment of the CT scanner prevents the staff from close evaluation of the patient as well as intensive resuscitation. In the instance of peritoneal signs, a rapid helical CT of the abdomen may be obtained, if the patient is stable, to guide laparotomy.

The majority of GSW also do not need a trip to the scanner, but rather need exploration as the track of the bullet is rarely a straight line. Multiple organs can be injured without hypotension with GSW, however the bowel leak is as life threatening. The following are diagnostic studies used to evaluate the abdomen:

- Focused assessment sonography for trauma (FAST) has become a useful resource in the early resuscitation of the trauma patient to identify both intra-abdominal hemorrhage and pericardial fluid.
  — Noninvasive, portable, rapid, serial ultrasound detection of intra-abdominal fluid (86-97% accuracy)(ATLS 2008)
    ▪ Able to identify as little as 100 mL fluid
    ▪ 200 to 500 mL of abdominal fluid is a positive examination
  — Performed by trauma surgeon or emergency physician in the trauma room
  — Evaluates four regions of the abdomen (Figure 8-1)

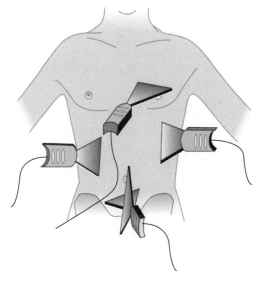

Figure 8-1   FAST examination. (Courtesy of SonoSite.)

- Pericardial
- Splenorenal
- Hepatorenal (Morrison pouch)
- Pelvic

— A negative study with instability, severe persistent abdominal pain, seat belt sign, hematuria, or associated injuries requires further evaluation; a positive study paired with hemodynamic instability requires operation

— Can be repeated

— CT scan for follow-up

— Limitations include
  - Body habitus (obesity)
  - Injuries without hemoperitoneum (30-40% of abdominal injury) (Myers 2007)
  - Retroperitoneal injury
  - Diaphragm, bowel

— May also be useful in identifying hemothorax

- Diagnostic peritoneal lavage (DPL) is 98% sensitive to abdominal injury and identifies blood, fecal matter, gut contents through the instillation of fluid into the abdomen and subsequent removal and analysis

  — Fast, portable, useful when the patient is hemodynamically unstable or no CT scan is available
    - Does not evaluate the retroperitoneum or diaphragm
    - Although uncommon with the advent of FAST, a DPL should still be available as a backup modality for abdominal assessment
    - It is also a rapid, useful tool for intensive care unit (ICU) or inpatient evaluation of the abdomen

  — If the patient has obvious signs of abdominal injury and is unstable, no study is needed. The patient needs rapid transport to the operating suite.

  — Limitations include
    - Morbid obesity

- Previous laparotomy
- Advanced cirrhosis
- Coagulopathy

— Procedure preparation

- Warm normal saline solution (NSS) or lactated ringer (LR) solution, 1 L bag with IV tubing (macrodrip without one-way valve)
- Foley catheter and gastric tube must be placed prior to DPL to decompress the bladder and stomach
- Peritoneal dialysis catheter is inserted (periumbilical) with a 20 mL syringe attached
  - Withdrawal of 10 mL of frank blood is sufficient evidence of hemoperitoneum
  - If no aspirate, instill 900 to 950 mL of warm LR (NSS is acceptable but causes cramping later)
  - Leave 50 to 100 mL in the bag to maintain the siphon effect during drainage
  - Drop the IV bag to the floor and allow the fluid to return
  - Return as much fluid as possible, however 40 mL is sufficient to send a sample to the laboratory

— Positive DPL results include

- Aspirate of gross blood
- >100,000 RBC/mm^3
- >500 WBC/mm^3
- Presence of any bile, amylase, bacteria, or fecal contents
- Positive DPL results in penetrating trauma have a lower threshold of >10,000 RBC/mm^3

— A positive DPL indicates a need for surgery

- CT—abdomen is only used if the patient is hemodynamically stable with an equivocal examination. Any unstable patient needs resuscitation and operative procedure. A FAST or DPL can be used to examine the abdomen, not the CT scan.

— Equivocal examination includes

- Head and spinal cord injury

- Inconsistent abdominal examination
- Distracting injury
- Multiple injury
- Alcohol or drugs affecting examination
— Helical multislice CT is a diagnostic tool that can be repeated and assists with the determination of nonoperative management of liver and spleen injury
  - Approximately 81% recognition of bowel and mesenteric injury (Ekeh et al. 2008), thus missed injuries can occur. Serial examination is necessary
  - Measure the grade of solid organ injury
  - Identify the presence of air indicating hollow viscus injury
— Contrast
  - Assess first for allergy
  - Hematuria is a sign indicating the need for IV contrast
  - Oral—may be used to assist with hollow viscus injury identification, however can induce vomiting
  - IV—used for vascular injury as well as renal perfusion
  - Head CT must be done prior to any administration of contrast
  - If a chest CT is anticipated, perform with the abdominal CT to decrease the dye load
  - After IV contrast, ensure that the patient is well hydrated to assist with excretion of the contrast
— Presence of chest injury or hematuria warrants an abdominal CT for evaluation if stable
— Evaluates the retroperitoneum and diaphragm which are not evaluated by FAST or DPL
— Limitations include
  - Missed injuries—diaphragm, small bowel
  - Body habitus—CT scanners have a limitation as to the weight the table can tolerate
  - Movement degrades images

- CT-cystogram is used for the evaluation of suspected bladder injury
  - If bladder injury is suspected, a CT-cystogram is more accurate than a simple CT abdomen with the Foley catheter clamped
  - If an abdominal CT is to be done and a bladder injury is suspected, include the CT-cystogram instead of a separate cystogram by plain film
  - CT-cystogram is accomplished with instillation of 300 mL water-soluble contrast
    - Stop instillation if the flow spontaneously stops, patient voids, or discomfort is experienced
- Retrograde urethrogram (RUG) is necessary when a urethral injury is suspected. It can be combined with a cystogram to evaluate the bladder
  - Identifies the extent of urethral injury
  - Assists the urologist in the placement of a Foley catheter with the suprapubic tube by determining the position and degree of urethral injury
  - Rapid evaluation that can be done during the secondary survey
- Angiogram is useful to identify significant vascular injury that can be managed by embolization in the interventional radiology suite.
  - Useful for nonoperative management of spleen and liver injury where any active extravasation can be controlled through embolization
  - Hemodynamically unstable patients to control vascular injury amenable to embolization

DOCUMENTATION

Documentation of abdominal injury includes the initial assessment of shape, tenseness, pain (site and intensity, radiation), and distention of the abdomen. Sites of any penetrating injuries should be labeled on the body diagram. A piece of x-ray film can be used to trace (with a permanent marker) the outline and size of the wounds which may later be useful in identification of a weapon. This is important for both stab and GSW. Following hospital policy, photographs can also be taken of the wounds. Use a measuring device to describe the size of the wound. Do not cleanse the area prior to photography. Areas of soot and gunshot burn are important to the forensic evidence collection. Include in the documentation, all studies done to determine abdominal injury as well as continuous documentation of hemodynamics, especially during any radiographic study like CT scan.

Documentation should also include the assessment prior to insertion of the gastric tube and Foley catheter. The size and placement of the tubes should be included. Documentation should then include continuous abdominal assessments for evidence of delayed presentation of injury, delayed peritonitis.

MANAGEMENT—HOLLOW VISCUS

Hollow viscus (stomach, small and large bowel) injuries can be as simple as a contusion, but more often involve perforation and leakage of the contents of the organ. This leakage is the source of contamination to the abdomen and sepsis if not managed appropriately.

Stomach

Injury to the stomach is relatively rare and usually is caused by penetrating trauma, primarily stabbings. Injury from blunt trauma is usually a sudden increase in intra-abdominal pressure, for example, impact to the stomach from handlebars, steering wheel, blast effect, or air bag. The stomach may also suffer injury when diaphragm laceration occurs and the stomach herniates through the tear. The chemical irritation from stomach acid leakage results in peritonitis and abdominal pain. Instability is usually caused by associated injuries. Vascular injury to the gastric artery can occur, especially with penetrating injury.

Signs and Symptoms of Stomach Injury

Penetrating injury overlying the stomach area
Rapid onset abdominal pain, epigastric, nonspecific
Hypotension
Hematemesis or bloody drainage from gastric tube
Tender abdomen
Signs of peritonitis
Abdominal x-ray—free air

Management

Management of a stomach injury requires laparotomy with direct repair or resection if necessary. The abdomen requires washout from the leakage of gastric contents. A gastric tube will usually remain for 3 to 4 days until peristalsis returns. Gastric ulcer prophylaxis should be provided with H_2 blockers and/or sucralfate. Potential complications include fistula or abdominal abscess from gastric leak. If the perforation is not well sealed, leak can continue resulting in peritonitis and abscess.

Duodenum and Small Intestine

Injury to the small intestine is similar to injury to the stomach. Being a hollow viscus, sudden increased pressure in the abdomen can result in rupture. Tears occur at fixed points in the gut. Seat belts worn inappropriately (high on the abdomen) can result in small bowel injury. A chance fracture of the lumbar spine with or without spinal cord injury can be associated with seat belt injury and hyperflexion of the abdomen.

Penetrating injury, particularly GSW can result in perforation or serosal injury to one or more sites. The blast effect from the GSW or an explosive device can result in contusion to areas apart from the sites of perforation or isolated injuries themselves. The duodenum is protected by its positioning in the retroperitoneum. However, a bullet does not follow a direct path and can easily traverse the abdomen to the retroperitoneal area. Duodenum injury can be associated with pancreas injury, bile duct, and vena cava tears including the pancreatic duct. These injuries should also be considered when evaluating the duodenum. Jejunum injury most often occurs near the umbilicus.

When examining the intestines during laparotomy, the surgeon palpates and visualizes the entire small bowel. Delayed rupture or presentation of the small bowel can occur from 48 to 72 hours after injury, especially the duodenum. Missed injury can also occur as small bowel injury is difficult to identify on CT or FAST examination.

Signs and Symptoms of Small Bowel Injury

Transient periumbilical pain
Pain increases as peritonitis develops
Seat belt sign—contusion/ abrasion
Nausea, vomiting
No bowel sounds
Inconsistent increase in amylase and lipase
Retroperitoneal signs—Cullen and Grey-Turner
DPL—amylase or bile, bacteria, fibers, gut contents, elevated
   WBC

Management

Small bowel and duodenal injury require surgical repair. At the time of laparotomy (celiotomy), the surgeon evaluates the entire length of bowel as injuries may occur in more than one site, especially with penetrating trauma. Injuries such as simple serosal tears and penetrating injury of <50% circumference with viable bowel may be managed with direct repair (Cayten et al. 1998). Small bowel and duodenal resection with primary anastomosis occur for larger injuries, multiple perforations in close proximity, severe mesenteric injury, or signs of ischemic bowel. The site of perforation frequently requires debridement. Resection is followed by primary reanastomosis. Hemoperitoneum without solid viscus injury is usually caused by mesenteric bleeding. As with any injury, bleeding is managed first, followed by the exploration of the bowel. Abdominal washout to remove bacteria and other leakage from the gut is part of the laparotomy procedure.

Perioperative antibiotics may be continued for up to 24 hours because of the bacterial spill into the peritoneum. Postoperative management includes observation for abscess, small bowel obstruction, or fistula formation. A gastric tube for drainage may be needed until peristalsis returns. Nutrition needs to be addressed early to assist wound healing and maintain gut integrity.

Colon and Rectum

Large bowel injury experiences the same effects of rapid increase of intra-abdominal pressure. The transverse colon is susceptible to penetrating injury because of its prominent location. Injuries to the colon result in significant fecal contamination and subsequent sepsis, causing a lethal injury if left unnoticed. Extraperitoneal rectal injury occurs with pelvic fracture, as well as penetrating injury. It can easily be missed and must be considered.

Signs and Symptoms of Large Bowel Injury

Peritoneal irritation, pain
Subcutaneous emphysema
Guaiac positive rectal exam (possible colon injury)
Gross positive rectal exam (rectal injury)
Absent bowel sounds
DPL—fecal matter, bacteria, fibers

Management

Colon injury requires surgery as with all hollow viscus injury. The exploratory laparotomy investigates the entire large bowel as with the small bowel. After control of any bleeding, direct repair or resection of the colon is undertaken. Abdominal washout is performed to remove fecal contamination. Delayed closure of the abdomen may be chosen as incisional infection is a known result of gross contamination.

Serosal tears can usually be managed with direct repair as long as there is viable bowel. Evidence of significant injury or ischemic bowel may require resection. Colostomy is frequent to allow the bowel to heal and to divert fecal matter from the site of injury, especially extraperitoneal rectal injuries. Choices in management during laparotomy are dependent not only on the site and extent of injury, but also the stability of the patient, presence of hypothermia and coagulopathy, and length of the operative procedure to achieve primary repair and anastomosis. Primary anastamosis is the optimal management of colon injury.

Rectal injury may be identified with water soluble contrast enema on CT. However even this can miss an injury. The surgeon may choose to perform a proctosigmoidoscopy at the time of laparotomy to view the rectum. Even the most diligent evaluation can miss a rectal injury that may present later as abscess or sepsis from leak. When rectal injury does occur, presacral drainage is placed at the time of laparotomy in addition to a diverting colostomy.

Postoperative management includes antibiotics to cover fecal soilage. The patient is monitored for peritonitis, abscess, and sepsis. The colostomy is observed for

- Color, moistness
- Retraction
- Prolapse
- Necrosis
- Stenosis
- Evidence of return of bowel function—note quality of stool

Consultation should be made to the enterostomal therapy nurse for evaluation and management of the colostomy.

The patient will require teaching regarding personal care of the colostomy at discharge as the takedown of the colostomy does not occur for several weeks to months. Colostomy takedown can occur within 2 weeks of injury if a contrast enema (non-barium) demonstrates distal colon healing and if the patient is without instability or sepsis (Cayten et al. 1998). Colostomy issues include management of the bag for containment, odor, stenosis, and gas.

A psychosocial consult may be necessary to assist the patient with the altered body image resulting from a colostomy. This may be particularly important if the cause of injury was a violent intentional crime. As with all trauma, the patient has a series of issues with which to deal, and the presence of a colostomy or even the laparotomy incision may be enough to warrant a consult to assist coping.

A gastric tube may be used to decompress the stomach while awaiting the return of peristalsis. Nutrition must be considered early and provided to promote healing. Oral or enteral nutrition is optimal. Of note, the colon is responsible for the synthesis of vitamins B and K. This should be taken into consideration when nutrition is being provided.

MANAGEMENT—SOLID VISCUS

Solid viscus injuries are the source of major bleeding as well as dysfunction of the organs involved. Early identification is essential as well as grading of the depth and extent of injury. The grading assists the surgeon with determining if nonoperative management can be implemented. Nonoperative management requires close monitoring for hemorrhage. In the case of multiple injuries, hypotension, coagulopathy, and hypothermia may rule out the option of nonoperative management even though the individual injury may be amenable to such.

Liver and Gallbladder

The liver is the largest solid organ and responsible for clotting factors (fibrinogen, prothrombin), protein synthesis, conversion of stores to glycogen, bile, and blood storage. The liver also plays a significant role in detoxification of blood, storage of iron and fat soluble vitamins A, D, E, and K. The liver also participates in the metabolism of carbohydrates, fats, and proteins. Up to 30% of the cardiac output is stored in the liver at any given time, resulting in a large pool of blood for hemorrhage. Injury can occur from direct impact, rapid deceleration, or penetrating events. The gallbladder is also susceptible to blast effect from GSW or explosive devices. It is a fluid-filled organ that responds as such to the pressure wave.

Signs and Symptoms of Liver and Gallbladder Injury

Right upper quadrant, lower right chest tenderness
May complain of referred right shoulder pain
Rebound tenderness, guarding, rigidity, peritoneal irritation
Increased pain with diaphragm excursion
Abdominal distention
Ecchymosis right lower chest, upper abdomen
Prothrombin time (PT) and partial thromboplastin time (PTT) abnormalities
Hypotension, dropping hematocrit

A brief description of the liver grading scale is listed in Table 8-1. A positive FAST for blood over the liver may lead to a CT scan of the abdomen if the patient is hemodynamically stable. The CT scan with both IV and oral contrast will assist with grading the injury and determining if other organ injury exists. If hemodynamically unstable, the patient is taken for laparotomy and possibly damage control surgery.

Management

Liver injury in general is amenable to nonoperative management. The choice is dependent upon hemodynamic stability. If nonoperative management is chosen, monitoring includes

Table 8-1   Liver Grading Scale

Classification	Description
I	Subcapsular hematoma, nonexpanding; minor subcapsular laceration without active bleeding
II	Minor subcapsular nonexpanding hematoma of <50% surface area; shallow capsular laceration (1-3 cm); nonbleeding penetrating wound
III	Hematoma >50%, expanding or ruptured; deep laceration >3 cm, may have duct involvement, blood loss >20%
IV	Burst fracture of <75% disruption involving 1 to 3 Couinaud segments
V	Massive parenchymal injury involving the vena cava or hepatic vein, >3 Couinaud segments
VI	Complete hepatic avulsion

Adapted from Association for the Advancement of Automotive Medicine. *Abbreviated Injury Scale (AIS) 2005.* Barrington, IL: AAAM; rev. 2008.

- Frequent monitoring of vital signs and hematocrit
  - Obtain a lactate on admission and repeat if elevated
  - Patient should be alert and cooperative with serial examinations
- Bed rest with a gradual increase in activity and diet
- Pain control
- Reassessment of the abdomen for peritoneal signs or changes
- Frequency of repeat CT scans depends upon patient progress
- Any signs of ongoing bleeding
  - Consider embolization to control bleeders
  - Plan laparotomy for hemorrhage control
- Successful nonoperative management results in a patient discharged without surgery

— Wear an "alert" bracelet regarding the presence of a liver injury

— Return to clinic within 2 weeks for first follow-up appointment

— Healing usually occurs within 3 months of injury

— Limit physical activity/sports during that time

— Normal activity resumes only after evidence of healing

• Failed nonoperative management guidelines include consideration of (Yanar et al. 2008)

— Increasing or uncontrolled lactic acidosis

— Transfusion required within the first 6 hours of injury

— Drop in hematocrit of 20% within the first hour

In the patient with severe (grade IV-VI) or multiple injuries, exploratory laparotomy occurs. Determination for laparotomy is surgeon dependent, but is driven by evidence of ongoing hemorrhage or coagulopathy. In patients with severe hemorrhage, damage, or coagulopathy, damage control surgery is undertaken (see below). Manual compression provides tamponade to the liver, followed by packing the area. Direct repair or sealing with a tissue glue may be used in some patients to stop bleeding. Efforts are made to save as much liver tissue as possible. Even when overt hemorrhage is controlled, ongoing oozing can continue because of coagulation disorders. Whether damage control or laparotomy is performed, a drain is placed postoperatively.

Retrohepatic vena caval injury is severe, results in hemorrhage, and is difficult to approach and control. The hepatic veins feed into the vena cava at this point. The majority of these injuries would have previously exsanguinated at the scene, but with rapid transport, may arrive to the operating suite and the injury discovered at that time. There are operative management options that include atrio-caval shunt, balloon shunt, vascular clamping, and damage control surgery. Rapid identification of the injury and the stability of the patient will determine survival. Control and repair of these injuries is difficult and carries a high mortality.

The gallbladder is usually managed by cholecystectomy, which is performed during the initial exploratory laparotomy unless the procedure becomes damage control surgery only. The cholecystectomy may then be done on the first relaparotomy. A simple bile duct injury may be repaired, however any complex injury is managed with cholecystectomy. Cholecystectomies are accompanied by drainage and monitoring for biliary fistula postoperatively.

Postoperatively, the patient must be monitored for development of abdominal compartment syndrome (ACS), hemorrhage, biliary fistula, and infection. ACS is discussed below. Postoperative care includes

- Monitoring for signs of renewed hemorrhage
- Monitor for infection, especially while packs are in place
- Monitor for biliary leak and adjust dressings to contain
  - Biliary drainage will damage skin around the drain site or fistula because of the enzymes present
  - Contain with an ostomy bag system to protect the skin
- Assess coagulation for abnormalities and anticipate administration of
  - Fresh frozen plasma, platelets, cryoprecipitate, vitamin K
- Administer packed red blood cells to replace blood loss
- Monitor for liver failure through assessment of ALT, AST, PT and PTT labwork

Spleen

The spleen is another commonly injured organ, especially from blunt trauma. The spleen functions in hematopoiesis, red cell and platelet destruction, and plays a primary immune function role by removing blood-borne bacteria. Hemorrhage can occur immediately or present as delayed rupture. With the use of CT scan, identification is early, allowing for continuous monitoring of the spleen as it heals. The presence of a pseudoaneurysm is most predictive of a delayed rupture (Ruffolo 2002). A subcapsular hematoma can increase in size with the capsule providing tamponade. However, even this can rupture under pressure, resulting in the delayed hemorrhage. Splenic injuries are graded based upon CT scan or visualization in surgery (Table 8-2).

Signs and Symptoms of Spleen Injury

Left upper quadrant tenderness/pain
Referred pain to the left shoulder (Kehr sign) especially when
   supine
Rigidity, distention, guarding, rebound tenderness
Hypotension, dropping hematocrit
Dullness to percussion over left upper quadrant (Ballance sign)

Management

Do not delay surgery in the presence of hypotension unresponsive to resuscitation. The surgeon will attempt to avoid splenectomy by surgical repair of the spleen. Embolization of the spleen is an effective means of controlling bleeders and preventing transfusion or splenectomy. Embolization is also effective in

Table 8-2   Splenic Injury Grading Scale

Classification	Description
I	Superficial, minor hematoma; simple capsular laceration, superficial
II	Subcapsular hematoma <50% surface area; simple capsular laceration <3 cm
III	Subcapsular hematoma >50%, expanding, ruptured or intraparenchymal to >5 cm depth; Parenchymal laceration >3 cm depth
IV	Severe stellate fracture, involving hilar vessels, devascularization >25%
V	Hilar disruption, total devascularization, avulsion

Adapted from Association for the Advancement of Automotive Medicine.
Abbreviated Injury Scale (AIS) 2005. Barrington, IL: AAAM; rev. 2008.

the presence of splenic artery pseudoaneurysm (Wei et al. 2008). If there are no hollow viscus injuries requiring laparotomy and the patient is hemodynamically stable, nonoperative management may be chosen. Management of the nonoperative splenic injury is similar to the nonoperative management of the liver (see earlier).

Despite the best attempts to protect the spleen, occasionally splenectomy is the only choice. The hemodynamically unstable patient with a splenic injury needs splenectomy to provide some stability. Grade IV and grade V injuries frequently require splenectomy to rapidly control hemorrhage.

Of note, up to 10% of blunt splenic injury will worsen after discharge. Approximately 20% of splenic injuries will not be completely healed by 3 months after injury (Savage et al. 2008). Close observation is necessary for delayed rupture. Otherwise, the discharge instructions for the salvaged spleen are the same as for nonoperative liver patients.

Because of the role of the spleen in immunity, all splenectomy patients require the administration of three vaccines to prevent postsplenectomy sepsis. The vaccines are

- Pneumococcus
- Meningococcus
- Haemophilus influenza B

Overwhelming postsplenectomy sepsis can occur from 1 to 5 years after splenectomy causing sepsis and disseminated intravascular coagulopathy (DIC). This syndrome has a mortality of up to 50% (Ziglar et al. 2004). Vaccination within a few days of splenectomy prevents this syndrome and protects the patient. In patients with splenic salvage, some surgeons choose to vaccinate these patients for additional protection. These patients should also be instructed that they may need antibiotics before dental work or future surgery. Other complications include infection, hemorrhage, extremely high platelet counts, and pancreatitis.

An unusual complication of splenectomy is pseudohyperkalemia. The false elevation of potassium occurs from release during cell destruction and clotting. It is usually associated with thrombocytosis, leukocytosis, and hemolysis (Johnson and Hughes 2001). Renal function will be normal. In patients with hyperkalemia after splenectomy with normal renal function, this syndrome should be considered and is self-limiting.

Pancreas

The pancreas provides the enzymes for digestion of proteins, fat, and carbohydrates. It also produces insulin and glucagon. The pancreas is housed in the retroperitoneum so is relatively protected and injury is difficult to diagnose (≥24-72 hour delay) (McQuillan et al. 2009). Injury is caused by direct blow, often the handlebars of a bicycle or steering wheel. Pancreatic injury can include the duct releasing enzymes into the abdomen as well, so this must be taken into consideration.

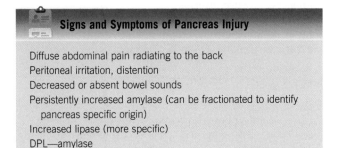

Signs and Symptoms of Pancreas Injury

Diffuse abdominal pain radiating to the back
Peritoneal irritation, distention
Decreased or absent bowel sounds
Persistently increased amylase (can be fractionated to identify pancreas specific origin)
Increased lipase (more specific)
DPL—amylase

CT scan can miss pancreatic injury for up to 8 hours after injury. If pancreas injury is suspected, CT should be repeated. An endoscopic retrograde cholangiopancreatography (ERCP) scan is more specific to the pancreas ductal injury.

Management

Low grade pancreatic injury is usually hemodynamically stable and heals on its own. Nonoperative management of isolated pancreatic injury on CT scan can result in missed small bowel injury (Duchesne et al. 2008). Injuries to the duct require operative intervention (Duchesne et al. 2008). Surgical intervention can include closed drainage, simple repair to distal pancreatectomy. All pancreatic surgery requires drainage to remove enzymes released into the abdominal cavity. The release of enzymes results in autodigestion. The most serious pancreatic injury with massive uncontrolled hemorrhage of the pancreatic head and irreparable ductal injury require a Whipple procedure (pancreaticoduodenectomy). The Whipple procedure is extensive and not usually an undertaking in which the trauma patient does well. It is a serious decision for the surgeon.

Complications after pancreatic injury include abscess (≤18%), pancreatitis, and fistula formation (14%) (Asensio et al. 2001). Acute pancreatitis is discussed below. Pancreatic injury may heal best with bowel rest. Tube feedings beyond the ligament of Treitz in the jejunum feeds the gut without pancreas involvement.

ABDOMINAL VASCULATURE

The majority of vascular injuries are managed at the same time as the organ with which it is associated. Pelvic vascular injury (iliac arteries and veins) are discussed under orthopaedic pelvic injury in Chapter 9. Abdominal vessels include the abdominal aorta, inferior vena cava, hepatic vessels, celiac axis, mesentery, and renal vessels. Injuries to vessels include contusion, laceration, intimal tear, and thrombosis. Several large vessels are housed in the retroperitoneum, where as noted previously, a large amount of hemorrhage can be hidden. Because these vessels are large, severe hypotension can occur rapidly and may not be controllable without surgery. Some repair of vascular injuries may require interposition grafting.

GENITOURINARY

Kidneys and Ureters

The kidneys are relatively fixed around the pedicle. Blunt trauma results from the torque against this area resulting in injuries to the kidney itself and the renal artery and/or vein. Penetrating injury occurs from a direct injury to the kidneys. Table 8-3 describes the grading system for renal injury. For the ureters, penetrating injury is the most frequent cause.

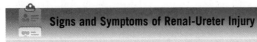

Signs and Symptoms of Renal-Ureter Injury

Flank contusion (Grey Turner sign)
Renal artery bruit
Upper abdominal, flank, lower rib tenderness
Costovertebral angle (CVA) tenderness
Gross or microscopic hematuria
Hypotension, dropping hematocrit

Table 8-3   Renal Injury Grading Scale

Classification	Description
I	Minor superficial hematoma, non-expanding; superficial laceration
II	Nonexpanding subcapsular hematoma; minor laceration <1 cm without urinary extravasation
III	Laceration >1 cm but not into the collecting system, no urinary extravasation
IV	Laceration into the parenchyma including the collecting system; contained hemorrhage of the renal artery and/or vein
V	Avulsion of the renal hilum; total destruction of the kidney

Adapted from Association for the Advancement of Automotive Medicine. *Abbreviated Injury Scale (AIS) 2005*. Barrington, IL: AAAM; rev. 2008.

Management

Renal injury is most often managed nonoperatively, ~95% (ATLS 2004). Nonoperative management is similar to nonoperative liver and spleen injury management and includes the addition of

- Monitor urine output
- Monitor blood urea nitrogen (BUN) and creatinine for renal function
- Monitor urinalysis

An intravenous pyelogram (IVP) or angiogram may show extravasation. Embolization can be used for renal artery and vein injury. CT evaluation provides the optimal method to determine the degree of renal injury. In the patient with perirenal hematoma, a magnetic resonance imaging (MRI) scan can discriminate between perirenal and intrarenal hematoma (Holevar et al. 2003). MRI does not involve iodine and assists when the CT is equivocal. Penetrating injuries to the kidney may benefit from both CT and angiogram for embolization.

Grade V injury requires surgical intervention. Every effort is made to preserve the kidney if possible. However if nephrectomy is necessary, a one-shot IVP identifies the presence of two kidneys. The shattered kidney that demonstrates perfusion and requires minimal transfusion may be managed nonoperatively. Care must be taken to closely monitor hematocrit. Embolization may be necessary. Grade III and grade IV injuries are at risk for delayed hemorrhage and need close monitoring, bed rest, and slow return to physical activity until healed.

Hematuria is not present in all patients with renal injury. In addition the degree of hematuria in no way relates to the degree of injury, however the presence of hematuria correlates with the likelihood of other intra-abdominal injuries (Holevar et al. 2003).

The adrenal glands are closely associated with the kidneys and can sustain injury as well. Adrenal hemorrhage as a whole is left to nonoperative management and will spontaneously resolve. The patient may or may not experience adrenal insufficiency.

Ureter injury may be missed on both IVP and laparotomy because of their position in the retroperitoneum. A helical CT scan with delayed images up to 5 to 8 minutes after contrast injection may increase sensitivity to ureter injury (Holevar et al. 2003). Ureter transection requires surgical repair and ureterostomy to divert urine flow. Stents may be placed to correct ureteral injury.

Complications of renal injury include hypertension, urinoma, infection (abscess), ureteral stricture, and obstructive hydronephrosis. Complications are rare but can occur up to 4 weeks after injury (McQuillan et al. 2009). Acute renal failure is not usually caused by renal injury but rather by ischemic injury from hypotension, acute tubular necrosis, or the systemic inflammatory response/sepsis. Grade III and grade IV renal injuries are associated with an urinoma caused by the extravasation of urine during the injury. Percutaneous drainage of the urinoma is essential to prevent further injury to the renal collecting ducts. During surgery for grade IV and grade V injuries, drainage of the urinoma is undertaken. Persistent extravasation of urine is a problem that can result in sepsis.

Hypertension after renal injury is caused by an excess of rennin excretion, infarct, and renal scarring. The incidence varies in range from <1% to 33% of patients and can occur as late as 10 years after injury. In most patients, the hypertension will resolve on its own or with a low-dose medication regimen.

Bladder and Urethra

The bladder and urethra are pelvic organs and injured by direct blow or secondarily by pelvic fracture. The bladder is more susceptible when it is full, especially from the seat belt. In children the bladder is in the intra-abdominal cavity and susceptible to any blow and again, especially when full. The bladder has both intraperitoneal and extraperitoneal components. Intraperitoneal injury usually involves the dome. Up to 25% of bladder and urethra injuries are associated with pelvic fractures and are missed initially (Ziran et al. 2005). Intraperitoneal bladder injury diagnosis can be delayed up to ~19 hours with a delay of up to 6 days for extraperitoneal bladder injuries. A high index of suspicion is necessary when considering these urinary injuries.

Posterior urethral injury is most often associated with pelvic fractures, although anterior urethra injuries are associated with straddle, GSW/penetrating, industrial, and self-inflicted instrumentation events. The urethra is injured more often in males because of length and exposure. The risk of urethra injury increases with both anterior and posterior pelvic fracture (Holevar et al. 2003).

Signs and Symptoms of Bladder Injury

Lower abdominal pain
Difficulty voiding
Hematuria
Rebound tenderness, guarding
Cystogram (CT cystogram)—positive extravasation

Signs and Symptoms of Urethra Injury

Blood at urinary meatus
Difficulty voiding, urge to void
Suprapubic pain, local pain
Butterfly-shaped contusion to perineum
Male—high riding or boggy prostate; scrotum hematoma/ swelling
RUG—positive extravasation

Management

Extraperitoneal bladder rupture is demonstrated by a flame-shaped extravasation of contrast on the cystogram (Figure 8-2). It is managed nonoperatively. A cystogram should be repeated

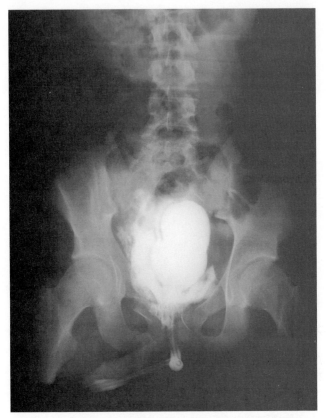

Figure 8-2 Extraperitoneal bladder rupture on cystogram.

later to determine closure of the rupture. A Foley catheter is adequate management for urine removal and results in fewer days of catheterization in comparison with management with a suprapubic tube (Holevar et al. 2004). Intraperitoneal bladder rupture requires operative repair and drainage of the extravasated urine. The pelvic hematoma is left intact.

With suspected urethral injury, a Foley catheter is not placed to avoid converting a partial injury into a full tear. Urethral injury that is anterior is managed nonoperatively with the placement of a catheter and suprapubic tube. Posterior urethral injuries can be managed with delayed perineal reconstruction or primary endoscopic realignment. Primary realignment is more simple, provides a shorter time to spontaneous void, and a decreased incidence of stricture, thus avoiding future surgical urethroplasty (Hadjizacharia et al. 2008). Complications of posterior urethral injury in males include permanent impotence and/or incontinence and urethral stricture. Psychosocial support is needed for alterations in self-image and sexual function.

Catheter care/perineal care prevents infection from the indwelling and suprapubic catheters. Adequate fluid intake to maintain urine output also prevents bladder infection. The patient and family will need instruction in catheter care. Antispasmodic may help with bladder spasm.

Male Genitalia

The testes, scrotum, and penis as an entity are rarely injured although they are susceptible to penetrating trauma. Rapid identification of testicular injury is essential to the salvage of the testicle itself. Penis injury, although rare, can also occur from strangulation and can result in amputation.

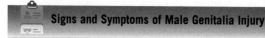

Signs and Symptoms of Male Genitalia Injury

Hematocele
Tender, enlarged scrotal mass/swelling
Scrotum fails to transilluminate
Scrotal avulsion may be present
Penis pain, swelling, discoloration, amputation
Penis will deviate away from the side of injury

Management

Testicular injury needs immediate surgical intervention to evacuate blood clots, examine the extent of injury, and repair. Occasionally orchiectomy is necessary if the injury cannot be repaired. Delay to treatment can result in testicular atrophy or infection.

Scrotal injury is amenable to repair or reconstruction. If avulsion of the scrotum is not able to be repaired, surgical implantation of the testes into the thigh allows preservation in this situation. The scrotum should be elevated on a towel roll and monitored to prevent decubiti with swelling. Swelling can also occur with pelvic fracture and no direct scrotal injury. The same care should be provided.

Penis injury has a high association with intra-abdominal injury. Total abdominal assessment should not be ignored in the presence of a penis injury. Penis injury can be managed nonoperatively with elevation, ice, and anti-inflammatory medication. Analgesia for pain is also essential. The hematoma may require surgical evacuation. In patients with amputation or partial amputation, surgical reattachment and monitoring for vascular stability is required. Complications include permanent deformity and/or inadequate erection. Psychosocial support may be needed for these alterations in self-image and sexual function.

SPECIAL SITUATIONS

Penetrating Abdominal Injury

Penetrating abdominal trauma can occur from stabbings, GSW, or impaled objects. Management of the impaled object is the most straightforward. The object should be stabilized until taken to surgery. In surgery, it is carefully removed with attention to injuries and bleeding. Repair then proceeds dependent upon the injuries identified. Figures 8-3 and 8-4 show injury that occurred when the victim fell through a glass shower door. The glass piece entered through the back and could be felt both anteriorly (where there was a small puncture) and posteriorly. Upon laparotomy to remove the glass, vascular injury was avoided and a small laceration to the jejunum was the only internal injury. The degree of

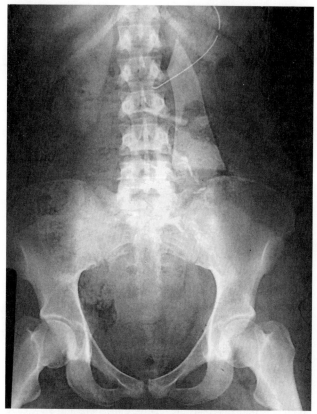

Figure 8-3   Penetrating injury of the abdomen with glass (A-P view).

injury cannot be predicted with impaled objects. Removal in surgery is the safe route to identify all possible injuries.

In the evaluation of penetrating injury from stabbing and GSW, hemodynamic instability and peritoneal signs are indications for laparotomy. In most patients, outside of tangential wounds, GSW are indications for surgery, especially because bowel injury is one of the most commonly associated injuries

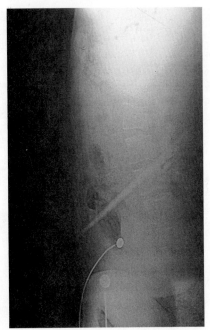

Figure 8-4 Penetrating injury of the abdomen with glass (lateral view).

and is not easily identifiable by CT, FAST, or DPL. Evisceration and retained foreign body are relative indications and may result in up to 50% nontherapeutic laparotomy (Clarke et al. 2008).

Other indications for laparotomy in penetrating abdominal trauma include an equivocal or unreliable examination such as those in head or spinal cord injuries, alcohol/drug presence, and sedation. If nonoperative management is chosen, serial examination is essential to identify changes and onset of peritoneal signs requiring laparotomy. Penetrating injuries to the right upper quadrant involve only lung, diaphragm, and liver. The surgeon may choose nonoperative management with a minimum of 24 hours of observation if the patient is hemodynamically stable with a reliable examination and minimal tenderness (Como et al. 2007).

Stab wounds are low velocity and frequently do not fully penetrate the abdomen. These are more amenable to observation as the likelihood of internal injury is lower. If the peritoneum is violated, the surgeon may choose to perform laparoscopy to identify injury. If negative, the wound is closed. If positive, the patient still needs a laparotomy for exploration and repair. If violation of the peritoneum is equivocal, laparoscopy can identify if the violation occurred or not. However laparoscopy does increase the patient's length of stay over nonoperative management (Leppaniemi and Haapiainen 2003). Anterior, flank, and posterior abdominal stab wounds can be explored locally to determine if fascia is penetrated. Flank and back wounds should also be evaluated with double contrast CT, both IV and a water-soluble enema.

In addition to identifying injury and performing necessary repair, a single dose of preoperative broad-spectrum antibiotics covering both anaerobic and aerobic bacteria should be administered. If after surgery no hollow viscus injury is found, no further antibiotics are necessary (Luchette et al. 2000). If hollow viscus injury is present, antibiotics should be continued for 24 hours.

Nonoperative management of any penetrating injury requires

- Close observation with serial examinations for peritoneal signs
- Monitoring hematocrit for evidence of bleeding
- Close monitoring of vital signs for any evidence of hemorrhage
- Local wound care

In the case of laparotomy for penetrating wounds, if the incision can avoid the actual wound, it allows the wound to remain for forensic evaluation (Lynch 2006). If cutting through the wound is inevitable, photographs of the wound prior to surgery will assist forensic evaluation of this exigent evidence. During the laparotomy, a search for the bullet also occurs. If the foreign body is found, it is picked up with the gloved finger or rubber-tipped forceps to avoid marking the bullet, which already carries the characteristics of the weapon from which it was fired. The bullet is placed in a cotton-lined specimen cup, labeled, sealed, and handed to police. A chain of custody form must be completed to maintain the integrity of the retrieval.

Laparotomy and Damage Control Surgery

Decision-making for laparotomy or laparoscopy is made by the surgeon and based upon the stability of the patient as well as the type of injury itself. Injuries to the abdomen that require laparotomy include

- Blunt trauma with hypotension, peritoneal signs, positive DPL, FAST
- Any penetrating trauma with hypotension
- GSW that enters the peritoneum
- Evisceration
- Hollow viscus injury, intraperitoneal bladder injury
- Peritonitis, evidence of free air
- Blunt rupture of the diaphragm

When the abdomen is opened for laparotomy, not only is an exploration performed but also immediate control of bleeding is undertaken. Packs are placed in the four quadrants to tamponade bleeding and then careful exploration is begun. It is essential that injuries are identified and then rapidly managed. The purpose of damage control surgery is to obtain "control" of hemorrhage and contamination while preventing or avoiding hypothermia and coagulopathy. This may mean leaving packs and delaying some procedures, for example, the colon is resected but reanastomosis and colostomy are left for the relaparotomy.

The patient is returned to critical care where he or she is warmed and resuscitation is continued. Any coagulopathy is controlled. The patient is critically ill throughout the initial surgery and upon arrival to the ICU. Often, because of the body's response to injury and inflammation, the belly may be left open as well with only temporary closure. In these patients, the gut is usually edematous and cannot be returned to the abdominal cavity. Leaving the abdomen open allows the gut to progress through the edema without the pressure of the abdominal wall, resulting in ischemia. The patient will return to the operating room (OR) for washout, reexploration, a staged procedure or repacking, and return. Over time, the procedures are completed, hemorrhage is controlled, and the gut returned to the abdominal cavity without loss from necrosis/ischemia.

During the time in ICU in the postoperative period

- Resuscitate to normalize base deficit or return lactate to <2.5 mMol/L
  — Continue to monitor for ischemia of the gut
  — Although the abdomen is open, ACS can occur
- Prevent hypothermia
- Administer coagulation products as needed
- Maintain/attain hemodynamic stability
  — Monitor for continued hemorrhage
  — Maintain ventilation, prevent hypoxia, acidosis
- Manage pain and sedation for comfort and ventilation

Abdominal Compartment Syndrome

Abdominal compartment syndrome (ACS) is like compartment syndrome in any part of the body. As pressure increases in a nonexpandable space, the pressure is reflected back upon the organs within the cavity. Decreased venous and arterial flow in this case, to the abdominal organs and vasculature as well as the diaphragm is affected. ACS affects lung expansion as the diaphragm attempts to push against abdominal pressure during inspiration. Table 8-4 describes the signs and symptoms of ACS.

Patients predisposed to ACS include those with acidosis, hypothermia, transfusion of RBC consisting of >10 units within a 24 hour period, coagulopathy, sepsis, and mechanical ventilation with positive end-expiratory pressure (PEEP) (An and West 2008) Common causes are abdominal surgery, massive fluid resuscitation, and hemoperitoneum (An and West 2008). ACS is classified by cause and it is also recognized that patients without abdominal injury and even nontrauma critical patients may experience ACS. The classification includes

Table 8-4   Abdominal Compartment Syndrome

Region	Signs and Symptoms
Abdomen	Ileus ↑ abdominal girth Tense, severe distention ↑ intra-abdominal pressure Bowel ischemia
Renal	↓ urine output ↓ GFR ↑ creatinine IAP >30 mm Hg—oliguria unresponsive to diuretics
Pulmonary	↑ peak inspiratory pressure ↓ tidal volume with decreased diaphragm excursion ↓ compliance Hypercapnia Prone to ARDS and pneumonia
Cardiac	↓ cardiac output Hypotension due to decreased venous return ↑ SVR ↑ CVP due to increased thoracic pressure
Liver	↑ LFT Coagulopathy

- Primary ACS—caused by injury, hemorrhage, visceral edema
- Secondary ACS—due to volume resuscitation, edema, ascites
- Recurrent ACS—after secondary ACS, further edema and ischemia

Definitions of ACS describe what is occurring with the intra-abdominal pressure (IAP). Pressures >12 mm Hg result in organ dysfunction. Pressures consistently >20 mm Hg result in organ failure.

- Normal IAP <7 mm Hg
- Intra-abdominal hypertension >12 mm Hg
- ACS >20 mm Hg

Abdominal perfusion pressure (APP) like cerebral perfusion pressure is an indicator of sufficient oxygenation to the organs within that cavity. APP is calculated in the same way

$$MAP - IAP = APP$$

APP is expected to be >60 mm Hg to maintain appropriate organ-saving perfusion. At this point APP may not be used as often as the IAP, however the concept and understanding of the effect of the pressure are well described by the arithmetic.

Measurement of IAP is best achieved through the Foley catheter, using the bladder as a pressure balloon to reflect (indirect measurement) the intra-abdominal pressure. The patient should be supine. The catheter is then connected to a manometer or transducer system. The process involves the instillation of ~50 mL NSS into the Foley after clamping the catheter. The pressure is read after zeroing the system to the midaxillary line. In some facilities, the symphysis may still be used to zero the system. There are commercial kits that connect directly to the monitor system which can then read the IAP by actuation of the valve attached to the system. The system is closed and demonstrates the pressure wave directly on the monitor (the wave is flat). It is important to remember that whether using a commercial product or not, any hospital can measure intra-abdominal pressure and identify this life-threatening situation early.

Management

The one method of management for ACS is surgical decompression of the abdomen. As with the brain and muscle compartments, room must be provided for the swelling. Decompressive surgery provides room in the abdomen which then allows arterial blood flow and resolution of ischemia that may have been occurring until that point. ACS is a life-threatening situation that must be rapidly identified and treated. Diligent monitoring of the critically ill patient must include abdominal evaluation. Once decompression has been achieved, reperfusion syndrome can occur, especially if ACS was initially unrecognized or allowed to progress. Volume loading the patient to washout the lactate will assist with reperfusion.

Once the abdomen is decompressed, typically it is left open for edema to subside and to prevent recurrent ACS. This is particularly important if acidosis, hypothermia, or coagulopathy is present. Reexploration for missed injury or bleeding will occur within the next few days. As the edema resolves, abdominal closure is the next order of business. There are a number of methods to accomplish closure

- Vacuum-assisted closure device (VAC)—may be attached at the time of the first surgery to gradually close the space
  - The device is changed approximately every 3 days or at the time of reexploration and washout
  - It may require up to three changes to bring the edges of the incision closed (Bee et al. 2008)
  - Delayed primary closure is usually possible
- Mesh
  - Checked daily and cinched to slowly bring the edges together over time
  - Delayed primary closure is usually possible
- Wittmann Patch (Star Surgical)
  - Consists of two adherent sheets sewn to the opposing fascia
  - Sequentially opposed decreasing the defect
  - Results in delayed primary closure
- Split thickness skin graft (STSG)
  - When delayed primary closure cannot be accomplished and a defect remains

Postoperative management for ACS is as with damage control surgery. This patient is critical and requires

- Prevention of hypothermia because open, exposed bowel even under a bag or mesh or VAC will rapidly cool the body
- Management of coagulopathy
- Prevention of acidosis
- Maintenance of ventilation and oxygenation
- Continued resuscitation, especially in light of reperfusion
- Skin monitoring to prevent breakdown

- Maintenance of the VAC device if used
- Provide nutrition for healing

Short-term goals include minimal to no organ dysfunction including ischemic bowel, decreasing bowel edema, and repair of injuries without infection. The long-term goal is delayed primary closure of the abdomen with minimal to no defect. Abdominal wall herniation is a possible complication later.

Acute Pancreatitis

Acute pancreatitis is not a common complication but may occur with pancreatic and duodenal injury, hypotension, and multiorgan dysfunction syndrome. Pancreatitis is an autodigestive state caused by premature activation of enzymes causing edema, hemorrhage, vascular damage, and fat necrosis. A mild inflammatory state may occur, which resolves within a few days. Necrotizing pancreatitis may present like sepsis, including hemodynamic instability.

Signs and Symptoms of Acute Pancreatitis

Abdominal pain radiating to the back
Pain increases with supine position
Nausea, vomiting
Fever, weakness
Abdominal distention, peritonitis
Dyspnea, bronchoconstriction
Tachycardia, vasodilation
Increased amylase initially, decreases within 24 hours
Increased lipase remains elevated up to 14 days (more specific)

Management

Mild interstitial pancreatitis can be managed with bowel rest, hydration, and pain management. Nutrition is always a concern with pancreatitis, and can be provided enterally via jejunal feeds beyond the ligament of Treitz.

For more severe pancreatitis, management includes nutritional needs, resting the bowel as well as maintaining hemodynamic stability.

- Monitor hemodynamics
  - Administer fluids
  - Fluid loss can be significant with the patient requiring hemodynamic support
- Manage pulmonary status
  - Patient is at risk for pleural effusions, ARDS, atelectasis, pneumonia
  - Provide pulmonary support; may require mechanical ventilation if pulmonary complications occur
- Nutrition
  - Nothing by mouth (NPO), bowel rest
  - Nasogastric tube; manage nausea and vomiting
  - Feed via jejunal tube past the ligament of Treitz
  - Total parenteral nutrition (TPN) if cannot provide enteral feeds
  - Hyperglycemia accompanies pancreatitis; strict glycemic control is necessary
- Antibiotics
  - Broad spectrum
  - Capable of penetrating the pancreas
- Pain management
  - Opiates

Acalculous Cholecystitis

After burns and major trauma, an uncommon and unexplained complication is acalculous cholecystitis. This complication causes the gallbladder to respond with inflammation in the same way it would in the presence of stones. Acalculous cholecystitis can also occur in patients on long-term TPN, usually >3 months.

An ultrasound will diagnose bile stasis and gallbladder ischemia. Necrosis and perforation can result from this condition.

Signs and Symptoms of Acalculous Cholecystitis

Abdominal pain/tenderness in right upper quadrant
Fever
Nausea, vomiting
Elevated WBC count
Elevated aspartate aminotransferase (AST)

Management

Care of the patient with acalculous cholecystitis requires cholecystectomy. If the patient is a high-risk surgical candidate, endoscopic gallbladder stent may be placed during ERCP to temporize the situation. Patients also benefit from

- NPO status with IV fluid resuscitation
- Antibiotic coverage for biliary and enteric coverage
- Manage hemodynamic instability
- Early identification and cholecystectomy

Acute Renal Injury and Renal Failure

Acute kidney injury (AKI) is a syndrome, not simply renal failure or acute tubular necrosis. The syndrome acknowledges that azotemia and oliguria are the body's normal response to decreased renal flow and volume depletion. Sustained AKI results in alterations in electrolytes, fluid balance, and acid-base balance. Injury to the tubules impairs the concentrating ability of the kidney causing nonoliguric renal failure. Acute tubular necrosis occurs when ischemia is followed by reperfusion as in coagulation disorders, systemic inflammation, and sepsis. Sepsis itself is the leading cause of acute renal failure (Kellum 2008).

The current criteria for defining acute kidney injury are described as the RIFLE criteria (risk, injury, failure, loss, and end-stage kidney classification) (Kellum 2008). The criteria evaluate creatinine, glomerular filtration rate (GFR), and urine output to determine the degree of damage to the kidneys.

- Kidneys at risk have an increased creatinine 1.5 times normal, a decreased GFR by at least 25%, and a urine output less than normal (0.5 mL/kg/hour) for 6 hours
- Kidneys demonstrating injury have a creatinine 2 times normal, a decreased GFR by at least 50%, and a urine output less than normal for 12 hours
- Renal failure is defined by creatinine 3 times normal, a decreased GFR by >75%, and a urine output <0.3 mL/kg/hour for 24 hours or anuria for 12 hours
- Kidney loss is persistent acute renal failure with complete loss of renal function for >4 weeks; which will result in end-stage renal disease

Renal failure is rooted in one of three sources: prerenal, intrarenal, or postrenal. Because of the significant hypotension after injury, the trauma patient is at significant risk for prerenal failure. Prevention of renal failure involves prevention of the common causes. In trauma, these causes would typically be injury itself, hypotension, rhabdomyolysis, nephrotoxic medications, infection, and possibly ureteral obstruction. Prerenal failure does not involve kidney damage. The source is completely outside the kidney.

Symptoms indicating prerenal failure include

- Increased BUN with less of an increase in creatinine
- Urine sodium <10 mMol/L
- Increased specific gravity >1.020
- May or may not have proteinuria
- Possible presence of myoglobin

Manage prerenal failure by securing hemodynamic stability, control coagulopathy, and hemorrhage control. Prerenal failure will correct itself through critical management of the trauma patient.

Intrarenal failure is caused by kidney damage, which includes trauma, infection, hypertensive disease, autoimmune response, nephrotoxins, and rhabdomyolysis. Management of intrarenal failure requires identification of the cause and removal of that cause. Identify any source of infection and evaluate antibiotics and other medications for nephrotoxicity. Monitor urine for myoglobin, especially in patients with crush injury, multiple injuries, or who may have had a prolonged period of immobility prior to arrival at the hospital.

Postrenal failure is associated with ureteral obstruction or issues with the bladder and urethra causing back pressure into the kidneys. Evaluation to identify obstruction includes

- Elevation of BUN and creatinine
- Urinary infection
- Radiographic evidence of obstruction

Treatment for postrenal failure involves removal of the obstruction. All types of AKI treatment involve maximizing perfusion and electrolyte balance, provide adequate nutrition, and prevent causes of renal failure when possible. As AKI progresses through initial dysfunction to healing, oliguria is one of the first signs along with alterations in electrolytes, creatinine, and GFR. Other systems are also involved including

- Altered level of consciousness
- Hypertension, tachycardia
- Pitting edema
- Pulmonary edema
- Nausea

The oliguric phase moves into a diuretic phase as renal function recovers. As with the oliguric phase, other body systems are affected as well including

- Continued altered level of consciousness, possible seizures, restlessness
- Hypotension from fluid loss, tachycardia, dysrhythmias
- Tachypnea
- Nausea

With the best efforts to remove the cause and balance hemo-dynamics, there are times when the kidneys need assistance through the AKI period. Some studies demonstrate that survival is improved and the incidence of sepsis and multisystem organ failure decreased if renal replacement therapy (RRT) is initiated when the BUN is <60 mg/dL (Palevsky 2008). Indications for RRT include

- Increasing vascular volume unresponsive to diuretics
- Increasing potassium unresponsive to medical management
- Unresponsive metabolic acidosis
- Uremic encephalopathy, pericarditis, uremic bleeding
- Progressive azotemia (Palevsky 2008)

The type of dialysis or RRT is dependent upon the state of the patient and his or her capabilities. Peritoneal dialysis is portable and simple; however it requires an intact peritoneum and a large number of critical trauma patients with AKI have had abdominal injury, damage control surgery, and/or ACS with decompression. It is also a slow process and thus less effective in severe and acute renal failure in trauma.

Continuous renal replacement therapy (CRRT) provides a dialysis circuit that is extracorporeal and managed by the critical care nurse 24 hours a day. The system may provide improved renal recovery over intermittent renal replacement therapy (hemodialysis) as it avoids rapid and severe fluid changes and does not cause hypotension during therapy (Uchino 2008). Intermittent therapy may lead to periods of renal ischemia which also lengthens renal recovery time (Uchino 2008). CRRT provides slow continuous solute removal reducing issues with medication and fluid administration. The setup may require anticoagulation which may be contraindicated in trauma patients. Continuous hemodynamic monitoring and maintenance is essential to prevent too rapid removal of fluid resulting in hypotension.

Hemodialysis is intermittent therapy daily or on a schedule tolerated by the patient and dependent on fluid and electrolyte balance. It is an effective and efficient means of lowering electrolytes and waste products in the body as well as excess fluid removal. It can, however, result in hypotension and periods of excess electrolytes and waste between treatments. The rapid fluid shifts can also result in seizures, nausea and vomiting, and altered level of consciousness. Medication administration must be carefully scheduled around treatments to prevent immediate elimination of a medication cleared by the kidney if administered to close to time of treatment.

With any choice of dialysis, medications cleared by the kidneys, primarily antibiotics, need levels monitored to ensure that a therapeutic level is attained but not a toxic one. Fluid balance is a continuous process between fluids administered, dialysate, and fluids recovered. This is a one-to-one patient in critical care requiring undivided attention to all details of care. Nutrition is essential to promote healing and renal recovery. Formulas designed specifically for the injured kidney are essential to this process. As renal recovery develops, labs normalize as does output. Total recovery, however, can take up to a year. In some patients, AKI is complete renal failure and remains permanent. These patients will require hemodialysis for their lifetime.

POSTRESUSCITATION MANAGEMENT AND REHABILITATION

Nutrition

Trauma induces a hypermetabolic state that is in place even before the patient arrives in the emergency department. The hypermetabolic state is initiated by

- Cortisol release
  - Guards against a reduction in blood glucose
  - Mobilizes amino acid release from muscle and liver
  - Increases enzymes needed for amino acid release for tissue repair
  - Decreases T lymphocytes, increasing risk of infection
- Endogenous opiates (pituitary)

— Encephalins and endorphins provide analgesia and inhibition of pain
- Vasopressin (pituitary)
  — Increases water absorption in distal renal tubules to maintain blood volume
  — Concentrates urine
- Renin-angiotensin system (kidney)
  — Angiotensin—releases aldosterone to increase sodium resorption with potassium and hydrogen ion excretion
  — Renin—causes vasoconstriction to maintain blood pressure
- Sympathetic nervous system
  — Releases epinephrine and norepinephrine causing
    - Pupil dilation
    - Tachycardia
    - Bronchial dilation
    - Mucous membrane arteriole constriction
    - Dilation of sweat glands
    - Decreases gastrointestinal (GI) motility

The goal of nutritional therapy is to support organ and cellular function, prevent malnutrition, protect protein mass, and promote healing. To meet these goals, nutrition needs must be met and initiated early. Multiple nutrients are required for health and healing. Briefly these include

- Protein
  — Supports enzymes; tissue growth/healing; immunity; gluconeogenesis
- Carbohydrates
  — Source of energy, especially for the brain/spine
- Fats
  — Required for fat-soluble vitamin absorption; cell growth/repair
- Vitamins
  — Fat soluble (A, D, E, K)

- Immunity; calcium absorption for bone mineralization; clotting factor synthesis
— Water soluble (C)
  - Supports formation of collagen; iron absorption; prevents oxidation of lipids and proteins; formation of dopamine
— Water soluble (B vitamins)
  - Metabolism of proteins and therapeutic drugs; gluconeogenesis; cell mediated immunity; synthesis of steroids
- Minerals (zinc, manganese, selenium, copper, iron)
  — Required for cell growth and repair; production of urea; oxygen transport
- Minerals (calcium, phosphorus, magnesium)
  — Bone mineralization; muscle contraction and nerve conduction; clotting
- Water
  — Necessary for delivery of nutrients throughout the body and removal of waste; required to maintain normothermia
- Fiber
  — Maintains colon health; maintains gut integrity to prevent bacterial translocation

From the time of arrival of the patient, one of the most important orders of business is assessment of nutritional needs and initiation of therapy as soon as the patient can tolerate feeds. Obviously oral nutrition is optimal; however the critical trauma patient is usually intubated and/or neurologically abnormal and thus unable to feed by mouth. Optimal nutrition is then by the enteral method with the goal of wound healing and sepsis prevention (Jacobs et al. 2004, Mazuski 2008). Feeding with TPN carries higher risk for sepsis than with enteral feeds.

For head-injured patients, early enteral feeds are also recommended with parenteral feeds as a second choice only (Jacobs et al. 2004). If enteral feeds in head-injured or seriously multisystem-injured trauma patients cannot be initiated with 7 days of arrival, TPN should be started until enteral feeds are tolerated. When >50% of enteral feedings is tolerated, the TPN should be weaned (Jacobs et al. 2004).

It is difficult to measure nutritional balance in the critically ill trauma patient as changes occur that affect labs, causing abnormality that may not be caused by nutrition alone.

- Albumin levels have a prolonged turnover (as long as 20 days) leaving them insensitive to acute needs
- Prealbumin can be affected by the administration of blood products, which also contain prealbumin; falsely altering the prealbumin level
- Urea nitrogen reflects severity of injury
- Nitrogen excretion peaks when total body protein loss peaks (~5-10 days after injury)
  — Include diarrhea, vomiting, fistula drainage into the estimation of nitrogen loss

Energy needs are determined starting with the resting energy expenditure. Basal metabolic rate (BMR) is the calculated energy needed to maintain the awake, resting state. It is expressed as kcal/minute with a kcal equal to the amount of energy needed to increase water temperature by 1°C (at 1 ATA). As caregivers, factors affecting energy expenditure should be taken into account.

- Increased energy expenditure—injury and healing, agitation, shivering, any physical activity or stressful procedure, autonomic hyperexcitability, hypertonia, fever
- Decreased energy expenditure—neuromuscular blockade, sedation, pain management, anesthesia, bed rest, therapeutic hypothermia (with prevention of shivering), SCI

The critically ill patient may tolerate slight underfeeding better than overfeeding, although the patient who needs to gain weight after the critical phase will need slight overfeeding. Feedings are available in a multitude of varieties including options for TPN that can be tailored to meet the individual patient's needs. Whichever feeding is chosen, it must be well-rounded and include protein, lipid, vitamin and mineral, as well as fluid needs. If the patient arrives with a preexisting problem with alcohol addiction, thiamine is usually added to the IV solutions as there is typically a deficiency of thiamine in this particular situation. The nutrition support team provides careful monitoring of the nutrients provided by monitoring

- Electrolytes
- Glucose—excess can result not only in hyperglycemia but in hypertriglyceridemia and hypercapnea
- Prealbumin levels
- Careful calculation of proteins administered
  - Refeeding syndrome occurs when normal or above normal amounts of protein are fed to a patient after a prolonged starvation mode
    - Feed these patients at 40% to 60% of the total calculated proteins
    - The pancreas and liver will not be able to tolerate a normal rate of protein administration after the prolonged lack of feeding
    - Evidence of refeeding syndrome include azotemia, dehydration, and metabolize acidosis
    - Overfeeding protein in tube feedings also results in the same

Feeding Methods

Enteral feeds, which are the optimal source of nutrition for the trauma patient, can be initiated through the gastric tube initially placed during resuscitation. This is not the optimal feeding tube, but can be used. The caregivers need to be aware that a rigid, large bore tube like a nasogastric tube may leave the cardiac sphincter slightly open predisposing the patient to regurgitation, esophagitis, and aspiration. Optimal feeding rules include

- Insertion of a narrow, weighted feeding tube that can remain in the stomach or be placed post-pyloric into the duodenum (minimum 105 cm length tube)
  — A flat abdominal plain film is done postplacement to identify the position of the tube
  — Coughing with insertion indicates improper placement; the tube must be immediately repositioned
  — Mark the tube for position at the nose (or mouth if oral), secure, and monitor for movement. Slippage out of the gut by ≥1 inch requires reexamination by radiograph for position check
  — Tubes should be cleaned, skin observed for pressure, and resecured daily to prevent skin breakdown
  — Tube placement check with instillation of air should be done routinely as well as after moving the patient (eg, to OR), change of shift, addition of new feeds
  — Flush the tube with water every 6 hours and with each tube feed change, administration of medications, and if tube feedings are held
    - Obstruction of the tube can be avoided by simple routine flushing with water and careful medication administration
    - Warm water flush may clear an obstruction from the tube
    - Choose suspensions, liquids, elixirs over syrups for medication administration to prevent obstruction
      ○ If crushing a medication be sure it is finely crushed and dissolved in ~30 mL of warm water
      ○ Do not crush or administer sustained release or enteric-coated medications through the feeding tube (or gastric tube)
      ○ Be aware of any medication-nutrient reactions and avoid mixing feeds with these medications (eg, phenytoin)
      ○ Hold feeds for these medications up to 30 minutes prior and up to 2 hours after administering the medication (check with pharmacy for medication specific holds)

- ○ Account for these holds in tube feedings when calculating total enteral intake
  - — If stopping tube feeds, flush the tube immediately after ending the feeds to clear the tube
- For feeds that will likely exceed 3 to 4 weeks (severe head-injured patients), a gastrostomy tube is placed into the stomach. If the patient does not tolerate gastric feeds or is experiencing pancreatitis, a feeding tube can be threaded through the percutaneous gastrostomy (PEG) into the jejunum (past the ligament of Treitz)
  - — Patients with postpyloric or jejunal feeds may still require a gastric tube to low intermittent wall suction to decompress the stomach
  - — Gastrostomy sites also need daily cleansing, skin observation for breakdown or leak, and redress the site with dry gauze
- If there is potential for feeding issues identified on the initial laparotomy, a jejunostomy feeding tube may be placed immediately in anticipation of needing to feed the jejunum directly
- Aspiration risk can be reduced by
  - — Elevation of the head of the bed (if allowed) to 45 degrees or >30 degrees (if allowed)
  - — Monitor gastric residuals
    - Check residuals every 2 to 4 hours, even after the patient appears to be tolerating the feeds
    - Gastric residuals >500 mL require a hold on the feeds
    - Reassess tolerance and rate of feeds
    - Assess for ileus
    - Absent bowel sounds or diarrhea are not reasons to withhold tube feeds (McQuillan et al. 2009)
  - — Monitor tube placement
  - — Pro-motility agents (eg, metoclopromide) decrease gastric reflux
  - — Balance narcotics with pain management
    - Narcotics slow bowel activity, causing constipation and ileus

- Tube feeds begin slowly to determine tolerance of the formula as well as volume
  — Initiate at ~25% of the goal rate (~20-40 mL/hour)
  — Increase slowly over the next 4 to 8 hours at a rate of 20 to 25 mL/hour until the full goal is reached
  — Full strength formula should be used
- Maintain glycemic control (Chapter 13)
- Monitor electrolytes and renal function

Parenteral nutrition is necessary when the patient cannot tolerate tube feedings and feeding has already been delayed up to 7 days. The patient must, however, be able to tolerate the fluid intake required to achieve nutritional support and have adequate access.

- Peripheral parenteral nutrition (PPN) can be administered via a peripheral line and is provided for a short period of time, <1 week
  — Extravasation, phlebitis, and thrombosis can complicate PPN administration
  — Less likely to cause hyperglycemia and other metabolic abnormalities as TPN
  — Change catheter sites every 72 to 96 hours
  — Check the bag with the orders for accuracy prior to administration
  — Store in the refrigerator until ~2 hours prior to administration; allow to warm to room temperature
- TPN is needed for the seriously ill trauma patient with longer term nutritional needs who is not tolerating enteral feeds
  — Increased incidence of sepsis and bacteremia
    ▪ Mitigated by isolating the line for TPN and using it solely for TPN (McQuillan et al. 2009)
  — Requires a central line due to the hyperosmolarity of the TPN
  — Check the bag with the orders for accuracy prior to administration; typical formula includes
    ▪ Amino acids, vitamins and minerals, glucose, electrolytes, trace elements

- Lipids are administered separately to supplement and complete the diet
- Insulin and H_2 blockers may also be included in the TPN formulation
— Store in the refrigerator until ~2 hours prior to administration; allow to warm to room temperature
— Check for particles, cloudiness, or any leak in the bag—do not administer
— Change tubing every 24 hours
— Lipid tubing should be changed every 12 hours
  - Infusion of lipids is done slowly usually over 12 hours
  - Symptoms of rapid infusion include tachypnea, wheezing, palpitations, cyanosis, headache
— Account for the lipids in medications (eg, propofol)

The final goal is to transition the patient to oral intake. Some patients, such as severe head injured patients, may leave the trauma center to a rehabilitation facility with gastric feeds still in place. For others, as they awaken, transition to extubation, and move toward intermediate care, they are ready to try oral intake. Factors to remember include

- Speech therapy consults evaluate not only speech and communication skills but swallowing as well
  — Assess prior to attempting oral feeds
  — Food texture affects swallowing ability
  — Initiate feeds with type and texture of feeds recommended by the therapist
  — As the patient improves, progress to regular diet as recommended by speech
- Wean enteral feeds as oral intake begins
  — Initiate night-only feeds if the patient is not hungry during the day to encourage appetite
- Once oral intake is initiated
  — Account for percentage and types of foods eaten
  — Provide more frequent, smaller meals if three larger meals are not tolerated well

— Provide supplements to add calories and nutrients

- The needs of the patient may exceed the actual amount of food required
- Smaller frequent meals with supplements may meet the ability of the patient to eat and the needs to be met
- May need to continue supplemental enteral feeds at night to meet nutritional requirements

For the patient with abdominal injury, a serious life-threatening situation exists at the time of arrival. Rapid decision making must occur to manage airway, breathing, and circulation and then determine the best course of action for managing the abdominal injury. In the best case scenario, nonoperative management is successful, without ileus, and nutritional balance is attained. In the most difficult, the surgeon must resort to damage control surgery, multiple reoperations for the open abdomen, and final closure. Potential complications such as hemorrhage, pancreatitis, ischemic bowel, and sepsis are as dangerous as the initial life-threatening injury.

 Critical Lifesavers

- For any patient who is hypotensive, a trip to the CT scanner is unacceptable
- Observe the urinary meatus for bleeding—indicates urethral injury; DO NOT place a Foley catheter
- Head CT must be done prior to any administration of contrast

REFERENCES

American College of Surgeons. *Advanced Trauma Life Support* (ATLS). 7th ed. Chicago, IL: American College of Surgeons; 2004.
American College of Surgeons. *Advanced Trauma Life Support* (ATLS). 8th ed. Chicago, IL: American College of Surgeons; 2008.

An G, West M. Abdominal compartment syndrome: a concise clinical review. *Crit Care Med.* 2008;36(4):1304-1310.

Asensio JA, Gambaro E, Forno W, et al. Duodenal and pancreatic injuries-complex and lethal injuries. *J Trauma Nurs.* 2001;8(2):47-49.

Association for the Advancement of Automotive Medicine. *Abbreviated Injury Scale (AIS) 2005.* Barrington, IL: AAAM; rev. 2008.

Bee TK, Croce MA, Magnotti LJ, et al. Temporary abdominal closure techniques: a prospective randomized trial comparing polyglactin 910 mesh and vacuum-assisted closure. *J Trauma.* 2008;65(2):337-344.

Cayten CG, Fabian TC, Garcia VF, et al. Practice management guidelines for penetrating intraperitoneal colon injuries. *J Trauma.* 1998;44(6):941-956.

Clarke S, Stearns A, Payne C, et al. The impact of published recommendations on the management of penetrating abdominal injury. *Br J Surg.* 2008;95(4):515-521.

Como JJ, Bokhari F, Chiu WC, et al. Practice management guidelines for nonoperative management of penetrating abdominal trauma. 2007. Available at: http://www.EAST.org. Accessed September 18, 2008.

Duchesne JC, Schmieg R, Islam S, et al. Selective nonoperative management of low-grade blunt pancreatic injury: are we there yet? *J Trauma.* 2008;65(1):49-53.

Ekeh AP, Saxe J, Waiusimbi M, et al. Diagnosis of blunt intestinal and mesenteric injury in the era of multidetector CT technology: are results better? *J Trauma.* 2008;65(2):354-359.

Hadjizacharia P, Inaba K, Teixeira PGR, et al. Evaluation of immediate endoscopic realignment as a treatment modality for traumatic urethral injuries. *J Trauma.* 2008;64(6):1443-1450.

Holevar M, DiGiacomo C, Ebert J, et al. Practice management guidelines for the evaluation of genitourinary trauma. 2003. Available at: http://www.EAST.org. Accessed September 18, 2008.

Holevar M, Ebert J, Luchette F, et al. Practice management guidelines for the management of genitourinary trauma. 2004. Available at: http://www.EAST.org. Accessed September 18, 2008.

Jacobs DG, Jacobs DO, Kudsk KA, et al. Practice management guidelines for nutritional support of the trauma patient. *J Trauma.* 2004;57(3):660-679.

Johnson CM, Hughes KM. Pseudohyperkalemia secondary to post splenectomy thrombocytosis. *Ann Surg.* 2001;67(2):168-170.

Kellum JA. Acute kidney injury. *Crit Care Med.* 2008;36(4):S141-S145.

Leppaniemi A, Haapiainen R. Diagnostic laparoscopy in abdominal stab wounds: a prospective randomized study. *J Trauma.* 2003;55(4):636-645.

Luchette FA, Borzotta AP, Croce MA, et al. Practice management guidelines for prophylactic antibiotic use in penetrating abdominal trauma. *J Trauma.* 2000;48(3):508-518.

Lynch V. *Forensic Nursing.* St Louis, MO: Elsevier Mosby; 2006.

Mazuski JE. Feeding the injured intestine: enteral nutrition in the critically ill patient. *Curr Opin Crit Care.* 2008;14(4):432-437.

McQuillan KA, Flynn Makic MB, Whalen E. *Trauma Nursing from Resuscitation Through Rehabilitation.* 4th ed. St Louis, MO: Saunders Elsevier; 2009.

Myers J. Focused assessment with sonography for trauma (FAST): the truth about ultrasound in blunt trauma. *J Trauma.* 2007;62(6):S28.

Palevsky PM. Indications and timing of renal replacement therapy in acute kidney injury. *Crit Care Med.* 2008;36(4):S224-S227.

Ruffolo DL. Delayed splenic rupture: understanding the threat. *J Trauma.* 2002;9(2):34-40.

Savage S, Zarzaur B, Magnotti L, et al. The evolution of blunt splenic injury: resolution and progression. *J Trauma.* 2008;64(4):1085-1092.

Uchino S. Choice of therapy and renal recovery. *Crit Care Med.* 2008;36(4):S238-S242.

Wei B, Hemmila MR, Arabi S, et al. Angioembolization reduces operative intervention for blunt splenic injury. *J Trauma.* 2008;64(6):1472-1477.

Yanar H, Ertekin C, Taviloglu K, et al. Nonoperative treatment of multiple intra-abdominal solid organ injury after blunt abdominal trauma. *J Trauma.* 2008;64(4):943-948.

Ziglar M, Bennett V, Nayduch D, et al. *The Electronic Library of Trauma Lectures.* Chicago, IL: Society of Trauma Nurses; 2004.

Ziran BH, Chamberlin E, Shuler FD, et al. Delays and difficulties in the diagnosis of lower urologic injuries in the context of pelvic fractures. *J Trauma.* 2005;58(3):533-537.

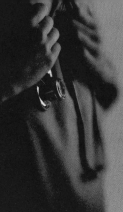

Chapter 9

ORTHOPAEDIC INJURY

INTRODUCTION

Because there are bones in every part of the body, fractures and other orthopaedic injuries are the most frequent injuries. The injuries range from simple sprains and strains of ligaments and tendons to severe open fractures and hemorrhage. Near every bone lies a nerve, artery, and vein, managing movement, nutrition, and oxygenation. This chapter discusses the management of orthopaedic injuries, several significant but less common musculoskeletal injuries, and some complications related to orthopaedic trauma.

ASSESSMENT

The assessment of orthopaedic injuries begins as all trauma assessment does. Attention to the mechanism of injury identifies potential injuries as well as the observations of the prehospital personnel who have likely identified some deformities and initiated scene management of them. The trauma primary survey begins with airway, breathing, and circulation, leaving the majority of orthopaedic injury for the secondary assessment. One caveat to this standard is the identification of loss of pulses in an extremity. As primary survey issues are managed concurrently with identification, so too the extremity without pulses. This may necessitate reduction of a fracture or joint dislocation or may be the indication of a vascular injury needing definition and operative management. The backboard initially provides some stability to extremity fractures. During the primary survey, the backboard may be sufficient to stabilize injuries that were not splinted at the scene. This is only a temporizing measure as the backboard has its own complications of skin breakdown.

History

The patient's history includes all of the expected measures regarding allergy, medications, past medical and surgical problems, last menstrual period, and last meal. If the patient is stable, the surgeons may elect to take the patient immediately to the operating room (OR) for fracture management. The time of last meal is important for the anesthesiologist intubating and managing the patient intraoperatively.

Other relevant history to the orthopaedic injury includes

- Mechanism of injury: blunt
  — Speed of vehicle
  — Restraint use
  — Passenger compartment intrusion and damage and the patient's position in relationship to the damage
  — Height of fall with or without any impact en route to the ground
  — If ground-level fall, especially of the elderly, was there an impact with an object; did they strike their head; in what position did they land; could they move afterward and if not how long since the fall
  — Sports: event resulting in injury, sport played, associated injuries
  — Assaults and being struck by objects
- Mechanism of injury: penetrating
  — Type of weapon
  — Distance from the weapon
  — Any blast effect

- Complaints of
  - Pain: type, intensity, relieved by positioning?
  - Tenderness to touch
  - Inability to move or bear weight
  - Guarding the extremity, limping
  - Swelling
  - Loss of function

- History of
  - Anticoagulants
  - Orthopaedic disorders (eg, osteoporosis, leg-length discrepancies, osteogenesis imperfecta)
  - Gait disorders (eg, stroke with residual deficit, Charcot-Marie-Tooth disease)
  - Orthopaedic injuries
  - Parathyroid disorders (loss of bone density)
  - Previous fractures/dislocations
  - Hardware placement. Total joint replacements

- Previous mobility status
  - Independent
  - With assistive device
  - With partial assistance
  - Totally dependent

Trauma Assessment

As with all assessment, begin with inspection. Note any skin injuries—abrasions, contusions, degloving, avulsions, lacerations. In the patient with lacerations, note any underlying deformity or the presence of bone or contaminants (leaves, dirt) in the wound itself. Visually identify

- Color, swelling, pain/tenderness, skin injuries

- Symmetry

- Open fractures—bone visible or missing, contaminants, bleeding

- Attitude—is the extremity when at rest, held in any particular position other than normal anatomic position
  - Abduction: abnormally rotated away from the body (externally), particularly in the lower extremity may indicate anterior hip dislocation
  - Adduction: abnormally rotated toward the midline (internally), particularly in the lower extremity may indicate posterior hip dislocation
- Limb-length discrepancies
  - Shortened: fracture and/or dislocation
  - Lengthened: in the upper extremity may indicate shoulder dislocation; may not be evident until the patient is standing upright and gravity affects the extremity
  - Muscle spasm may also appear as shortening as the limb "self-splints"
- Deformity
  - Angulation
  - Swelling
  - Valgus—outward angulation of the distal end of a bone or joint
  - Varus—inward angulation of the distal end of a bone or joint
- When identifying phalanges
  - Count from the thumb or great toe as #1 and the small finger or toe is #5
  - This provides consistency between providers rather than naming fingers and toes (eg, pinky, baby toe)

Inspection is performed simultaneously with palpation. As each extremity is visualized, the bones are palpated for integrity, step offs, angulation. At examination, inspection and palpation are compared for symmetry between the extremities.

- Palpate the bones for integrity
- During palpation note
  - Tenderness
  - Guarding

— Temperature

— Crepitus (multiple bone fragments or the ends of the bone touching each other)

— DO NOT manipulate bones with crepitus or perform multiple examinations, which may result in continuous grating of the bone ends. Protect the bone from movement with a splint after initial examination

— Manipulation is carefully done in limb-threatening situations (loss of pulses), placement of splints, and for fracture/dislocation reduction

• Pulses

— Palpation of pulses occurred in the primary survey as discussed in Chapter 2

— Capillary refill should also be assessed for all extremities and should be <2 seconds

— Immediate action is taken for any extremity without a pulse or with a weakened pulse by reducing any deformity and placing in a splint

— Any further evaluation for vascular injury should be planned early

— Recheck pulses continuously to

  ▪ Identify any new changes in pulse quality

  ▪ Reassess the limb after immobilization to ensure pulses are attained and maintained

  ▪ Any loss of pulses after splinting or placement of a traction device requires removal of the splint and repositioning, then reassess

• Neurologic status—when palpating, check for motor strength and sensory status

— When assessing for spine injury, perform motor and sensory examination for all extremities (Chapters 4 and 5)

— An extremity with deformity or possible injury should be checked for

- Sensation to pinprick
- Proprioception
- Sensation to light touch
- Note any paresthesias described by the patient, such as numbness, tingling, "pins and needles," burning
— This examination is done before and after placing a splint, traction device, or reduction procedure to ensure that neither motor nor sensory examination is lost
— If there are changes to the examination after device placement, as above, remove, reposition, reassess
  - Alterations in sensation, motor, or pulses after manipulation is a sign of nerve or vascular injury
  - Femoral nerve—knee extension, anterior knee sensation (pubic rami fractures)
— Specific nerve functions and sources of injury include
  - Radial nerve—thumb and finger extension, dorsal web space sensation #1 (humerus fracture, anterior shoulder dislocation)
  - Ulnar nerve—#2 abduction, sensation to #5 (elbow fracture/dislocation)
  - Median nerve—thenar contraction and flexion distal interphalangeal (DIP) #2, sensation #2 (wrist dislocation, humerus fracture)
  - Axillary nerve—deltoid motor, shoulder sensation (anterior shoulder dislocation, humerus fracture)
  - Myocutaneous nerve—elbow flexion, lateral forearm sensation (anterior shoulder dislocation)
  - Sciatic nerve—hip abduction (acetabulum fracture)
  - Peroneal nerve—ankle eversion and dorsiflexion, foot sensation (proximal fibula fracture, knee dislocation)
  - Posterior tibial nerve—toe flexion, foot sole sensation (knee dislocation)
  - Gluteal nerves—hip abduction/extension (acetabulum fracture)

- Range of motion (ROM)
  - ROM examination is most often performed by the physician and predominantly the orthopaedic surgeon and frequently in the OR under anesthesia
  - Flexion, extension, rotation are tested
  - If the patient can participate in active ROM, passive ROM need not be tested
  - Major joints are assessed, unless an obvious deformity is present and then reduction of the joint is usually attempted with conscious sedation in the emergency department (ED)
  - This may not be performed on all joints in the ED based on the stability of the patient at the time. During resuscitation, all joints are protected from abnormal movement or unsupported movement, which could worsen an injury if present

- Muscle strength
  - Assessment of muscle strength should reveal bilateral symmetrical strength
  - See description in Chapter 4, Head Injury

During the secondary survey, joints or bones that require immobilization should be managed at the time of identification of the injury. Displaced fractures and dislocations are reduced in the ED to provide proper alignment for immobilization, pain reduction, and relief of pressure on the vessels within a joint (preventing avascular necrosis particularly in the hip). Plain radiographs usually follow to define the fracture and/or dislocation. Some specific fractures, for example, the pelvis, require specific views, such as inlet/outlet and judet. In some patients, computed tomography (CT) is used to evaluate complex fractures that require three-dimensional reconstruction or improved visualization to determine operative management. In addition, some sprains, strains, and dislocations, particularly the knee and shoulder, are best seen on magnetic resonance imaging (MRI). Angiography or CT-angiography will be necessary to identify vascular injuries. In some patients, embolization during angiography may be incorporated to manage vessel bleeding, particularly in the pelvis.

In the multiple-trauma patient, fractures can be missed in up to 6% of patients (Ward and Nunley 1991). One purpose of the tertiary survey, which must include the initial ambulatory period for the patient, is to identify previously unnoticed orthopaedic injuries (Chapter 2). Injuries are most often missed because of

- Orthopaedic injury in the same extremity

- Hemodynamic instability

- Altered level of consciousness

- Splints that obscure a deformity

- Poor initial radiographs

- Failure to recognize subtle signs and symptoms

DOCUMENTATION

Proper documentation of the orthopaedic injuries includes

- Diagram all skin injuries and any association with fractures

- Include direction of dislocation (anterior, posterior, inferior, etc)

- Document pulses, motor, and sensory examinations
  — Repeated frequently in the injured limbs

- During and after reduction
  — Conscious sedation documentation as per hospital protocol
  — Success of reduction
  — Pulses, sensory, and motor examination
  — Reassessment of pain; relief
  — Paresthesias

- Document radiographs taken before and after reduction

- Frequent reevaluation to document that there is no change
  — If a change occurs, document time and immediate interventions to rectify the situation

MANAGEMENT

Lacerations into Joint

Consideration that a laceration near a joint extends into the joint is part of the assessment. The evaluation is usually performed by the orthopaedic service. When a laceration penetrates a joint, there is the potential for ligamentous injury or injury into the meniscus. The wound is evaluated in surgery with arthroscopy and any injuries repaired at that time including irrigation of the joint to prevent infection and remove foreign bodies. A drain is usually placed for a short period and depending on contamination, the wound may not be closed primarily.

In the patient with a bullet in the joint, the bullet is removed because of the presence of lead. When in contact with synovial fluid in the joint the bullet leaches lead into the body, resulting in lead poisoning. The bullet is removed by arthroscopy when possible.

Sprains and Strains

Sprains involve ligaments and therefore joints. A stretching and tearing occurs to varying degrees. Pain, swelling, heat may be present around the joint. Diagnosis is made by examination of ROM. Radiographs may be taken to rule out fracture or dislocation associated with the ligamentous injury. Some ligaments require surgical repair, such as in the knee. The surgery is frequently done arthroscopically. The ankle requires maintenance of flexibility. Ambulation with an air splint provides optimal healing without loss of function. Severe sprains may require a period of nonweight bearing with crutches. Wrist sprains are supported with bracing in functional position. All sprains require follow-up exercises to retain mobility. Removal of constricting clothing, elevation, and the periodic application of ice is helpful in decreasing swelling as well as increasing comfort. Pain management is also important.

Strains involve muscle and tendon overuse or overexertion. An internal laceration of the muscle can occur but is infrequent.

In the abdomen, the rectus abdominis can rupture, resulting in herniation of abdominal organs. The lower spine is vulnerable when lifting improperly, for example. Muscle strain is managed with muscle rest, muscle relaxants, and progressive physical therapy. Rehabilitation includes proper lifting techniques. In the patient with rectus abdominis rupture, laparotomy is likely to rule out internal organ injury and repair the muscle defect.

Upper extremity

Upper extremity sprains most often involve the wrist after a fall onto outstretched hand. Other injuries include rotator cuff tears and labral tears of the shoulder from falls, tears during lifting/twisting motion, and frequently after dislocation/relocation.

Signs and Symptoms of Shoulder Sprains

Rotator Cuff
Pain, tenderness when reaching overhead, behind the back, lifting, pulling with the injured arm
Pain with sleeping on the side of injury
Weakness at shoulder
Loss of ROM at shoulder
Tendency to protect the injured arm
Pain which can be continuous if severe injury

Labrum
Pain, tenderness when reaching overhead
Locks, pops, grinds with movement of the shoulder
Shoulder "feels" unstable
Loss of ROM
Loss of strength

Lower extremity

Lower extremity sprains most commonly involve the knee and ankle joints. The ankle is injured by inversion or eversion usually when landing on the ankle incorrectly (eg, stepping off a curb). Knee sprains are more complex involving the anterior cruciate ligament, medial collateral ligament, lateral collateral ligament. The medial meniscus is a segment of cartilage within the knee joint.

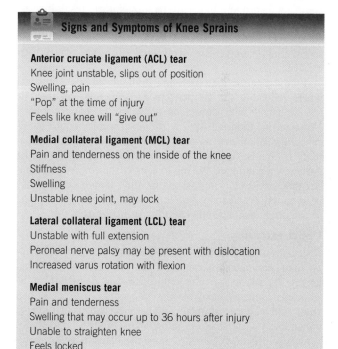

Signs and Symptoms of Knee Sprains

Anterior cruciate ligament (ACL) tear
Knee joint unstable, slips out of position
Swelling, pain
"Pop" at the time of injury
Feels like knee will "give out"

Medial collateral ligament (MCL) tear
Pain and tenderness on the inside of the knee
Stiffness
Swelling
Unstable knee joint, may lock

Lateral collateral ligament (LCL) tear
Unstable with full extension
Peroneal nerve palsy may be present with dislocation
Increased varus rotation with flexion

Medial meniscus tear
Pain and tenderness
Swelling that may occur up to 36 hours after injury
Unable to straighten knee
Feels locked

Dislocations

Dislocations involve joints. The complex bone and ligament structures form the joint, allowing for varying degrees of mobility dependent upon the joint involved. When a joint dislocates it can be partial (subluxation) or a complete dislocation. The joint may also spontaneously reduce itself. In other patients, the dislocation is obvious and will need closed reduction urgently. The nerves and vessels passing through the joint can be injured during the dislocation, resulting in temporary to complete disruption. Injury to the hip joint can result in avascular necrosis of the femoral head if the hip is not reduced emergently. Pulse checks and sensorimotor examination are essential to determine the involvement of the vascular or neural structures.

Immobilize the joint as found until arrival at the hospital where reduction can be performed. Reduction can then be accomplished with conscious sedation in many patients. However due to muscle spasm, some reductions require surgical manipulation and may also require internal fixation for stability. Do not be surprised to see the orthopod standing on the gurney when reducing the hip to achieve the correct angle and strength for the reduction. Traction, either skin or skeletal, may be required to maintain the reduction especially with muscle spasm. Reduction can relieve both spasm and pain.

Upper extremity

Dislocations in the upper extremity can include sternoclavicular joint, acromioclavicular, shoulder, elbow, wrist, and phalanges. The sternoclavicular joint dislocation is rare but can be associated with a lateral blow to the upper arm, a crushed chest, and with sternal fractures. The acromioclavicular joint is vulnerable to lateral blows, falls, sports injuries, and motor vehicle collision (MVC) with T-bone mechanisms as the shoulder is the most prominent joint and is struck first. Anterior dislocations of the shoulder are most common (Lin 2006). Other joint dislocations of the lower arm occur frequently with falls and may also occur in combination with fractures (Table 9-1).

Upper extremity dislocations are amenable to closed reduction and splinting or a sling for the shoulder. Some dislocations may require surgical repair. Vascular and nerve injury must be evaluated and managed.

Table 9-1 Named Fractures

Name	Bones-Joint	Description of fracture/dislocation
Bankart	Shoulder	Anterior glenoid labrum tear
Barton	Radius	Intra-articular distal radius fracture with dislocation of carpals
Bennet	Carpal-metacarpal joint #1	Fracture-dislocation at the intra-articular base of the thumb
Bimalleolar	Tibia/fibula	Lateral and medial malleolus fracture
Both bone forearm	Radius/ulna	Both radius and ulna fracture
Boxer	Metacarpal neck #5	Metacarpal head is free of attachments and in hyperextension
Chauffeur	Radius	Radial styloid fracture
Colles	Radius	Dorsal angulation distal radius (silver fork deformity) fracture
Essex Lopresti	Radius	Radial head fracture with dislocation of distal radioulnar joint
Galeazzi	Radius/ulna	Distal radius shaft fracture with radial-ulnar dislocation
Hill-Sachs	Humerus	Compression fracture posterior humeral head after anterior dislocation

(Continued)

Table 9-1 Named Fractures (Continued)

Name	Bones-Joint	Description of fracture/dislocation
Jones	Metatarsal #5	Base of metatarsal #5 fracture ~1.5 cm distal to the tuberosity
Lisfranc	Metatarsal	All 5 metatarsals may be dislocated (homolateral) and are often associated with cuboid fracture; 1 to 2 metatarsals dislocated (isolated); displacement sagittal and coronal (divergent) may be associated with navicular fracture
Maisonneuve	Tibia/fibula	Distal tibia/fibula fracture from external rotation with proximal third fibula
Mallet	Phalanges	Displaced distal phalanx fracture with flexion
Malgaigne	Pelvis	Both pubic rami and sacrum and/or SI joint fracture vertically oriented with superior displacement; pelvic floor rupture with ligamentous disruption; unilateral or bilateral
Monteggia	Radius/ulna	Proximal ulna shaft fracture with radial head dislocation
Nightstick	Ulna	Isolated midshaft ulna fracture
Open book	Pelvis	Pubic symphysis diastasis with sacro-iliac joint disruption from anterior-posterior compression

Pilon	Tibia	Distal metaphyseal tibia fracture with medial malleolus, anterior margin of the tibia, transverse posterior tibia involvement
Plafond	Tibia	See Pilon
Rolando	Metacarpal	Three-part fracture of the base of the metacarpal, intra-articular
Smith	Radius	Volar (downward) angulation distal radius fracture
Tillaux	Tibia	Salter Harris III tibial epiphysis fracture occurring before entire epiphyseal plate is closed
Trimalleolar	Tibia/fibula	Lateral, medial, and posterior malleolus fracture
Torus	Radius/ulna Tibia/fibula	"Buckle" fracture in children; crumpling of distal cortex but not the volar cortex; periosteum and cortex are intact opposite the fracture site

Signs and Symptoms of Acromioclavicular Joint Dislocation

Displaced clavicle in grade II and III separations
Pain, tenderness
Decreased ROM of shoulder
May be visible deformity, dropped shoulder, flat clavicle

Lower extremity

Lower extremity dislocations include the hip, knee, ankle, metatarsals, and phalanges. Hip dislocations occur in MVC when the knee is driven into the dashboard forcing the femur out of the joint. It may be associated with both femur and acetabular fractures. Because of the vascular structures that can be trapped here, immediate reduction is essential. Knee dislocations bear the same severity of vascular injury. They do not result in avascular necrosis like the hip, but rather direct injury to the popliteal artery and peroneal nerve.

Because of the weight-bearing role of the lower extremities, the patient will be nonweight bearing for several weeks after dislocation unless operatively stabilized. Even with internal fixation, weight bearing is a gradual progression to allow the joint to heal. In some situations a total joint replacement is the best option for repair. In the patient with the posterior hip dislocation, once reduced avoid

- Flexion

- Adduction

- Internal rotation

An abduction pillow is used to prevent dislocation from occurring. If the joint does not maintain reduction, a traction pin may be placed to keep the hip joint in alignment until definitive surgical management. Knee dislocations require immediate reduction followed by angiogram to evaluate the popliteal artery.

Lost or decreased pulses with knee dislocation require an immediate consultation to orthopaedics and vascular surgery. There is a high association of limb loss with any delay to treatment. The arteriogram can be performed in the OR to prevent delay. An examination under anesthesia can be performed to evaluate the ligaments and/or repair vascular injury at the same time.

Signs and Symptoms of Lower Extremity Dislocation

Hip
Pain
Muscle spasm
Paresthesias (neurovascular injury)

Hip: anterior
Superior dislocation—hip extension, external rotation, palpable
    femoral head; femoral artery, vein, or nerve may be involved
Inferior dislocation—hip abduction with external rotation and flexion

Hip: posterior
Shortened, internally rotated, and adducted
May be associated with acetabulum fracture and/or femoral head

Knee
Absent or weak pulses (popliteal artery injury)
Peroneal nerve palsy
Ligamentous disruption

Pelvis

The pelvis most often suffers fracture, however in addition to the fracture, or independently, the sacroiliac joint or the symphysis pubis may become dislocated. If both are involved, the pelvic ring becomes unstable. These dislocations are referred to as diastasis (widening) of the joints (Figure 9-1). Open book fracture demonstrates both a symphysis diastasis and sacroiliac joint diastasis.

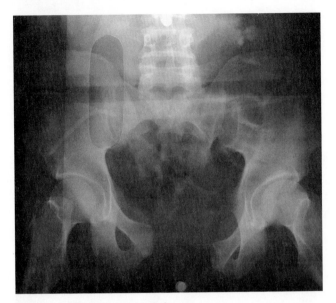

Figure 9-1 Pelvic open book fracture.

An open book pelvic fracture is not an open fracture, but rather a splaying of the pelvis as if a book had been "opened" at the pubis hinging on the sacroiliac joints in the posterior pelvis. Profound blood loss can occur with this fracture pattern. Aggressive fluid resuscitation including blood products is necessary.

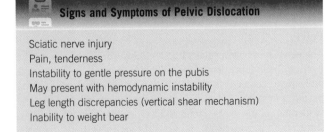

Signs and Symptoms of Pelvic Dislocation

Sciatic nerve injury
Pain, tenderness
Instability to gentle pressure on the pubis
May present with hemodynamic instability
Leg length discrepancies (vertical shear mechanism)
Inability to weight bear

One of the most immediate treatments for pelvic dislocation is to close the ring. Because the vascular structures associated with the pelvis can result in hemorrhage and exsanguination, closing the ring may tamponade the bleed as a temporizing measure as well as stabilize the joints and fractures decreasing pain and continued injury to the vessels and nerves. Rapid stabilization includes

- Place a sheet under the pelvis, wrap it around to the front and tie tightly or use towel clips to close; check pulses

- Pelvic binder—various types of pelvic binder stabilizers are available using corset-like methods of tying the pelvis closed rapidly

- C-clamp or external fixator may also be placed by the surgeon with revision later

- Frequent assessment of hemodynamic stability

- Administration of crystalloid and blood products

- Interventional radiology to manage vascular injury

The patient may not need immediate definitive fracture or joint stabilization in surgery. What is essential is the closure of the ring and management of vascular injury in resuscitative period.

Fractures

Fractures involve the bones and can occur in multiple types, some of which are unstable. In addition, a fracture line may cross into the intra-articular bone thus involving the joint. Fracture complexes have been described by various physicians over time and may still be referred to or described by that name. Table 9-1 describes the named fractures and the pattern of injury involved. Table 9-2 defines the different types of fractures that occur.

Fractures, unless displaced, may not be obvious when looking at the extremity. The patient may complain of pain, or crepitus may be noted on palpation. Radiographs are taken to

Table 9-2   Types of Fractures

Type	Description
Linear/transverse	Simple fracture across the bone
Hairline/fissure	Simple fracture without displacement through the outer layer of bone only
Oblique	Fracture at a diagonal across the bone, unstable
Spiral	Twisting fracture parallel to the bony axis, unstable
Comminuted	Multiple bony fragments at the site of fracture; unstable
Butterfly fragment	Slight comminution fracture with a fragment shaped similar to a butterfly
Wedge	Fracture creating a "wedge" of bone separated from the main bone
Displaced	Two ends of the bone fracture are no longer in anatomic alignment with each other
Overriding	Two ends of the bone fracture are no longer in anatomic alignment with each other and they have shifted (shortened) the ends to be alongside each other
Compound/open	Fracture through the skin or a penetrating injury entering the skin and fracture the bone; direct connection of the bone with the external environment
Impacted	Where the bony ends of the fracture are wedged together

identify the type of fracture and the degree of displacement or comminution. A CT scan may be needed to better define the complex fractures prior to fixation. A fracture may not be noted until the patient is well enough to use the extremity and then complains of pain or loss of ROM. This is particularly true of critical patients who, for example, may complain of foot pain when attempting to walk, which then prompts radiographs to identify the foot fracture heretofore unknown.

Signs and Symptoms of Fractures

Swelling, tenderness
Guarding, refusing or unable to move or bear weight
Ecchymosis
Deformity—visible, palpable
Crepitus
Pelvis: crepitus or instability with gentle pressure applied to the pubic symphysis
Open fracture—wound directly in contact with the fracture below; bone may be protruding
Contamination in open wound (eg, dirt, leaves, foreign bodies)
Paresthesia (nerve injury)
Decreased pulses or pulselessness (vascular injury)

If a fracture is identified, a splint should be placed to maintain alignment, decrease movement, and decrease pain until definitive management. Reduction of displaced fractures is done during secondary survey under conscious sedation if needed. The splint is then placed to maintain alignment. Splints and casts should immobilize one joint above and one below the fracture site. See specific fractures for splinting recommendations in the next section. Traction splints are used in lower extremities to assist with reduction and alignment.

Pulses and a sensorimotor examination need to be checked before and after splint placement and repeated frequently. Any alterations require immediate reassessment, loosening, or replacement of the immobilization device. Definitive treatment through internal or external fixation is used in some fractures whereas others are amenable to closed reduction and nonoperative management as noted below.

Upper extremity

Fractures of the upper extremity involve the clavicle, scapula, humerus, radius and ulna, bones of the wrist (carpals), metacarpals, and phalanges.

Management

Management of upper extremity fractures includes

- Identification of fractures through assessment and radiographs

- External splinting or at a minimum temporarily immobilize the patient until evaluation and splinting can occur

- Clavicle fracture
  — Components: head (proximal) end, acromial (distal) end, or midshaft (70-80%)
  — Nonoperative management: sling placement
  — Operative management: closed reduction with internal fixation (CRIF) or open reduction with internal fixation (ORIF)
  — If displaced midshaft, there is a high incidence of malunion and nonunion (Canadian Orthopaedic Trauma Society 2007); improves with operative fixation
  — Postoperative issues include irritation, prominence of fracture site, or mechanical failure
  — Improved satisfaction with appearance after operative management (Canadian Orthopaedic Trauma Society 2007)

- Scapula fracture
  — Components: body, glenoid, coracoid, acromial process
  — Nonoperative management, sling for comfort
  — Evaluate joint and associated ligaments for involvement
  — Assess axillary nerve function

- Humerus fracture
  - Components: humeral head (proximal), surgical and anatomical neck, greater tuberosity, diaphysis (shaft), supracondylar, condyles (distal)
  - Majority (80%) proximal humerus nondisplaced or minimally displaced (Lin 2006)
  - Assess radial and axillary nerve function; radial pulse
  - Hill-Sachs lesion: assess for rotator cuff injury
  - Minimally displaced proximal humerus can be managed with splint/fracture-brace
  - Displaced proximal humerus: operative management
  - Midshaft: closed reduction with nonoperative management in fracture-brace
  - Supracondylar humerus fractures are frequent in children falling while playing and are usually managed with operative fixation
- Radius and ulna fracture
  - Components: radial head/neck (proximal), capitulum (proximal) diaphysis (shaft), distal end/styloid process; Ulna olecranon process (proximal), coronoid (proximal), diaphysis (shaft), distal end/styloid process
  - Can be caused by air bag deployment (forearm and distal radius/ulna)
  - Assess radial, ulnar, and median nerve function, finger ROM
  - May fracture individually or together (both bones forearm)
  - Nondisplaced ulna: cast
  - Displaced ulna shaft: operative management
  - Radius shaft: operative management
  - Galeazzi and Monteggia complex fracture-dislocations need operative management
  - Distal radius (Colles, Smith, Bartons) with minimal displacement: sugar tong splint or short-arm cast
  - Distal radius/ulna displaced: operative management; may require external fixator

- Carpals and metacarpals fractures
  — Components: bones of the wrist: scaphoid (navicular), lunate, triquetrum (cuneiform), pisiform, trapezium, trapezoid, capitate, hamate; metacarpals
  — Metacarpals form the body of the hand
  — Most commonly injured carpal is the scaphoid (Lin 2006)
  — Assess for snuffbox tenderness (snuffbox: dorsal hand, abduct thumb, visible depression at the junction of the wrist and base of first metacarpal); pain with dorsiflexion; radial deviation
  — Closed reduction and splinting for nondisplaced fracture
  — Scaphoid: long-arm cast with thumb spica
  — Displaced: operative management
- Phalanges
  — May be caused by air bag deployment
  — Most often managed nonoperatively through splinting
  — Complex may require internal fixation/Kischner wires for stability

Lower extremity

Fractures of the lower extremity involve the femur, patella, tibia/fibula, bones of the ankle (tarsals), metatarsals, and phalanges.

Management

Management of lower extremity fractures includes

- Identification of fractures through radiographs
- Splinting through immobilization to the backboard for the immediate arrival of the patient
- The backboard should be removed as soon as possible to prevent skin breakdown
- Femur fracture (includes "hip" fracture)
  — Components: head (hip), neck (hip), greater/lesser trochanters (hip), diaphysis (shaft), condyles

— "Hip" fractures occur most often in the elderly caused by a simple ground level fall; have a 20% mortality at 1 year and up to 50% do not return to independent living (Lin 2006)

— Risk factors for hip fractures—caffeine, alcohol, osteoporosis, age >50 years (increases with each decade), white females, smokers, low body weight, psychotropic medications

— May be placed in Bucks (skin) traction for comfort until surgery

— Displaced proximal femur: best managed with prosthesis (hip replacement)in the elderly or low demand patient because of increased risk of osteonecrosis and nonunion

  ▪ In the younger patient, urgent ORIF will decrease the risk of avascular necrosis

— Potential complications for the proximal femur: heterotrophic ossification, peroneal nerve injury, infection, loosening prosthesis, leg length discrepancies

— Initial management at the scene and during resuscitation

  ▪ In-line traction (Hare or Sager device) provides reduction for the fracture along with relief of pain and muscle spasm

  ▪ Should not be used with distal femur fractures and any fracture below the femoral shaft

  ▪ Pulses should be checked before and after placement of the traction device

  ▪ Temporary measure until definitive management with surgery or placement of a Steinman pin for skeletal traction

  ▪ A critical patient may be placed briefly in skeletal traction until stable enough for operative management

— Shaft: requires operative management with CRIF, ORIF, or external fixation

  ▪ Within first 24 hours intramedullary nail (IMN) or external fixation with later conversion to IMN if the patient is unstable/critical (Pape et al. 2007)

  ▪ Stable patients may have shorter ventilator times if IMN placed

- Reamed versus unreamed IMN show no difference in the incidence of acute respiratory distress syndrome (ARDS) between the two (Canadian Orthopaedic Trauma Society 2006)
- In young children, a hip spica may be placed for femoral shaft fractures

— Supracondylar femur, lateral and medial condyles, and/or tibial plateau fractures involve the knee joint and are amenable to nonoperative management if nondisplaced; displaced require operative fixation

- Ligaments of the knee also may be involved
- Function of the knee joint is central to rehabilitation
- Support with a Bledsoe hinged knee immobilizer during rehabilitation (may be used for proximal tibia fractures)

- Patella fracture
  — Single bone
  — May require ORIF for stability
  — May be associated with ligamentous injury

- Tibia and fibula fracture
  — Components: head (proximal), condyles/tibial plateau (proximal), diaphysis
  — Common injury in motorcycle crashes, pedestrians struck
  — Proximal tibia as above distal femur fractures
  — Tibia shaft usually requires operative management and as with femoral shaft ORIF, CRIF, or external fixation especially for complex fracture stabilization
  — Plafond or pilon fracture of the tibia is at the distal shaft above the malleoli
  — Independent proximal or shaft fibula fractures may not require surgical treatment
  — Figure 9-2 demonstrates a complex comminuted tibia and fibula shaft fracture
  — Monitor for compartment syndrome

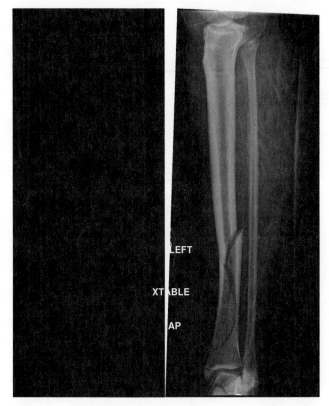

LEFT

XTABLE

AP

Figure 9-2   Complex tibia-fibula comminuted shaft fracture.

- Malleoli fracture ("ankle" fracture)
  — Components: medial malleolus (tibia), posterior malleolus (tibia), lateral malleolus (fibula)
  — Bimalleolar and trimalleolar are unstable and are usually treated with operative management if displaced

— Stable ankle fractures may be treated in a weight-bearing cast

— Function of the ankle joint is an essential component of the rehabilitation of this injury

• Tarsals and metatarsals fracture

— Components: calcaneus, talus, scaphoid (navicular), cuboid, cuneiform, metatarsals

— Calcaneus is vulnerable with falls from a height landing on the feet

— Calcaneus usually requires nonweight bearing and may result in long-term arthritis with the best healing

— Talus has a tenuous blood supply resulting in nonunion and avascular necrosis

— Foot fractures may be managed with casting or a walking boot to ORIF/CRIF based on the stability and complexity of the fracture

— Lisfranc injuries are fracture-dislocations of the forefoot involving the tarsal-metatarsal joints; fracture may not always be present

  ▪ Commonly caused by the foot trapped in the brake/gas pedal, caught in stirrup (original cause), football injuries

  ▪ May self-reduce to near-normal position

  ▪ May be missed initially and identified when the patient becomes ambulatory

  ▪ Initial findings are often subtle and may require a standing or stress view films to identify; high index of suspicion is essential because of mechanism

  ▪ Monitor for compartment syndrome

  ▪ Managed with ORIF and casting

  ▪ Frequently associated with arthritis and stiffness of the foot

• Phalanges fractures

— If displaced, reduce and immobilize by taping to fellow toe

  ▪ Monitor for tightness as swelling occurs

  ▪ If patient is nonambulatory because of other injuries, the toe should heal without specific intervention

— Also heals with weight bearing as tolerated
— A fracture boot or sturdy shoe may be necessary for support
— Complex toe fractures may be surgically managed similar to fingers with Kirschner wires

Pelvis

Pelvic fractures involve three bones with multiple components that make up the pelvis. These include the sacrum/coccyx and the two innominate bones forming the sacral ala, iliac wings, ischium, pubic rami (inferior and superior), and acetabuli. The sacrum and coccyx are part of the distal spinal column although they are an integral part of the pelvis. The ligaments at the sacroiliac joints provide stability. The pelvis carries the weight of the body, the major vessels of the iliac system, and is involved in the distribution of nerves to the lower extremities.

Pelvic fractures can hemorrhage very quickly due to the large vessels that travel through and around the pelvic bones. The pelvic cavity and retroperitoneal cavity can hold large amounts of blood, providing a place for the blood to pool without external evidence, such as ecchymosis. Bleeding with pelvic fractures should be assumed until proven otherwise.

Management

- Identify fractures; radiographs (include Judet, inlet and outlet views when able); spiral, thin cut CT scan with three-dimensional reconstruction (IV contrast)
  — During assessment of the pelvis, DO NOT compress the iliac wings OR rock the pelvis as this can displace fractures and/or increase hemorrhage
  — The pelvis is a ring; if one fracture is identified, there should be a high index of suspicion for a second fracture

- If a pelvic fracture is suspected, close the pelvic ring as with dislocations above to decrease the volume of the pelvic cavity
  — Tie a sheet around the pelvis
  — Apply a C-clamp or external fixator

- If posterior instability, an anterior fixation device may stabilize the front of the pelvis but open the unstable ligaments in the posterior component
- External fixation can be accomplished prior to laparotomy
— If no other choice, the military antishock trousers (MAST) or pneumatic antishock garment (PASG) (depending on which name is used locally) may be applied in this and only this situation
  - Even though the MAST are being applied for pelvic ring control only, the appropriate technique for inflation and deflation must still be followed
  - Inflate legs then pelvis; monitor pulses
  - Deflate gradually starting with the pelvis and progressing to the legs
  - Anticipate hypotension with removal and be prepared with fluid resuscitation
  - Placement makes the approach to the femoral artery for angiography very difficult to impossible
  - If prolonged use, compartment syndrome and ischemia can occur
  - This technique is used only when there is no other option
- Angiography
  — Consider angiography for pelvic bleeding (DiGiacomo et al. 2001) when
    - Recurrent hypotension despite resuscitation
    - Arterial extravasation on CT (IV contrast) (Figure 9-3)
    - Other sources of ongoing hemorrhage already ruled out
    - Pelvic bleeding that could not be controlled during laparotomy
  — If able, embolization prior to operation decreases mortality (Lopez 2007)
  — Fracture pattern does not help with determining vascular involvement (Sarin et al. 2005)
  — Embolization is accomplished with gelfoam or coils

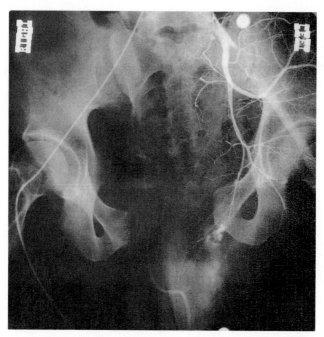

Figure 9-3   Pelvic open book fracture with arterial extravasation.

• Acetabulum fracture
  — Types include anterior column, posterior column, both column, hemitransverse, and T-type
  — Both column and hemitransverse acetabulum fractures require the most transfusions (Magnussen et al. 2007)
  — May be associated with dislocation of the hip, especially in MVC where the femur is driven backward into the acetabulum upon impact with the dashboard
  — Reduction of dislocation must be conducted in a timely fashion; delays have poor outcomes and are associated with avascular necrosis of the femoral head

— Not all acetabulum fractures require ORIF as some do not involve the weight-bearing components

— Posterior wall fractures, especially intra-articular, show good outcome with ORIF (Moed 2007)

- Ilium and ischium fracture

    — Pelvic fractures are classified by compression and direction of fracture pattern; the following have major ligamentous involvement and instability

        ■ Anterior-posterior compression grade II to III (eg, crush)

        ■ Lateral compression grade III (eg, MVC with T-bone mechanism)

        ■ Combined compressive forces

        ■ Vertical shear (eg, fall from height landing on feet or one foot)

    — Anterior-posterior compression and vertical shear fracture patterns require the highest transfusion rates (Magnussen et al. 2007)

    — All pelvic fractures do not necessarily require surgical repair unless unstable ligamentous involvement or displacement/comminution

- Pubic rami fracture

    — Straddle injuries, ground level or low level falls in the elderly

    — Pubic rami fractures without any other fracture are usually managed nonoperatively

    — "Open book" pelvic fractures involve widening of the symphysis pubis with or without sacroiliac diastasis

    — Suspect urethral/bladder injury

Vascular Injury

Vascular injury can occur with any extremity fracture or dislocation. Diligent assessment of pulse presence and quality and any changes in the pulses is an integral part of identification of these injuries. Color and capillary refill are also cues to issues with circulation.

- If a vascular injury is suspected, a CT-angiogram and/or arteriogram are performed to confirm the injury.
- If possible, during the angiogram, embolization with gelfoam or coils is undertaken to halt the extravasation.
  — Figures 9-1 and 9-3 demonstrate an open book pelvic fracture and the angiogram of the iliac artery demonstrating extravasation. This injury was embolized with coils, which halted the hemorrhage and stabilized the patient.
- In the instance of partial or circumferential transection, the artery or vein needs operative repair. The patient requires rapid transfer to a trauma center and from there, into the operating suite. Management in the operating room includes
  — Direct suture repair
  — Reverse saphenous vein graft
  — Interposition graft
- Postoperative management includes frequent monitoring of the limb distal to the repair for
  — Pulses
  — Capillary refill
  — Color
  — Temperature
- Rehabilitation begins with protection of the repair/graft and initiating physical therapy
  — Therapy activity and weight-bearing status are coordinated between the vascular and orthopaedic surgeons
  — Specifics for management of venous congestion associated with replantation is discussed under amputations below
- Potential complications include
  — Graft occlusion
  — Amputation
  — Hemorrhage
  — Compartment syndrome

Management of Orthopaedic Injury

The management of fractures, dislocations, and sprains is dependent upon several factors including

- Associated injuries

- Hemodynamic stability

- Vascular injury

- Associated dislocation

- Comorbidities and functional status prior to injury

Priority injuries are associated with bleeding, such as intra-abdominal injury and vascular injury. The order of surgery is determined by the surgeons and may include a combination of surgery, interventional radiology, and temporary orthopaedic measures to stabilize the fracture or joint. The goal is early stabilization to enable early mobilization. This is however, temporized by the hemodynamic stability of the patient. If attempted early, the addition of the orthopaedic procedure may overwhelm the body's ability to cope. Thus, if unstable, the orthopaedic injuries may undergo staged repair. There is no evidence to require antibiotics in closed fractures. In operative orthopaedic patients, antibiotics are given 1 hour prior to incision and discontinued within 24 hours after operation.

- Casting and splinting
  — Assess skin prior to splinting/casting: clean, dry, without open wounds
  — Assess pulses before and after
  — Monitor frequently for swelling, paresthesias, color, temperature, pulses
    ▪ Indicates a tight cast that needs to be bivalve (splitting)
    ▪ Bivalving should relieve the symptoms
  — Weight bearing after splinting/casting is determined by the surgeon
  — Progression from casting to splinting occurs as the fracture heals

— Splints
  - Types include vacuum, air, premolded, any rigid padded object, malleable
  - Vacuum splints allow the wound/extremity to be seen, however can exert excess pressure on the extremity; be particularly careful when changing altitudes (increased pressure on ascent, loss of air in the splint on descent)
  - Air splints (eg, Aircast) are particularly useful for ankle sprains
  - Premolded are acceptable initial splints; must be padded; must be refitted to the appropriate molded shape of the extremity
  - In the field any solid long object can be used as long as it is padded, eg, the author has used a flipper attached by weight belts when rescuing an injured snorkeler in the open ocean
  - Pillows are particularly good ankle splints
  - Body splinting is also an effective maneuver for the lower extremities by padding between the legs and tying the legs together
  - Remove daily and cleanse skin
  - Check for pressure points
  - Place gauze or elastic wrap from the distal extremity toward the heart to hold splint in place
  - Keep splint clean
  - Allows easy access to wounds or incisions
— Casts
  - Keep dry
  - Padding is placed under the cast material
  - Check edges to assure no pressure points
  - Elevate to the level of the heart (not above) and avoid pressure on the cast while it sets (to prevent deformity)
  - Hip spica casts also need to be monitored around the abdomen for tightness especially after eating

o Ileus may occur

o If the patient is bed bound, avoid complications of immobility and superior mesenteric artery syndrome (see special situations section)

- Traction
  — Although used infrequently, traction plays a role presurgery in some instances
    ■ Hare or Sager traction devices are useful for transport of femur fractures
    ■ Relieves muscle spasm and decreases pain
    ■ Provides stability during transport and initial resuscitation
  — Bucks traction (skin traction) may be applied to the hip fracture patient prior to surgery to provide comfort
  — Skeletal traction with a Steinman pin may occasionally be needed if femoral surgery is delayed caused by hemodynamic instability
    ■ Patient is taken for more definitive fixation as soon as possible
    ■ Cleanse the pin sites with a 50% mixture of hydrogen peroxide and normal saline twice daily
  — Potential complications are severe because of immobility associated with the traction
    ■ Pneumonia, atelectasis
    ■ Skin breakdown both at pressure sites and associated with the pin sites
    ■ Venous thromboembolism
    ■ Ileus

- CRIF and ORIF
  — Closed reduction may be all that is necessary, followed by immobilization with a splint or cast
    ■ May be accomplished in the ED under conscious sedation
    ■ May also be all that is needed to restore pulses as well and should be first-line therapy when pulses are absent
    ■ Follow the management and monitoring of casting/splinting

— CRIF is used when the support of the internal hardware is needed
  - Includes intramedullary nails
  - Surgical incision care is standard
— Open reduction is necessary when the surgeon needs to visualize the fracture site or is unable to reduce the fracture closed
  - Also allows for exploration of vessels and nerves
  - Complex fractures can be managed with plate/screw fixation
— Timing of fixation is dependent on the patient's ability to tolerate the procedure
  - Long initial surgery of >6 hours increases risk for ARDS and multisystem organ failure (MSOF) (Pape 2005)
  - Early fixation must be done rapidly
  - In head injury, repeat head CT prior to surgical fixation
  - The presence of any infection precludes placement of hardware
  - In addition, hardware cannot be placed into an infected or contaminated body part
— Decision to move forward with surgical fixation is tempered by (Pape et al. 2005, Scalea 2008)
  - Hemodynamic instability—shock, need for transfusion, BP <90 mm Hg; low urine output
  - Lactate >2.5 mMol/L, abnormal base deficit
  - D-dimer abnormal (early disseminated intravascular coagulation [DIC]); coagulopathy
  - Head injury with increased intracranial pressure (IICP), Glasgow coma scale (GCS) <9
  - Platelet count <90,000/mm^3
  - Hypothermia—temperature <36°C and particularly if <32°C
  - Bilateral pulmonary contusion on initial chest x-ray
  - Multisystem trauma with abdominal/pelvic injury
  - Normalized preoperative glucose levels
  - Estimated operative time >8 hours

— Simultaneous operative teams maximize the patient's tolerance of multiple surgeries as well as minimizes initial operative time

  ▪ There is evidence for an increase in ARDS for patients with head injury who receive early fixation (within the first 24 hours) (Scalea 2008)

— Unstable patient who is unresponsive to resuscitation needs early temporizing measures, such as external fixation with later internal fixation within 7 days is optimal (Scalea 2008)

  ▪ This is referred to as damage control orthopaedic management

— Rehabilitation is dependent upon the patient's overall severity of injury as well as bone injury

  ▪ Early mobilization is key but also dependent upon the severity of the associated injuries

  ▪ There is evidence that the presence of some hardware may result in chronic pain syndrome and later removal of the hardware

• External fixation

— Frame device external to the body with pins entering the bone designed to span the fracture and/or joint

  ▪ Frame provides stability, especially for severely comminuted, complex fracture and/or dislocation

  ▪ Rapidly applied

  ▪ Allows access to wounds and access to other injuries such as vessels

— Converted later to internal fixation or may remain as the definitive treatment

— A unique version of external fixation formerly used for leg length discrepancies is the Ilizarov device; a circular external fixator, which provides stability especially for severely unstable fractures (Figure 9-4)

— Pin care: 50% hydrogen peroxide and sterile saline, twice daily

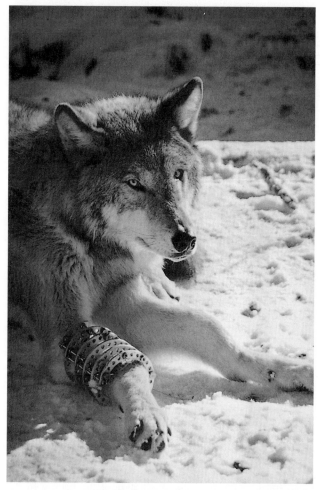

Figure 9-4   Ilizarov external fixation device. (www.wolfsanctuary. net)

— Examine the frame daily for stability
— Monitor pin sites for signs of infection—redness, warmth, drainage, odor

- Recombinant human bone morphogenic protein
  — Protein allograft used for osseous repair in place of autogenous bone graft
  — Healing rate similar to autogenous bone (Jones 2005)
  — Eliminates pain and blood loss from the site of bone graft harvest (eg, iliac crest)
  — Decreases surgical time by eliminating the harvest procedure
  — Chronic donor site pain is a long-term complication of autogenous bone graft harvest
  — Nonallergenic

- Fracture blisters
  — Vesicles or bullae that occur in the swollen areas over fractures
  — Most often tibia, ankle, elbow
  — Fractures undergoing operative fixation within 24 hours of injury appear to have the lowest incidence of fracture blister (Varela et al. 1993)
  — Usually develop within 24 to 48 hours after fracture
  — Blister fluid is a sterile transudate; leave blisters intact acting as a sterile biological dressing for the tissue underneath the blister
  — Will delay surgery to prevent complications, such as wound infection

Open Fracture Management

Open fractures involve a communication of the bone with the external environment. It may occur when the bone passes through the muscle, subcutaneous, and skin layers resulting in an open skin wound. A GSW or impaled object can also result in an open fracture as the foreign body passes through the skin and results in

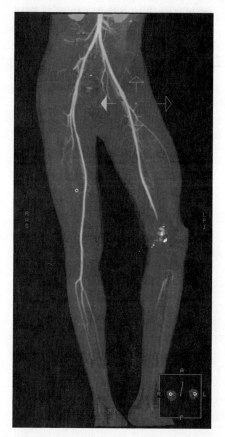

Figure 9-5 Gunshot wound with popliteal artery extravasation.

fracture. Both open fractures and penetrating injury causing open fractures can result in nerve and vascular injury (Figure 9-5).

The wound may be simple or extensive tissue destruction (mangled extremity) and may or may not include contaminants (eg, dirt, clothing). Open fracture involves management of both the fracture, open wound, and the foreign bodies present. Vascular and nerve injury needs attention. The open pelvic fracture requires assessment of the rectum and vagina for penetration. The open pelvic fracture into the vagina or rectum is the most contaminated open fracture. The wound is always in a contaminated environment, which makes it difficult to heal and keep clean. A diverting colostomy is likely one of the temporizing measures to heal the rectal wound. The vagina wound requires monitoring for infection.

To provide consistent descriptors for open fractures, Gustilo et al (1976, 1984) defined a grading for open fractures, which includes

- Grade I—open wound <1 cm; wound is clean
  — Average time to healing, 20 to 28 weeks

- Grade II—open wound >1 cm without damage, avulsion, flap, moderate comminution
  — Average time to healing, 28 weeks

- Grade III—open wound with extensive soft tissue damage, open segmental fracture, amputation, bone loss
  — Grade IIIa: coverage is adequate regardless of the size of the wound
  — Grade IIIb: extensive loss of tissue, periosteal stripping, bone exposure, massive contamination
  — Grade IIIc: open fracture with an associated vascular injury requiring repair to obtain limb salvage
  — Average time to heal 30 to 35 weeks
  — May need to consider amputation for grade IIIc

Because of the contamination as well as the presence of the open wound, the fracture has potential for infection and necrosis of both tissue and bone. Management is focused on all components of this complex injury.

- Open wound
  — Place a sterile dressing over the open wound to prevent further contamination

— A tourniquet may be used if hemorrhage cannot be controlled in any other way to salvage the limb or life (Kortbeek et al. 2008)

- Must occlude arterial circulation
- Threatens the limb
- Length of time must be monitored closely
- Transient nerve palsy may occur
- Increased length of tourniquet time increases the possibility of fasciotomy (Kragh et al. 2008)

— Isolated venous injuries with active hemorrhage after penetrating trauma should be explored and the bleeding controlled; repair if the patient is stable and the time to repair will not interfere with the patient's stability (Arrillega et al. 2002)

- Fasciotomy may be necessary when both arterial and venous injuries are present

— Early closure decreases the likelihood of nosocomial infection and is safe with thorough debridement (Okike and Bhattacharyya 2006)

— Thorough surgical irrigation and debridement must be arranged early in the treatment (preferably within 6 hours) and may be done bedside if the patient is unstable

- Decreases bacterial load
- Removes foreign bodies
- High-pressure lavage causes macroscopic bone damage; low-pressure lavage should be used
- Suggested liters of fluid for irrigation increases with the grade of open fracture, such as 3 L for grade I, 6 L for grade II, 9 L for grade III
- Normal saline solution (NSS) with an antiseptic is the most effective irrigant (Okike and Bhattacharyya 2006)
  ○ Soap causes the least injury to osteoblasts
  ○ May be wound healing issues if bacitracin is added

— Second irrigation and debridement usually occurs within 24 to 48 hours

— Daily wound care until closure
— Further management depends on timing and type of closure by delayed primary suture repair, split thickness skin grafting, or flap coverage
— Observe the wound for signs of infection: redness, swelling, heat, foul odor, purulent drainage
— Administer tetanus
— Vacuum-assisted closure accelerates wound healing through increased local blood flow enhancing granulation
  ▪ Sterile dressing
  ▪ Change every 72 hours
• Fracture stabilization is as discussed above except that there also may be a wound that requires care
— External fixation allows optimal access to the wound instead of a cast
— Consider early intramedullary nail
— May need to consider amputation in the severely mangled extremity, especially in the presence of hemodynamic instability
— Use of bone grafting or recombinant human bone morphogenic protein (rhBMP) may assist healing, resulting in decreased time to union
  ▪ Decreased hardware failure
  ▪ Decreased incidence of secondary intervention
• Antibiotics
— Preoperatively, the first dose should be given as soon as possible and cover gram positive organisms (Luchette et al. 2000)
  ▪ Grade III open fractures must also cover gram negative organisms
  ▪ If the injury occurred on a farm or has fecal contamination (anaerobes), high-dose penicillin is necessary
— Grade I and grade II open fractures require antibiotics through 24 hours after closure (monotherapy)

— Grade III open fractures require antibiotics through 72 hours after injury or up to 24 hours after closure, whichever comes first (cephalosporin and aminoglycoside)
— The organisms responsible for infection in the majority of patients are nosocomial, not the organisms present at the time of injury (Okike and Bhattacharyya 2006)
— Increased risk of infection occurs with
  ▪ Age >80 years
  ▪ Use of nicotine
  ▪ Diabetes, malignancy, pulmonary disease, immunodeficiency
— Fluoroquinolones affect osteoblasts
— Local antibiotic beads (aminoglycoside eluting poly-methylmethacrylate) placed into the wound decrease the rate of infection (Okike and Bhattacharyya 2006)

SPECIAL SITUATIONS

Pediatric Fractures

Pediatric fractures are sometimes difficult to diagnose as the epiphyseal growth plates may appear as fractures. Comparison films of the uninjured limb may be used to determine if what is visible is the open growth plate or a fracture. The immature bones of children can tolerate deformation without fracture. However because of the difference of the bone structure, children experience specific fractures that are not usually present in adults. Healing fractures that involve the growth plates can result in deformity or length discrepancies.

Types of pediatric fractures are described in Table 9-3. Pediatric fractures may result in overgrowth of bone during healing caused by the increased blood supply to the injured extremity. This may result in limb length discrepancies. Remodeling occurs in young children and those with growth plate fractures, which has the benefit of healing even with an imperfect reduction. Remodeling can also result in overgrowth of bone causing deformities.

Table 9-3   Pediatric Fractures

Fracture	Description	Management
Buckle/torus	Buckling near the metaphysis from compression without actual fracture	Heals 4 to 6 weeks
Greenstick	Incomplete fracture due to angulation; fibula and ulna vulnerable to greenstick when tibia and radius fracture	Heals 4 to 6 weeks
Growth plate: Salter Harris types I–V	I—epiphysis completely separated from metaphysis	I—heals ≤3 weeks; excellent prognosis; may not be evident on x-ray if nondisplaced and may be diagnosed by index of suspicion
	II—traverses the growth plate but exits the opposite metaphysis; periosteum torn	II—easily reduced
	III—growth plate is already partially closed; traverses the growth plate then exits the epiphysis	III—intra-articular and involves the growth plate usually requiring operative reduction
	IV—joint surface through the growth plate and exits the metaphysis; vertical split of the epiphysis	IV—if unreduced, healing results in partial growth arrest, joint stiffness, deformity; requires ORIF; may still result in growth disturbance
	V—crush of growth plate; negative radiographs	V—may not be evident until growth arrest has occurred

Most pediatric fractures are managed with closed reduction and casting under general anesthesia or conscious sedation. Intra-articular fractures require anatomic reduction and may also require ORIF. Femoral fractures may be managed with a spica cast. The management of open fractures is the same as for adults and may include the use of external fixation as well.

Amputations

Microsurgery has advanced so that limbs previously lost are now replantable. Lower extremities remain difficult because of the dependent position, however replants of upper limbs have been found to be successful. Replantation success is dependent upon several factors

- Hemodynamic stability of the patient

- Physiologically capable of tolerating the prolonged replant procedure

- Viable body part
  - Warm ischemic time <6 hours
  - Cold ischemic time <12 hours
  - Digits may be viable up to 8 to 10 hours if warm, and possibly up to 20 to 28 hours if kept cold

- Rapid transfer to the replant facility

- Contamination of the wound

- Ragged or "clean" cut at the site of amputation
  - A guillotine-type amputation has a higher success rate of replantation

- Treatment of the part from the scene

- Level of amputation; upper versus lower limb

Amputations may be full or partial. When a severe injury occurs, severing the nerves, vessels, soft tissue and causing open bone fracture, a near amputation is diagnosed and the injured part is treated the same as a full amputation regarding rapid transfer to the operating suite for microsurgical repair.

Management

The management of the patient as well as the amputated part is essential to the success of replantation, or more importantly, survival. Most amputations result in hemorrhage that is self-limiting when the arteries constrict themselves and retract. Occasionally this is not the case and is the one situation where a tourniquet may be used to attempt to stop the bleeding. Direct pressure is also first-line therapy for hemorrhage. It is important that the amputation does not become the focus of resuscitation to the detriment of other injuries. The primary and secondary survey must be conducted as usual to ensure an airway with ventilation and circulatory control. A hemorrhage from the site will be controlled during the primary survey. Overall management includes

- Primary and secondary surveys with appropriate intervention as needed

- Stabilize fractures as part of the secondary survey; this includes the amputation site

- Place a sterile dressing over the wound to prevent any further contamination

- Amputated part
    — Wrap in sterile gauze
    — Place in a resealable bag or container in an ice slush
    — Prevent direct contact of the part with the ice water or ice
    — NEVER use dry ice
    — Goal: maintain the temperature of the tissue for as long as possible
    — Bring the part with the patient to the receiving facility
    — If the part is not immediately located, transport the patient and bring the part as soon as it is found

- If the receiving hospital is not a replant center, arrange immediate transfer to the appropriate trauma center for replant evaluation

- If an amputation is necessary because of the severity of original injury or as a life-saving procedure, the psychological effect is overwhelming for the loss of the body part
  — Psychological support must be provided
  — Caregivers must be accepting of the appearance of the patient
  — The most severe amputation is a hemipelvectomy, or removal of half of the pelvis and frequently bladder and/or genitalia as well
  — Early rehabilitation assists the patient in understanding the level of function still available to them despite the amputation
  — Phantom pain is a very real sensation of the presence of the missing limb, including
    - Itching
    - Burning
    - Pain
    - Wet-dry sensation
    - Moving sensation
  — Prosthetic fitting and use occurs when the stump of the amputation is healed
    - Physical therapy and the orthotics and prosthetics professionals design and work with the patients for fit and function of the prosthesis

After replantation is complete, management focuses on the survival of the replanted part. Survival can be complicated by venous congestion, obstruction of arterial inflow, infection both aerobic and anaerobic. Considerations for care include

- Warm room to prevent vascular constriction from the environment (78°F)

- NO caffeine or smoking, which both result in vascular constriction

- Elevation of the replant at the level of the heart to promote both arterial inflow and venous output

- Assess temperature of the replant directly

- Assess capillary refill or pinprick for bleeding
- Assess sensation; motor is usually restricted until healing has occurred, then rehabilitation of the replant is initiated
- Administration of dextran to prevent clotting by decreasing platelet adhesion
- Arterial occlusion—pale, slow capillary refill, cool, pruny
  — Hyperbaric therapy can oxygenate tissue without the benefit of full arterial flow and may be a treatment option with arterial repair
  — Repair of the arterial occlusion or thrombectomy is necessary
- Venous congestion—dusky, blue, more brisk capillary refill, pinprick bleeding rapid
  — Relief can be accomplished with thrombolytics
  — Leeching is a viable alternative and assists the replant through the venous congestion
- In the case of the unstable patient, the surgical choice may be amputation initially or if the replant appears to be failing
  — The stress of the failing replant can increase lactic acid and overwhelm the unstable patient with inflammatory mediators
  — The failing replant is also a potential source of infection
- Leeches
  — Relieves venous congestion through feeding and releases hirudin, which continues slow oozing for up to 1 to 2 hours after the leech is removed
  — Hirudin is a selective thrombin inhibitor and prevents fibrinogen from clotting
  — Attach the temperature probe to the digit
  — Isolate the area with sterile towels to prevent the satiated leech from wandering away
    - A clear small sterile container over the leech and area also works
  — Treatment is not painful

- Pick up the leech with a sterile glove and carry to the patient's bedside in a sterile container
- Attach the leech just distal to the anastomosis
— If there is difficulty with attachment, add a drop of 5% dextrose to the site
— Allow the leech to feed undisturbed
— Remove the leech when it is satiated and has detached on its own
  - Premature detachment can result in its teeth being left in the wound
  - If early removal is necessary, place salt over the anterior sucker
— Destroy the leech after one feeding by placing in a container of alcohol
  - Flush the leech in a body waste disposal unit
— Volume loss of up to 1 to 2 g/dL Hgb can occur; monitor Hgb/Hct

Forequarter Amputation

A unique situation is the forequarter amputation (Figure 9-6). This scenario occurs when the shoulder is torqued away from the body, such as a motorcyclist clipping the mirror of a vehicle pulling the arm and shoulder posterior. In the process of the mechanism, the shoulder is dislocated and the surrounding soft tissue, subclavian artery and vein, and brachial plexus are torn or stretched. Essentially, an internal amputation has occurred, leaving the skin intact, but all of the internal structures are severely injured and separated.

If the artery is transected, the arm will be pulseless. However, the artery may be intact with an intimal tear leaving the extremity with normal pulses. The suspicion of a brachial plexus injury is high and the dislocation may not be evident on radiographs. As shown in Figure 9-6, a brachial plexus injury was diagnosed; however, the extent of the shoulder injury was not evident until the patient stood upright for ambulation with physical therapy.

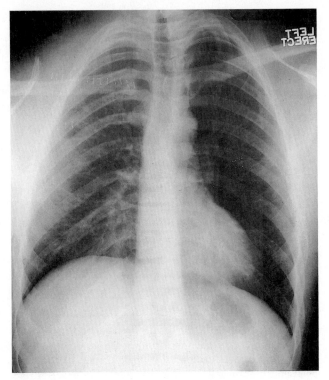

Figure 9-6   Forequarter amputation.

Gravity then pulled on the shoulder joint, dropping the shoulder and clavicle, which made the full extent of the injury obvious. On arteriogram, extravasation from a branch of the subclavian was obvious and repaired.

The decision for treatment is up to the patient. Obviously arterial and venous injuries require repair. However the brachial plexus injury is usually permanent. The arm will most likely never again be functional. It will require sling support for comfort. The dislocation may also need repair depending on the degree of displacement.

In some cases, the patient may elect amputation and placement of a prosthesis, which will result in a more functional limb.

Morel-Lavalle Lesion

The Morel-Lavalle lesion occurs in the thigh over the greater trochanter from a crush-like mechanism. The lesion is a separation of the skin and associated subcutaneous and fatty tissue away from the fascia leaving a space within the tissue, an internal degloving. Signs and symptoms include

- Soft fluctuant area

- Swelling

- Loss of cutaneous sensation

- Contusion may be present and may be tense if the area of the lesion is large

- Skin is hypermobile

- In severe lesions, necrosis and sepsis may occur

A Morel-Lavalle lesion is difficult to diagnose in the obese. Diagnosis can be made with ultrasound or MRI.

Management

Treatment requires operative intervention as percutaneous drainage may increase the opportunity for deep tissue infection. When present with fracture, it is important to manage the soft tissue injury and allow it to heal prior to internal fixation of the fracture.

- Irrigation and debridement

- Suture the space closed thus removing dead space within the deep tissues

  — Prevents recurrent fluid collection

- If necrotic fat or other tissue is present, debridement is necessary

- Monitor for sepsis

- Superficial skin loss may occur

Compartment Syndrome

When the tissues within a fascial compartment swell beyond the capacity of the fascia, compartment syndrome occurs. The swelling that occurs exceeds the normal capillary perfusion pressure resulting in collapse of the capillaries. The elevated pressure within the compartment will result in tissue and muscle necrosis unless relieved. Compartment syndrome can occur in any compartment of the body, including the abdomen (Chapter 8). Crush injury of soft tissues and vascular structures can also result in compartment syndrome. Other common mechanisms associated with compartment syndrome include snakebites, electrical burns, MAST/PASG, immobilization of the limb (eg, trapped after a fall, unable to get up for hours). Compartment syndrome is also seen after delayed revascularization of an extremity (reperfusion injury). Compartment pressures >55 mm Hg can cause irreversible muscle and soft tissue necrosis.

The most common sites are the calves and forearms. Periods of hypotension can potentiate compartment syndrome. An open fracture does not eliminate the possibility of compartment syndrome. The syndrome should be suspected with any extremity injury and especially in the presence of hypotension.

Signs and Symptoms of Compartment Syndrome

Pain out of proportion to the injury
Sensitive to touch, movement, pressure
Throbbing
Pain on passive ROM of the distal limb (pain with stretch)
Limb may be kept in flexion by the patient
Pallor (uncommon)
Paralysis
Palpable tenseness
Paresthesias
Pulselessness (LATE sign and uncommon)
Compartment pressures >30 to 40 mm Hg (normal <20 mm Hg)

Management

Prevention of compartment syndrome begins with simple routine measures

- Maintain alignment

- Immobilize the fracture/dislocation

- Do not elevate above the heart, causing a relative hypotension in the extremity
  — Elevate injured extremities to the level of the heart, not above

- Frequent monitoring of sensation and pulses

- Monitor casts, splints, traction devices for swelling, pulses

Compartment syndrome, if allowed to progress for up to 4 to 6 hours, will result in irreversible cellular death. Cellular death can cause metabolic acidosis, hyperkalemia from the intracellular fluid, release of myoglobin causing rhabdomyolysis and renal failure, and multisystem organ failure.

If suspected, measure compartment pressures with a side port/slit catheter needle or with a pressure measuring device. Diastolic blood pressure minus compartment pressure should be >30 mm Hg. Management includes

- Remove any offending device (eg, bivalve the cast, remove the splint)

- Maintain hemodynamic stability to prevent hypotension

- Fasciotomies can be performed at the bedside if the patient is unstable or preferably in the operating suite
  — The fasciotomy releases the pressure within the compartment and allows the muscle and soft tissue room for swelling
  — Often four-compartment fasciotomies are required to effectively release the compartments
  — Leave wounds open until swelling decreases; apply sterile dressings or preferably a vacuum-assisted closure device to maintain moist open areas

- When swelling decreases, closure can be delayed primary closure or split thickness skin grafts
  — Vacuum-assisted closure devices shrink the wound with the goal of closure without grafting
  — Other closure devices exist, which can be used to tighten the edges slowly, bringing the edges of the wound together until closure is obtained

- Hyperbaric oxygen therapy assists with oxygenation of tissue and promotes wound healing

A serious complication that can occur when the fasciotomies are performed is reperfusion syndrome. Reperfusion goes hand in hand with rhabdomyolysis, which can occur from cell death without compartment syndrome. Reperfusion occurs when the arterial blood flow is restored to the ischemic tissue. Lactic acidosis occurs as the lactate in the dying tissue is released back into the circulation. Hyperkalemia results from the intracellular potassium released into the circulation. The hyperkalemia should be self-limiting. The myoglobin released from the damaged skeletal muscle, however, is flushed through the kidneys, causing acute tubular necrosis from obstruction. Management includes

- Monitor creatinine kinase (5 times normal is indicative of rhabdomyolysis)

- Measure myoglobin in the urine
  — Suspicion for myoglobinuria should be high with tea-colored urine

- Administer intravenous fluids to maintain urine output at ~100 mL/hour

- Include bicarbonate in the IV fluids to alkalinize the urine, which moves myoglobin out of the tubules

- Mannitol may be added to the IV fluid to increase urine output

Heterotrophic Ossification

After fracture, spinal cord injury, and head injury, heterotrophic ossification (HO) can occur. HO is the overgrowth of extra bone within the soft tissue usually greater than 1 month after injury. It most commonly occurs within the hip. In patients with head injury, the shoulders and elbows are most frequently involved. For spinal cord injury patients, the knees are the most likely site, but will always be a joint below the level of spine injury. HO becomes disabling causing immobility of the joints involved.

Signs and Symptoms of Heterotrophic Ossification

Localized inflammation
Painful, palpable mass within soft tissue near large joints
Swelling
Radiographic confirmation

Management

Management includes control of both the bone growth and the inflammation.

- Nonsteroidal anti-inflammatory drugs (NSAIDs) administration preferably indomethicin

- Radiation therapy
  — Administered as a single dose postoperatively as a preventative measure
  — Posterior hip dislocation with femoral head fracture may be a contraindication as there is potential for avascular necrosis and nonunion

- Surgery
  — Likely recurrent HO
  — Some suggest delaying operation up to 12 months (*Duke Orthopaedics presents Wheeless' Textbook of Orthopaedics*)
  — Resection once ossification matures

Avascular Necrosis

Avascular necrosis (AVN) results from loss of blood supply. The femoral head is particularly susceptible during posterior hip dislocation.

Signs and Symptoms of Avascular Necrosis

Hip—pain in the groin radiating down the thigh; worse with walking
Wrist—pain in wrist with finger weakness; worse with movement
Knee—pain in the knee; commonly the distal femur
Shoulder—pain in the proximal humerus; stiffness

Diagnosis includes the use of radiographs and MRI, which demonstrate bony changes, identifying avascular necrosis. If untreated or undiagnosed, the bone will degenerate and collapse, resulting in disability. Severe AVN may require surgery.

Management

Management of AVN is focused on stopping the degenerative process and managing the pain to regain function. However, prevention is key and that begins with rapid identification of dislocation and immediate reduction. This is particularly important in the hip.

- Medications
  - NSAIDs for inflammation and pain
  - Bisphosphonates may be promising in slowing the progression of degeneration as well as treat pain
- Nonweight bearing (NWB) or touchdowm weight bearing (TDWB) status decreases stress on the joint with gentle ROM
- Electrotherapy—electrical stimulus applied to the area to encourage bone growth
- Surgery
  - Osteotomy: reshaping to adjust the areas of stress, relieving pressure on the area of AVN

— Total joint replacement
— Bone graft (vascularized fibula) to encourage new bone growth
— Core decompression

Fat Embolism Syndrome

The source of fat embolism is the fatty marrow within the bones, which is released into the bloodstream upon fracture or movement of the fracture edges of bone. Another theory holds that chylomicrons (free fatty acids) are released during trauma, which coalesce and result in the same fat embolism syndrome (FES). It develops rapidly within 12 to 48 hours but up to 96 hours after injury. Any bone can be the source of the fat emboli. FES can be life threatening if the ventilation issues are not recognized and treated.

Signs and Symptoms of Fat Embolism Syndrome

Confusion, restlessness, agitation
Respiratory distress, tachypnea
Hypoxemia (PaO$_2$ <60 mm Hg)
Hemoptysis, productive cough
Chest pain
Fever 38°C to 40°C
Persistent tachycardia
Intermittent nonpalpable petechiae on the chest, axillae, oral
    mucosa (diagnostic, but appear and disappear rapidly)
Retinal hemorrhages
Renal dysfunction
Jaundice
Decreased hemoglobin and/or platelets (<50,000/mm^3)
Oliguria, lipuria (fat in the urine)

Management and Prevention

Prevention of FES is part of the initial stabilization of every trauma patient. The prevention of FES involves immobilization of fractures from the scene, minimal manipulation, and early reduction and fixation. Since the primary organ system involved in FES is the lungs, early recognition and ventilatory support is paramount. During the evaluation, other causes of these symptoms must be ruled out including

- Diffuse axonal injury—petechial hemorrhages in the brain on CT or MRI

- Rule out pulmonary embolism as a cause of the respiratory symptoms

- Rule out infection as a source of fever

- Rule out hemorrhage as the cause of dropping hemoglobin and platelets

- Treat FES by
    — Maintaining adequate ventilation including intubation
    — Maintaining hemodynamic stability
    — Corticosteroids may have some benefit in maintaining respiratory stability through treatment of inflammation
    — Early fixation of fractures

- May take up to a year for complete lung healing to occur

Superior Mesenteric Artery Syndrome

Superior mesenteric artery (SMA) syndrome occurs when a patient is on bed rest for a prolonged period of time particularly in the supine position and particularly when the patient is thin. When body casts were used frequently to treat pelvic or vertebral fractures, SMA syndrome was more frequent. However, the providers should be aware of the syndrome in patients with spica casts, supine positioning for bed rest because of multiple fractures, and elderly thin patients who are bed bound. SMA syndrome occurs when the SMA and the duodenum are compressed against the aorta. The compression results in obstruction of the duodenum.

Signs and Symptoms of Superior Mesenteric Artery Syndrome

Loss of appetite
Initially increased flatus and belching
Epigastric pain
Abdominal pain after eating (up to 4 hours)
Vomiting
Decreased bowel sounds
Tympanic upper abdominal quadrants
Lethargy
Radiograph—distended bowel on abdominal plain films; CT is also helpful in making the diagnosis

Management and Prevention

As with all posttrauma complications, prevention is key. Frequent turning, small protein meals, and prevention of constipation are routine management activities that can prevent SMA syndrome in the patient on bed rest. Of course, these activities prevent other complications as well. In addition, turning the patient to the right after eating encourages peristalsis. Management of the syndrome includes

- Maintaining electrolyte balance and nutrition

- Treat constipation

- Jejunal feedings may be necessary to rest the duodenum

- Monitor weight

- Metoclopramide may assist with peristalsis

- If medical management fails and surgery is necessary, release of the ligament of Treitz or duodenojejunostomy may relieve the duodenal dilatation and obstruction

- Prevent dehydration

- Delayed or missed diagnosis can result in dehydration, hypokalemia, as well as death

POSTRESUSCITATION MANAGEMENT AND REHABILITATION

For the orthopaedic trauma patient, rehabilitation is paramount. From the initial arrival and stabilization, through fixation, the goal is always return to preexisting function. Every orthopaedic injury, however slows that process until the bone or joint is healed. Patience through the rehabilitation, as well as adherence to the exercise program designed for the patient, is essential to healing in alignment, prevention of nonunion, hardware failure, and stability of the bone at the end of the healing time. Both physical and occupational therapy are key rehabilitation specialists involved in the patient's care. In addition, early involvement of the physiatrist enables the design of a rehabilitation program from the beginning. Early rehabilitation focuses on balance, exercises, strengthening, and transfers. Progress to ambulation with assistive devices and regaining control of activities of daily living (ADL) is part of the process.

Follow-up studies of orthopaedic patients have shown that after sacral fractures impaired mobility still exists at 1 year for up to 63% with 91% having some degree of sensory deficit from the fracture (Totterman et al. 2006). Voiding, bowel and sexual function impairment remain for up to 50%. For patients with preexisting psychiatric diagnoses, impaired functional outcome results in posttraumatic psychopathology, which peaks at 2 months and improves by 6 months (Sutherland et al. 2006).

Sequelae identified after intramedullary nailing of the tibia demonstrate a low percentage of venous stasis (18%). Persistent sequelae include arthritis (33%) and muscle atrophy (27%). The study followed patients for up to 14 years and identified that few had any ROM of the knee issues, although 73% had moderate pain in the knee (Lefaivre et al. 2008).

In a study of self-reported disability versus observed disability, most observers rated the disability of the patient lower than what was perceived by the patient themselves (Dowrick et al. 2006). This is important to note as therapy is initiated and then continued in aftercare. The patient's perception of disability will affect their motivation to participate in activities.

Rehabilitation after hospitalization is dependent upon the ability of the patient to participate as well as associated injuries. If severe head or spinal cord injury is present, the rehabilitation center of choice will likely be a center with a neurologic focus. The orthopaedic trauma will be rehabilitated at the same time. For the elderly with limited endurance or limited preexisting mobility, a short-term stay at a skilled nursing facility will provide the physical and occupational therapy needed to return to independent living. Of note, a single "hip" fracture in the elderly is frequently the singular reason for loss of independent living. Prevention of falls is essential.

Acute inpatient rehabilitation provides ~8 hours per day of active therapy. The patient needs to be able to tolerate 2 to 3 hours at a time to participate. For patients with good mobility but are homebound, follow-up therapy can be provided by home health. For patients mobile enough to leave the home and tolerate a car ride, outpatient therapy is provided until the patient is independent.

Various tools and assistive devices are used to improve mobility including

- Crutches—requires coordination, upper body strength, and no upper extremity injury

- Cane—provides stability as the patient progresses from crutches and is allowed to weight bear on the injured extremity

- Quad-cane—cane with four "feet" instead of one that provides more stability as a base

- Walker—requires weight-bearing upper extremities; a platform may be attached if an upper extremity is injured and is partial weight bearing; requires the ability to lift the walker

- Front-wheel walker—easier for the elderly as it does not require lifting and provides a wide base of support

- Wheelchair—for nonweight-bearing patients or mixed upper and lower extremity injuries; if upper extremities are uninjured, the patient may be able to "wheel" without assistance

- Bracing is used to support joints including a hinged "Bledsoe" brace for knee injuries, which can maintain the knee in functional position

- For some knee injuries, continuous passive ROM may be used very early in treatment to prevent freezing of the knee joint

    Weight-bearing status applies to both upper and lower extremities as both weight bear to a degree. Definitions include

- NWB—nonweight bearing, no weight at all on the extremity

- TDWB or TTWB—touch down or toe touch weight bearing, 10% of normal weight is placed on the extremity

- PWB—partial weight bearing, <50% of normal weight is born by the extremity

- WBAT—weight bearing as tolerated, as much weight as the patient can tolerate

- FWB—full weight bearing, 100% weight bearing is allowed

    Specific rehabilitation goals (estimates dependent on individual healing) include

- Hip
    — Exercises, transfers, balance, and ambulation begin day 1 after surgery
    — Ambulation with assistive device
    — Home physical therapy (PT) 2 to 8 weeks after discharge

- Pelvis
    — If stable, WBAT
    — Unstable requires surgical fixation first then a determination of weight-bearing status by the orthopod

- Ankle
  - Weight-bearing cast for 4 to 6 weeks
  - Displaced requires NWB for 4 to 6 weeks, followed by a walking cast for 2 weeks
  - ROM and strengthening is provided when healed
- Foot
  - Short-leg cast with NWB for 6 weeks, then a walking cast for 12 weeks
- Shoulder
  - Sling with elbow ROM
  - Shoulder ROM restricted per orthopaedic surgeon's decision and degree of instability
  - Strengthening and passive ROM activities begin at 2 weeks
  - Increase to active ROM at 6 weeks
- Proximal humerus
  - Initiate exercise at 1 week
  - Remove sling after 3 weeks
- Humerus shaft
  - Initiate ROM
  - Fracture brace for 6 weeks
- Radius-ulna
  - Long-arm cast or splinting usually < 3 weeks at 90 degrees flexion with conversion to a brace at 2 weeks
- Distal radius
  - Short-arm cast for 4 to 6 weeks, followed by a splint for 1 month
  - Maintain shoulder and finger ROM
  - Weight bearing is allowed at 6 weeks if callus formation is present
- Scaphoid (upper extremity)
  - Healing varies from 6 weeks to 6 months

— A nondisplaced fracture at 2 months should be considered for ORIF

All listed goals are viable if the patient participates appropriately in therapy and callus formation is evident at the time of decision to change to a splint or brace and then to full weight bearing. Smoking, alcohol, poor nutrition, and comorbidities affect the healing of bones and will delay return to optimal function. The patient must also strictly follow the weight-bearing status of the extremity to avoid "undoing" the healing that has begun. Vitamin D and calcium in the diet are essential components of healing bone.

Evaluation by social services and case management is necessary to determine the structure and safety of the home to which the patient will return. Issues to consider include

- One story or multistory home
- Steps both inside and to enter the home
- Bathroom on entry level
- Can a bedroom be set up on the entry level?
- Does the patient need a hospital bed?
- If going home with a wheelchair
  — Is there access to home entry (ramp or no stairs)?
  — Will the wheelchair fit through bathroom/bedroom doors?
- Are there safety rails in the bathroom for the toilet and shower?
- Safety hazards removed
  — Throw rugs
  — Poor lighting
  — Clutter
- Assistive devices needed, such as durable medical equipment (commode, raised toilet seat)
- Is there a phone?

- Is there running water?
- Is there heat and electricity?
- Does patient live alone?
  — Need food delivered?
  — Need 24-hour assistance?
  — Home therapy?
- How will patient be transported home?
- Does patient understand the use of the devices?
  — Splints: on/off periods of time
  — Off for showering?
  — Off in bed?
  — Halo devices and external fixators are meant to be in place at all times and are not to be removed by the patient or family

Overall, the orthopaedic healing is dependent upon patient resuscitation and stability, participation in therapy, and gentle progress toward return to function in the hospital, in acute rehabilitation, and at home for up to months after injury.

 Critical Lifesavers

- **At every examination inspection and palpation are compared for symmetry between the extremities**
- **Any loss of pulses [motor or sensory examination] after splinting or placement of a traction device requires removal of the splint and repositioning, then reassess**
- **[To close the pelvic ring] Place a sheet under the pelvis, wrap it around to the front and tie tightly, check pulses**
- **During assessment of the pelvis, DO NOT compress the iliac wings OR rock the pelvis as this can displace fractures and/or increase hemorrhage**

REFERENCES

Arrillega A, Bynoe R, Frykberg ER, et al. Practice management guidelines for penetrating trauma in the lower extremities. 2002. Available at: http://www.east.org. Accessed October 17, 2008.

Canadian Orthopaedic Trauma Society. Nonoperative treatment compared with plate fixation of displaced midshaft clavicular fractures: a multicenter randomized clinical trial. *J Bone Joint Surg Am.* 2007;89(1):1-10.

Canadian Orthopaedic Trauma Society. Reamed vs undreamed intramedullary nailing of the femur: comparison of the rate of ARDS in multiple injured patients. *J Orthop Trauma.* 2006;20(1):384-387.

DiGiacomo JC, Bonadies JA, Cole FJ, et al. Practice management guidelines for hemorrhage in pelvic fracture. 2001. Available at: http://www.east.org. Accessed October 17, 2008.

Dowrick A, Gabbe B, Williamson O, et al. A comparison of self-reported and independently observed disability in an orthopedic trauma population. *J Trauma.* 2006;61(6):1447-1452.

Duke orthopaedics presents Wheeless' Textbook of Orthopaedics. Heterotrophic ossification. Available at: http://www.wheelessonline.com. Accessed October 17, 2008.

Gustilo RB, Anderson JT. Prevention of infection in the treatment of one thousand and twenty five open fractures of long bones: retrospective and prospective analyses. *J Bone Joint Surg Am.* 1976;58:453-458.

Gustilo RB, Mendoza RM, Williams DN. Problems in the management of type III (severe) open fractures: a new classification of type III open fractures. *J Trauma.* 1984;24:742-746.

Jones AL. Recombinant human bone morphogenic protein-2 in fracture care. *J Orthop Trauma.* 2005;19(10):S23-S25.

Kortbeek JB, Al Turki SA, Ali J, et al. Advanced trauma life support: the evidence for change. *J Trauma.* 2008;64(6):1638-1650.

Kragh J, Walters T, Baer D, et al. Practical use of emergency tourniquets to stop bleeding in major limb trauma. *J Trauma.* 2008;64(2):S38-S50.

Lefaivre K, Guy P, Chan H, et al. Long-term follow-up of tibial shaft fractures treated with intramedullary nailing. *J Orthop Trauma.* 2008;22(8):525-529.

Lin CD. Orthopedic rehabilitation. In: Cooper G, ed. *Essential Physical Medicine and Rehabilitation.* Totowa, NJ: Humana Press; 2006.

Lopez PP. Unstable pelvic fractures: the use of angiography in controlling arterial hemorrhage. *J Trauma.* 2007;62(6):S30-S31.

Luchette FA, Bone LB, Born CT, et al. Practice management guidelines for prophylactic antibiotic use in open fractures. 2000. Available at: http://www.east.org. Accessed October 17, 2008.

Magnussen R, Tressler M, Obremskey WT, et al. Predicting blood loss in isolated pelvic and acetabular high-energy trauma. *J Orthop Trauma.* 2007;21(9):603-607.

Moed, R. Improving results in posterior wall acetabular fracture surgery. *J Trauma.* 2007;62(6):S63.

Okike KB, Bhattacharyya T. Trends in the management of open fractures: a critical analysis. *J Bone Joint Surg Am.* 2006;88A(12): 2739-2748.

Pape HC, Giannoudis P Krettek C, et al. Timing of fixation of major fractures in blunt polytrauma: role of conventional indicators in clinical decision making. *J Orthop Trauma.* 2005;19(8):551-562.

Pape HC. Rixen D, Morley J, et al. Impact of the method of initial stabilization for femoral shaft fractures in patients with multiple injuries at risk for complications (borderline patients). *Ann Surg.* 2007;246(3):491-499; discussion 499-501.

Sarin E, Moore J, Moore E, et al. Pelvic fracture pattern does not always predict the need for urgent embolization. *J Trauma.* 2005;58(5):973-977.

Scalea TM. Optimal timing of fracture fixation: have we learned anything in the past 20 years? *J Trauma.* 2008;65(2):253-260.

Sutherland AG, Alexander D, Hutchison J. The mind does matter: psychological and physical recovery after musculoskeletal trauma. *J Trauma.* 2006;61(6):1408-1414.

Totterman AS, Glott T, Madsen JE, et al. Unstable sacral fractures: associated injuries and morbidity at 1 year. *Spine.* 2006;31(18): E628-E635.

Varela CD, Vaughan TK, Carr JB, et al. Fracture blisters: clinical and pathological aspects. *J Orthop Trauma.* 1993;7(5):417-427.

Ward WG, Nunley JA. Occult orthopaedic trauma in the multiply injured patient. *J Orthop Trauma.* 1991;5(3):308-312.

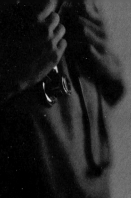

Chapter 10

BURN AND EXTERNAL INJURY

INTRODUCTION

One of the most successful injury prevention programs in the country has been for burn prevention. However, despite the progress made by the burn centers and fire protection agencies, ~500,000 burns occur each year (White and Renz 2008). Of these, 40,000 patients will be hospitalized with ~50% requiring burn center care. Identification of the severe and specialty burns must occur early in the resuscitation of the patient to arrange for rapid transfer to the appropriate facility.

Burns occur from flame/thermal injury, chemical, radiation, and electrical events. Radiation burns are discussed in Chapter 15. Thermal events can be caused by flame, heat or cold exposure, scalds, hot objects, and steam/hot gases. Burns from scalds remain a frequent injury from child abuse. The children tend to be young (~2.4 years) with a relatively large burn surface area (13%) (Thombs 2008). A high level of suspicion for abuse is maintained in these cases. Scald burn depth is determined by temperature, duration of contact, and thickness of the skin exposed.

The skin is the largest organ of the body and has many functions. Skin enables sensation of pain, touch, temperature, and pressure. It provides thermoregulation primarily through sweat. The sebaceous glands of the skin secrete sweat. It also protects from heat and cold, bacteria, and chemicals. All of these properties are disrupted to some degree when a burn occurs.

BURN

Assessment

Assessment for burn patients follows the same pattern of management as of the trauma patient with additional considerations specific to management of the burn. It is possible for the burn patient to have concomitant trauma. Using the resuscitation process for trauma (Chapter 2) ensures both rapid management of the burn as well as identification and management of associated injuries. Motor vehicle collisions (MVC), jumping from burning buildings, blast injuries, and industrial events can all result in serious associated trauma.

History

The history of the burn event should begin with the source of the burn injury and any associated mechanisms as noted above. In addition, past medical history, age, allergies, medications, alcohol or drugs, and environmental exposure are essential in the history collection. When transferring a burn patient to the burn center, providing this information is necessary for the burn center to prepare for the incoming patient. Increased mortality from burn injury is predicted when associated with human immunodeficiency virus-acquired immunodeficiency syndrome (HIV-AIDS), renal or liver disease, and metastatic cancer (Thombs 2007). Increased length of stay can be predicted in the presence of dementia, peptic ulcer disease, neurologic disorders such as paralysis or stroke, cardiac dysrhythmias, renal disease, or psychiatric illness (Thombs 2007). Circumstances of injury that are essential to the big picture of the burn itself include

- Type of burn event
  - Flame: clothing involved?
  - Other thermal: scald, hot object, hot liquid
  - Chemical: identify if possible, alkali vs. acid, exposure or ingestion
  - Electrical: voltage, current direct or alternating

— Cold: note if exposure to a wet environment is involved

— Blast exposure: includes chemical/tar explosions

- Duration of exposure
- Temperature in the event of cold or scald exposure
- Enclosed space?
- Loss of consciousness
- Associated mechanism of injury in addition to the burn
- History consistent with the injury and between informants—possible abuse

— Length of time between event and seeking medical assistance

- Events that occurred immediately after the injury

— How was the burn extinguished?

— Decontamination of chemical?

— Cardiopulmonary resuscitation (CPR) at the scene? Other prehospital procedures, such as oxygen, intubation, intravenous lines (IV)

Trauma assessment: burn specific

Principles of trauma primary assessment are undertaken to determine both the impact of the burn injury as well as any associated injuries (Chapter 2). Burn events may include mechanisms other than the burn, such as motor vehicle collision (MVC) or fall. Primary assessment includes

- Airway

— Insert an endotracheal tube using rapid sequence intubation (RSI) for signs of inhalation injury, airway compromise, respiratory difficulty, or hemodynamic instability

— Inhalation injury occurs most often with a fire in an enclosed space

  ■ Inhalation injury includes inhaling superheated air, the product of combustion and soot. Products of combustion are described in Table 10-1

  ■ Patients smoking with oxygen in place results in a direct airway burn and inhalation of heated air

Table 10-1   By-products of Combustion

Source	Irritant	Toxin
Polystyrene—foam		Carbon monoxide (CO), styrene
Acrylic	Acrolein	Hydrogen cyanide (HCN)
Nylon (carpeting, clothing)	Ammonia	HCN
Acrilon (carpeting)	Acrolein	HCN
Polyvinyl chloride (PVC) (wall coverings, flooring, insulation, pipes)	Hydrochloric acid (HCl), phosgene	CO
Wallpaper, lacquered woods	Acetaldehyde, formaldehyde, oxides of nitrogen	Acetic acid
Polyurethane (furniture)	Isocyanates	HCN, ammonia, halogen acid
Rubber		Sulfur dioxide

- Early identification of inhalation injury and early intubation prevents airway loss. Inhalation injury can take up to 24 hours to present (ATLS 2004)
- Insidious onset of edema 24 to 48 hours, even up to 72 hours after injury; vigilant airway assessment is necessary to prevent crisis
— Hypopharyngeal edema can progress to complete airway obstruction.
- Mortality increases by 20% when inhalation injury is present (TNCC 2007)
- Children <2 years and the elderly >60 years suffer increased mortality directly related to smoke inhalation (Osborn 2003)

Inhalation Injury Signs and Symptoms

Soot oral or nasal passages; within airway (carbonaceous sputum)

Facial burns, singed facial and nasal hairs

Productive cough

Hoarse voice

Stridor, expiratory wheezes, retractions

Shortness of breath

Increased secretions, difficulty swallowing

Swollen tongue, reddened mucous membranes

Increased carbon monoxide level

Fiberoptic bronchoscopy for direct airway assessment—redness, edema, sloughing, carbonaceous material

- Breathing—affected by past medical history, presence of the by-products of combustion, inhalation injury, and carbon monoxide (CO)
  - CO poisoning occurs during combustion and the inhalation of CO. Hemoglobin has an affinity for CO that is >240 times the affinity for oxygen The affinity for CO shifts the oxyhemoglobin curve left
    - Smokers commonly have a CO level of 7%
    - CO levels of 20% to 30% result in headache and nausea, altered mental status, difficulty concentrating, tightness over the forehead
    - CO levels of 30% to 40% result in severe headache, confusion, altered judgment, irritable
    - CO levels of 40% to 60% results in coma
    - CO levels >60% result in apnea, death within hours
    - CO levels >80% result in death within 1 hour; CO levels >90% result in death within minutes
  - Transcutaneous CO monitors are useful for rapid determination of elevated CO

Signs and Symptoms of CO Poisoning

Singed nasal hair, soot, carbonaceous sputum
Headache
Nausea, vomiting
Dizziness
Tachypnea
Loss of dexterity
Subtle memory loss, confusion, progresses to coma, irritability
Cherry red mucous membranes are rare
Pulse oximetry readings are usually normal

- Circulation
  - Pulses should be assessed in all extremities, especially in the presence of a circumferential burn
  - Circumferential burns of the chest impair breathing by preventing chest wall expansion
    - Immediate escharotomies may be necessary to prevent respiratory distress
    - High Fowler position may also assist with respirations in these patients
  - Hemodynamic and urine output monitoring
    - Tachycardia, tachypnea may be present
    - Unable to regulate temperature
  - Check for associated injury that may result in blood loss
  - Burn shock occurs with total burn surface area (TBSA) >20%
    - Disruption of capillary integrity results in protein leak
    - Capillary stability is usually restored within 24 to 36 hours (Ziglar et al. 2004)
- Extent and depth of burn
  - Rule of nines: determines the percentage of TBSA that has sustained burn. It is necessary for determining the need

for and amount of fluid resuscitation as well as management of the burn wound. Figure 10-1 describes the rule of nines for children (<3 years) and adults

— Rule of palms: the palm (including fingers) of the patient is equal to 1% of the patient's body surface area. This method of determination of TBSA is particularly useful for scattered burns

— Depth of burn: is described by the layers of the skin involved. Table 10-2 describes the differences among burn depths

Documentation

Documentation of the burn wound includes all trauma documentation and in addition, the burn depth and extent. A method of documentation of both extent and depth is the burn estimation chart (see Table 10-3). The chart enables the provider to specifically determine TBSA by depth and complete the resuscitation formula. It provides one concise place for burn information. As the burn can progress over the initial 48 hours caused by inflammatory mediators and initial management, the burn estimation chart should be repeated to monitor the progression.

Emergent Management

Resuscitation

Personal protective equipment (PPE) is essential to protect the patient from infection. Minimize activity in and out of the room to maintain temperature as well as decrease exposure.

• Intubation should be considered for patients with inhalation injury, altered level of consciousness, and hemodynamic instability

— Deliver humidified oxygen at 100%

— Apply pulse oximetry and CO detector if appropriate; be careful with false-positive readings in the presence of CO

— Obtain arterial blood gas (ABG) with carboxyhemoglobin level

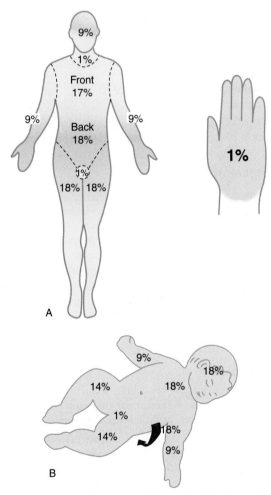

Figure 10-1   Rule of nines, adult (A) and infant (B). (Adult illustration by Maggie Reynard. Infant illustration, with permission, from Auerbach PS. *Field Guide to Wilderness Medicine,* 5th ed. Mosby, 2003.)

Table 10-2 Burn Depth

Depth	Superficial	Superficial Partial Thickness	Deep Partial Thickness	Full Thickness
Epidermis	Minor edema, erythema, pain, blanches Peeling 24-48 hours 3-5 days healing	Significant edema, red, moist, fluid filled blisters, weeping, intense pain, sensitive to air flow	Flat, dehydrated, very thin skin, mottled, waxy white, dry; no blanching	White, charred, eschar, dry, pain/sensory decreased or none, loss epidermal appendages, leathery
Dermis—blood vessels, nerve endings, sweat glands, hair follicles, new cell regeneration		Into upper dermis 10-14 days healing	Into subcutaneous tissue 21-28 days healing	
Subcutaneous fat, muscle, bone				No healing, requires grafting

Table 10-3 Burn Estimation Chart

Area	<1 year	1-4 years	5-9 years	10-14 years	15 years	>15 years	PT	FT	TOTAL
Head	19	17	13	11	9	7			
Neck	2	2	2	2	2	2			
Anterior trunk	13	13	13	13	13	13			
Posterior trunk	13	13	13	13	13	13			
R buttock	2.5	2.5	2.5	2.5	2.5	2.5			
L buttock	2.5	2.5	2.5	2.5	2.5	2.5			
Genitalia	1	1	1	1	1	1			
RUE, upper	4	4	4	4	4	4			
LUE, upper	4	4	4	4	4	4			
RUE, lower	3	3	3	3	3	3			
LUE, lower	3	3	3	3	3	3			

R hand	2.5	2.5	2.5	2.5	2.5	2.5
L hand	2.5	2.5	2.5	2.5	2.5	2.5
R thigh	5.5	6.5	8	8.5	9	9.5
L thigh	5.5	6.5	8	8.5	9	9.5
R leg	5	5	5.5	6	6.5	7
L leg	5	5	5.5	6	6.5	7
R foot	3.5	3.5	3.5	3.5	3.5	3.5
L foot	3.5	3.5	3.5	3.5	3.5	3.5

R, right; L, left; RUE, right upper extremity; LUE, left upper extremity; PT, partial thickness; FT, full thickness.

— Restlessness and anxiety are usually associated with hypoxia or hypovolemia; assess for these prior to medication administration and administer oxygen first

— Bronchodilators may be necessary in airway burns

— Steroids should not be used

— If cyanide poisoning is suspected (see Table 10-1) administer the antidote to cyanide as described in Chapter 15

• CO poisoning

— Apply 100% oxygen until CO level is <10%

— Half-life of CO is 250 minutes on room air

— Half-life of CO is 40 minutes on 100% oxygen

— Hyperbaric oxygen (HBO) should be considered if available; the half-life of CO is 23 minutes in a hyperbaric chamber at 3 atmospheres absolute (ATA) (48 fsw [feet of seawater])

— A patient with CO >25% or any signs and symptoms of CO poisoning should receive HBO

— HBO forces oxygen into plasma and into cells providing oxygenation without the need for hemoglobin while the gradient forces out the CO

• Two large bore IV are placed for fluid resuscitation.

— If possible, avoid placement through the burn. However, if the only option is through the burned area, placement of the IV is the priority.

— Fluid resuscitation is initiated for burns >20% TBSA. Initiation involves careful calculation of fluids needed based upon TBSA and body weight (kg). This is an estimate of the total fluid needs of the patient.

— Administer warm lactated ringer (LR)

— Burn formulas for the first 24 hours after the burn

$$2 \text{ to } 4 \text{ mL} \times \text{TBSA\%} \times \text{weight (kg)}$$
$$\text{Example: } 4 \times 40\% \times 70 \text{ kg} = 11{,}200 \text{ mL LR}$$

— Pediatric fluid resuscitation formula = 3 to 4 mL × TBSA% × weight (kg)

— Administer one-half total in the first 8 hours, followed by one-half total over the next 16 hours

— Timing for fluid resuscitation begins at the time of the burn, not the time of patient arrival

— Inhalation burn, high voltage electrical burn, associated injury, dehydration prior to injury, presence of alcohol, and delayed resuscitation result in increased fluid requirements (Kramer et al. 2007)

— An additional maintenance IV that includes dextrose should also be maintained during fluid resuscitation in children because of rapid loss of glycogen stores (ABA 2007)

- First 10 kg body weight = 100 mL/kg over 24 hours
- Second 10 kg body weight = 50 mL/kg over 24 hours
- Each kg >20 kg = 20 mL/kg over 24 hours
- Example: for a 25 kg child = 1000 mL + 500 mL + 100 mL (1600 mL maintenance IV D5LR over 24 hours)

— Continuous monitoring to avoid over-resuscitation, which is evidenced by

- Pulmonary edema
- Cerebral edema
- Abdominal compartment syndrome (ACS) mortality >80% (White and Renz 2008)

- Place a nasogastric or orogastric tube to prevent aspiration
  — Burn patients are prone to ileus
  — Particularly in children with uncuffed ETT
- Insert a Foley catheter and monitor urine output
  — Minimum adult urine output = 0.5 to 1 mL/kg/hour
  — Minimum pediatric (<30 kg) urine output = 1mL/kg/hour
  — Diuresis can occur with glycosuria, hypertonic saline or dextran administration
  — Oliguria is a sign of inadequate fluid resuscitation; fluid infusion must be increased
  — Burns to the penis require Foley catheter placement

- Warm the patient
  — Warm room
  — Warm blankets
  — ALL fluids administered through a fluid warmer
- Extremities with decreased pulses or circumferential burns require emergent escharotomies to relieve pressure from the burn and prevent muscle necrosis, nerve ischemia, and rhabdomyolysis. This includes the torso.
  — Monitor distal pulses hourly
  — Assure pulselessness is not due to hypovolemia
  — Use electrocautery
  — If compartment syndrome is suspected, measure the muscle compartment pressures (Chapter 9)
  — If necrotic muscle is present, debridement is necessary to decrease the incidence of rhabdomyolysis
- Pain should be managed initially with short-acting narcotics and closely monitor hemodynamics
- Elevate extremities above the heart to decrease edema
  — Active range of motion (ROM) hourly also decreases edema

Wound care

Burn wounds are characterized by three zones of injury

- Zone of coagulation (central)
  — Nonviable tissue
  — Necrosis
  — Unable to regenerate
- Zone of stasis (surrounding the center)
  — Occluded capillaries, decreased perfusion
  — Edema
  — Salvageable
- Zone of hyperemia (surrounding stasis zone)
  — Increased blood flow caused by inflammation

- Inflammatory response
  — Histamine: increases capillary permeability (arterioles)
  — Prostaglandins: increases capillary permeability (arterioles)
  — Thromboxane A: platelet aggregation
  — Leukotrienes, cytokines: inflammation
  — Bradykinin: increases permeability of venules
  — Oxygen free radicals (OFRs): damage to endothelial cell microcirculation

  Immediate wound care involves

- Stop the burning process. Chemical burns are discussed under special situations.
- Remove clothing and jewelry. Edema will occur. Removal of jewelry is necessary before edema begins.
- Cover the burns with clean, dry sheets and blankets for warmth
- Do not break blisters if they are not contaminated
- DO NOT apply soaks or ice as it will increase the depth of the burn. Wet soaks will result in hypothermia, causing vasoconstriction and cellular death
- In the case of tar burns,
  — Cool the tar
  — Dissolve the tar with antibacterial or other petrolatum based product. The presence of the tar causes increased depth of the burn as it retains heat and a chemical burn in addition.
- Synthetics burn and melt onto the skin
- Do not apply ointments, creams, or dressings. Dressings will be done at the burn center. If applied prior to burn center arrival, the dressings will be removed for wound assessment.
- If transfer to a burn center is delayed >24 hours, initial debridement should be undertaken at the referring facility
  — Large blisters
  — Cleanse with diluted chlorhexidine or a gentle soap and water

— Apply thin layer of silver sulfadiazine

— Continue to pursue transfer

Transfer criteria

The American Burn Association recommends transfer to a designated burn center for the following burn patients (ABA 2007)

- TBSA ≥ 10% partial thickness burn
- Full thickness burns in any age group and any TBSA
- Inhalation burn
- Electrical burn/lightning injury
- Chemical burn
- Burns with associated trauma
  — If the trauma is more severe or life threatening, transfer to a trauma center first
- Pediatric burns in a non-pediatric hospital
- Burns to hands, feet, face, genitalia, major joints
- Past medical history (PMH) including, for example, diabetes mellitus, hypertension, peripheral vascular disease, chronic obstructive pulmonary disease (COPD), congestive heart failure (CHF), myocardial infarction (MI)
- Burns that will require long-term rehabilitative care, special situations such as social or emotional needs requiring intervention
  — Past medical history that could prolong recovery or increase complications

Ongoing Management

Management of the burn patient is complex and involves all body systems. Prevention of complications is foremost in all levels of care.

- Pulmonary care
  — Early intubation to manage airway burn as well as prevent acute lung injury from the inflammatory mediators of the systemic inflammatory response syndrome

— Early tracheostomy results in shorter ventilation time to extubation (Ipaktchi and Arbabi 2006)
— Chest escharotomy for circumferential thoracic burn
— Acute lung injury/airway burn
  ▪ Extracorporeal membrane oxygenation may be helpful in children
  ▪ High-frequency jet ventilation or low tidal volumes with permissive hypercapnea in the adult patient
  ▪ Nitrous oxide may assist with hypoxic vasoconstriction, improving $\dot{V}/\dot{Q}$ mismatch
— Ventilator-associated pneumonia (VAP)
  ▪ Decreases ciliary action, secretory clearance, and increases plasma leak
  ▪ Bronchoscopy has been shown to decrease unnecessary antibiotic administration and the incidence of VAP (Ipaktchi and Arbabi 2006)
— CO poisoning
  ▪ After the initial management with oxygen or HBO, residual side effects may be present for up to 40 days, including
    ○ Personality changes
    ○ Seizures
    ○ Chronic headache
    ○ Parkinson-like movements
— Increase-head of the bed to decrease edema in the head and neck
• Resuscitation
  — Monitor urine output
  — Monitor for rhabdomyolysis
    ▪ Associated mortality >70% (White and Renz 2008)
    ▪ Increase IV fluids to maintain urine output 1 mL/kg/hour (75-100 mL/hour)
    ▪ Mannitol (12.5 g) added to each liter of fluid; may result in hypovolemia; should be added when myoglobinuria is not clearing with fluids (rare)

- Myoglobin is more soluble in alkaline urine; add sodium bicarbonate to each liter of fluid to increase urine pH >6

— Monitor potassium and creatine phosphokinase (CPK)

- Persistent increased potassium may require renal replacement therapy

— Studies show that in >58% of patients complete resuscitation requires more than the recommended 4 mL × TBSA% × weight (kg) (Ipaktchi and Arbabi 2006)

— Avoid overresuscitation that can result in ACS and pulmonary edema

— Hypertonic saline (7.5%) may modulate systemic inflammatory response syndrome from reperfusion and restore intravascular volume

- Use in early resuscitation
- Maintain serum sodium 160 mMol/L

— Resuscitation is adequate when

- Heart rate <120
- BP >100 mm Hg
- Urine output sustained at 0.5 mL/kg/hour

— Prevent hypothermia

— In the case of associated trauma, maintain hematocrit at 30% to 35% by administering packed red blood cells

- Wound care
  — Do not administer prophylactic antibiotics
  — Avoid sun exposure
  — Manage pain before dressing changes as vasoconstriction decreases wound healing
    - Low-dose narcotics
    - Nonsteroidal anti-inflammatory drugs (NSAIDs)
    - Biofeedback
    - Imagery
    - Distraction

- Antidepressants
- Anxiolytics to assist sedation
— Superficial burns
  - After wound cleansing, apply aloe vera until wound healed or unperfumed lotion
  - May be associated with fever, chills, vomiting if the TBSA is large
  - Administer NSAIDs
— Superficial and deep partial thickness burns
  - Cleanse with antibacterial soap (chlorhexidine)or soap and water, remove debris and devitalized tissue
    - Prevents further destruction by infection
  - Use a warm OR and warm tub room
  - Leave blisters intact as they form a biological dressing, healing the skin beneath
  - Debride large blisters
  - Apply antimicrobial creams in a thin layer
    - Silver sulfadiazine
      - Broad-spectrum antimicrobial
      - Relieves pain
    - Sulfamylon
      - Antimicrobial for Gram-positive and Gram-negative organisms
      - Penetrates eschar
      - May develop metabolic acidosis from carbonic anhydrase metabolism
      - Burning pain with application for ~20 to 30 minutes
    - Triple antibiotic ointment for the face
      - Face is very vascular and heals quickly
      - Keep moist
      - Shave facial hair
      - Use ophthalmic antibiotic ointment for eye injury; keep moist

- o Remove topical antimicrobials completely at each hydrotherapy session
- Dressings
  - o Following application of cream, apply gauze to cover burns
    - Prevents further fluid loss
    - Wrap each finger and toe with a separate gauze
  - o Silver-nylon dressings covered with gauze
    - Requires less frequent dressing changes
    - Silver ion imbedded in the dressing is antimicrobial
  - o Vacuum-assisted closure (VAC) device
    - Assists with wound closure
    - Facilitates removal of exudates
    - Expedites granulation
    - Conforms to the shape of the wound
- Prevent contractures with splinting and physical and occupational therapy
  - o Monitor splints to prevent skin breakdown
- Granulation tissue is easily injured
— Full thickness burns
  - Require skin grafting
  - Daily cleansing with antibacterial soap
  - Daily debridement of loose, dead tissue
    - o Prepares wound bed for grafting
  - Wound care is the same as for superficial/deep partial thickness burns
  - Tangential excision
    - o Begin early to remove dead tissue and promote healing
    - o Sequential removal of skin layers until viable dermis is reached
    - o Bleeding occurs
  - Grafting
    - o Full thickness skin graft (FTSG) includes the entire dermis
      - Applicable for small TBSA

- Split thickness skin graft (STSG) includes partial layer of dermis
  - Heals within 10 to 14 days
  - Meshing increases surface area to cover by 2 to 9 times
  - Sheet graft for face, hands, neck, joints in children, upper torso of women
  - Sheet grafts might collect blood, bacteria, and serous fluid
- Harvest site should be covered with fine mesh petrolatum-impregnated gauze
  - Allow to dry
  - Gauze separates from wound when healed
- VAC dressing may be used to cover the harvest site to increase healing
- Biologic dressings include cadaver or pig skin used in the same way as grafting to cover the burn and decrease fluid loss
  - Amputation
    - Amputation may be necessary if digits or extremities are unsalvageable
    - The wound is allowed to declare itself prior to amputation to determine the site for amputation
- Nutrition
  — Burn patients are in a hypermetabolic state with tachycardia, hyperthermia, and protein catabolism
    - Impairs wound healing
    - Increases chance of sepsis
    - Immunodeficient
    - Metabolic rate returns to normal when all burns are healed
    - Loss of appetite
  — Initiate early feeding within 24 hours if TBSA >40%
    - Encourage by mouth if not intubated; difficult to obtain all necessary calories by mouth

- High-carbohydrate, high-fat meals with appropriate proteins
- Use tube feedings as a first choice before resorting to total parenteral nutrition
- Aggressively monitor glucose to prevent hyperglycemia
- Some research suggests an immune enhanced diet that includes
  - Arginine
  - Glutamine
  - Omega-3 fatty acids
  - Antioxidants—vitamins E and C
- Prevention of complications decreases mortality. In patients with >40% TBSA, there is a 75% death rate if infection occurs (Murray 2007). In the initial 48 hours, typically the source of infection is Gram-positive organisms, followed by Gram-negative organisms and fungal infections within the first week after burn (Murray 2007).
  — Infection
    - Cellulitis
    - Exudate
    - Increased pain
    - Fat necrosis
    - Early rapid separation (fungal infection)
  — Do not administer antibiotics unless a known infection is present
  — Early excision of eschar decreases burn infection
  — Early colonization occurs, primarily Gram-positive cocci
  — Monitor for rhabdomyolysis and treat to prevent acute renal failure
  — Hyperkalemia
  — Prevent complications (Chapter 13)
    - Prevent gastric ulceration by administering H_2 blockers or proton pump inhibitors (PPIs)

- Prevent decubiti by frequent turning and monitoring splints
- Prevent deep venous thrombosis (DVT) through administration of low molecular weight heparin (LMWH) or subcutaneous heparin, sequential compression devices

Special Situations

Chemical burn

Chemical burns are dependent upon the agent, duration of contact, amount of agent, and concentration of the agent. In taking the patient's history, these questions should be asked to determine the next step in cleansing the wound.

Management of the chemical burn

- Wear PPE for personal protection from the chemical and protection of the burn patient
- Brush off all dry chemicals thoroughly
- Follow with copious irrigation for a minimum of 20 to 30 minutes
  — Increase flush time if the chemical is an alkali
  — Collect flushed water to dispose
- If the eye is involved
  — Flush thoroughly at least 15 minutes
  — If alkaline provide continuous lavage for up to 8 hours
  — Protect the opposite eye from runoff during irrigation
  — Consult an ophthalmologist
- Volatile forms are inhaled; monitor for inhalation burn
- Do not attempt to neutralize frequently as heat is produced during the process (exothermic)
- Specific chemicals
  — Hydrofluoric acid—deep penetration and necrosis; requires topical calcium gluconate gel
    - Found in glass etching, rust removers
    - Causes hypocalcemia, hyperkalemia, severe pain

- Prolonged QT interval, peaked T wave, ventricular dysrhythmias
- Low concentrations may have delayed symptoms occurring 6 to 18 hours after exposure
— Acids cause coagulation necrosis and protein precipitation (pH <2)
  - Found in bathroom cleaners, pool chemicals
— Alkali cause liquefaction necrosis and loosens tissue (pH >11.5)
  - Found in drain and oven cleaners, fertilizers, industrial cleaners
  - Oral ingestion requires lavage
— Lye: DO NOT flush; activated by water
— White phosphorus: DO NOT flush; explodes with water contact
— Lime: DO NOT flush—brush off, then use a dry towel
— Organic compounds: use rubber gloves
  - Phenols, gasoline, creosote
  - Systemic toxicity may be delayed up to 24 hours, coagulation necrosis
  - Phenols—irrigate with lipid soluble solvent (polyethylene glycol or ethyl alcohol)
  - Gasoline and petroleum derivatives—cause delipidation
  - Anhydrous ammonia—fertilizer, refrigerant; may be used to manufacture methamphetamines; blisters; irrigate with water; intubate if inhaled
— Tar
  - Cool the burn
  - Use petroleum-based ointment (triple antibiotic ointment or mineral oil) to dissolve

Electrical burn

Electrical burns are dependent upon voltage, current, duration of contact. Electricity will take the path of least resistance through the body. Heat from the transit moves deeply into the tissue, burning the patient from the inside out.

- Low voltage injury occurs at ≤ 600 volts
- High voltage injury is any exposure > 600 volts. The involuntary contractions that occur during contact can be severe enough to result in fractures or falls with resulting associated trauma
- Direct current forces the person away from the source usually resulting in superficial injury.
  — High voltage direct current may have direct contact (most common), an arc to a grounded victim, or a flash burn caused by the 2500°C to 4000°C arc near the victim (may result in clothing catching fire)
  — Defibrillation is an example of direct current
- Alternating current results in tetany with intermittent tonic muscle contractions mimicking a seizure
  — No definitive entrance and exit sites
  — Household current
- In order of resistance highest to lowest
  — Nerves
  — Blood vessels
  — Muscle
  — Skin
  — Tendon
  — Fat
  — Bone
  Management of electrical burns
- Secure a patent airway and initiate CPR
- Check electrocardiogram (ECG); monitor cardiac activity for 24 hours
- Significant predictors of cardiac involvement include
  — Vertical path
  — Magnitude of TBSA

- Wound care is the same as above dependent on depth and extent of burn
  — Identify entrance and exit wounds
  — The burn follows the path between the two wounds
  — Assume the burn is more extensive than it appears at first glance
  — The exit may involve traumatic amputation from the explosive exit of the electricity
- Myoglobin is released from damaged cells causing rhabdomyolysis
  — Obstructs renal tubules causing acute renal failure
  — Maintain urine output >100 mL/hour
  — Dark, tea-colored urine with positive myoglobin in urinalysis
- Neurologic injury includes
  — Cerebral dysfunction
  — Respiratory depression
  — Spastic paralysis
  — Assess cervical spine for injury, especially after a fall
- GI hemorrhage or bowel necrosis can occur
  — Symptoms may be delayed 3 to 4 days
- Vascular injury includes clot formation and vessel rupture

Lightning injury

- Lightning injury is dependent upon the distance between the individual and the strike zone; lightning itself flows around the skin causing a flashover effect
  — A fern-like burn pattern is common
  — Any metal overlying the skin may super-heat and burn the skin
- Lightning strike mortality is 30%, however of the survivors, 70% suffer complications (ABA 2007)
  — "Hair standing on end" and blue halos around objects are signs of an imminent strike
  — A direct strike has a high mortality
  — A side-flash occurs when an object nearby is struck

— Step voltage occurs when the current travels through the ground after a ground strike

Signs and Symptoms of Lightning Injury

Respiratory arrest if brainstem is involved
Cardiac dysrhythmias include supraventricular tachycardia (SVT), ventricular fibrillation (V fib), bundle-branch blocks, ventricular or atrial ectopy
Loss of consciousness, confusion, impaired concentration
Headache
Lower extremity paralysis
Cyanosis and cold below waist from parasympathetic nervous system (transient for a few hours)
Superficial burn, feathery and spider-like
Tympanic membrane rupture
Blurred vision, retinal detachment, cataracts
Fractures or dislocations from the shock wave

— Secure the airway and initiate CPR
— Long-term complications
  ■ Transient hypertension
  ■ Amnesia, short-term memory deficit
  ■ Cataracts
  ■ Vestibular dysfunction, sensorineural deafness
  ■ Retinal detachment, optic nerve damage

Frostbite

Frostbite is determined by exposure, humidity, wind chill, and the presence of wetness. It is more likely to occur at temperatures $\leq 10°C$. Temperatures $< -5°C$ result in cell damage that is unrecoverable. Vasoconstriction alternates with vasodilation (hunting response) but ultimately fails if prolonged.

Frostbite, like burn, has varying degrees of depth and extent (Table 10-4). Ice crystals form within the cell along with microvascular occlusion. Vasoconstriction results in sludging and thrombosis, decreased flow and stasis. Approximately 90% involve the hands and feet. It is essential to check the patient for hypothermia. Homelessness, age, past medical history of cardiac disease, diabetes and immunosuppression, and the

Table 10-4   Degrees of Frostbite

Depth	Signs and Symptoms	After Rewarming
Frostnip	Pain, pallor, numbness	Reverses with rewarming
First Degree	Numbness, erythema, white/yellow, edema, blue mottling, firm	Mottled, cyanotic, painful, pruritic, burning; Desquamation 5 to 10 days later
Second Degree	Clear, milky fluid-filled blisters, erythema, edema	Deep red, hot/dry, edema 2 to 3 hours Blisters fill with clear fluid 6 to 12 hours after injury
Third Degree	Blue, blisters with hemorrhagic fluid, necrosis skin and subcutaneous tissue	Early anesthetic to severe throbbing within 1 to 2 weeks; edema over the first week Demarcation 1 to 6 months later
Fourth Degree	Gangrene, mummified, necrosis, may involve bone; full-thickness loss	Deep red, mottled, cyanotic, anesthetic, dry gangrene

presence of alcohol are factors in frostbite. Other types of frost-bite include

- Chilblains—chronic damp exposure
  - Primarily face, hands, feet, anterior tibia
  - Pruritic, red-purple lesions to ulceration and hemorrhagic lesions
  - Followed by formation of scar and fibrous tissue
  - Administration of calcium channel blockers may be helpful
  - Elevate
  - Rewarm slowly to room temperature
  - Experience with previous mild frostbite can result in chilblains later
- Trench foot—chronic wet exposure in temperatures above freezing (1.6-10°C)
  - Black, deep tissue destruction
  - Alternating vasodilation and vasoconstriction (spasm)
  - Anesthetic
  - Within 24 to 48 hours becomes hyperemic, painful burning
  - Blistering, edema, redness, ecchymosis, ulceration progresses to cellulitis, gangrene
  - Elevate, rewarm in warm dry air
  - As with chilblains, subsequent exposure results in vasospasm

Management of frostbite includes

- Remove from the cold environment; remove all constricting clothing
- Pat dry, cover, keep warm
- Assess for associated injury; monitor for hypothermia
- Administer warm IV fluids for dehydration
- Pad between fingers and toes with sterile dressings; prevent maceration
- Elevate
- Place foot cradle to keep bed covers off feet

- Administer antiprostaglandins (ibuprofen)
- Immerse in circulating water bath at 40°C to 42°C until the skin is pliable and erythematous (~20-30 minutes)
  — Initiate rewarming ONLY if the entire process can be completed (Auerbach 2007)
  — Do not partially rewarm
- DO NOT massage; DO NOT use dry heat
- Administer pain medication and tetanus
  — As the tissue warms, the extremity is extremely painful
- Leave blisters closed as they provide a biological dressing unless infected
- Twice daily whirlpool cleansing and dressing changes
- Avoid vasoconstricting substances such as caffeine and smoking
- Low molecular weight dextran or heparin may prevent clot formation
- Apply silver sulfadiazine every 12 hours after rewarming and cleansing
- DO NOT debride tissue on first treatment
- Takes weeks to months to demarcate before surgical intervention or amputation
- Long term consequences include
  — Ischemic neuritis, chronic pain; consider pain clinic
  — Permanent increased vasomotor tone
    - Excess sweating
    - Abnormal sensitivity to cold (decreased)
    - Neuropathy
    - Decreased nail and hair growth
    - Raynaud phenomenon
    - At risk for reinjury
- Begin exercise during whirlpool after edema is resolved
  — Nonweight bearing until full resolution of edema

POSTRESUSCITATION MANAGEMENT AND REHABILITATION

Rehabilitation after a burn injury is extensive. Not only are the burn wounds healing, but activities of daily living (ADLs) and movement are impaired. Full active rehabilitation begins when there is <20% TBSA left open (Osborn 2003)

Rehabilitation includes

- Exercise
  - Increase strength and endurance
  - Decrease contractures, increase circulation and pulmonary function
  - Decrease edema
  - Active-assistive exercises
  - Provide exercise at regular intervals
  - Include periods of rest between exercise activities
- Stretch
  - Increase ROM, decrease contractures
  - Should be gentle, slow, and sustained
- Splinting
  - Occurs early in burn care to prevent contracture
  - Splint in functional position, joint extension
  - Anatomic, protecting joints and skin
  - Pad the splints to allow healing of the burn and prevent breakdown
- Pressure garments
  - Assist with refiguring skin
  - Protection
- Sensory
  - Evaluation of sensation of burned skin
  - Retraining
- Psychosocial support
  - Depression and self image issues

- ■ Provide psychiatry consult
  — Preexisting psychological history or anxiety predisposes the burn patient to depression at 1 year from injury (Dyster-Aas and Willebrand 2008)
  — Affective disorders or substance abuse predisposes the burn patient to posttraumatic stress disorder (PTSD) at 1 year from injury (Dyster-Aas and Willebrand 2008)
- • Vocational rehabilitation
  — Plan for return to home and occupation
  — If a change in occupation is necessary because of disability, vocational rehabilitation assists with identifying appropriate opportunities

Long-term management of the skin includes continued plastic surgery repair as needed. Maintaining skin moisture is essential and can be accomplished with aloe vera or unscented lotions. Protection from injury is provided by the pressure garments as well as reshaping the skin and decreasing scar formation. The new skin must also be protected from the sun through clothing coverage and SPF formulas. The protection of the skin is a long-term commitment.

EXTERNAL INJURY

Skin injuries are the most common of all injuries and the least severe. Despite the simplicity of the wound, inaccurate and conflicting documentation of the wounds abound. Each skin injury has distinct characteristics and should be documented appropriately. If given the opportunity, photographs should be taken of the wounds. Always take a total body photo first. Then focus on the wounds involved and photograph with and without a measurement tool. Follow hospital protocol for consent for photography, label, and enter the photos into the medical record. With increasing issues of reimbursement related to wounds acquired during the hospital stay, many facilities are documenting all wounds on arrival both for healing and legal purposes.

Forensic Wound Evidence

Wound-related forensic evidence collection is part of the provider's role

- In all cases of suspected or known abuse or assault, photographs should be taken with and without a sizing marker (eg, a ruler or coin).
- If the wound is from a stabbing or gunshot (GSW), a piece of x-ray film can be used to trace the shape/size of the wound with a permanent marker. Patterned injuries can be traced in the same way.
- Skin injuries are exigent wounds, that is, they will heal and no longer be available for evidence. Documentation is essential.
  - Patterned injuries (Figure 12-2) and bite marks are very specific tools for determining the implement causing the injury or the person inflicting the bite
  - Human bites are most often associated with sexually-based assaults; remember to evaluate for sexual assault and call the sexual assault nurse examiner
  - Swab a bite mark with a cotton-tipped swab moistened in sterile water followed by a dry swab moving from the outer area to the central area of the bite; store in a sterile container and follow evidence chain of custody
- Never describe a wound using the terms "entrance" or "exit" unless you are a forensic nursing/medicine specialist. This is not the responsibility of the caregiver, and can provide inaccurate documentation in court that can be used to support the perpetrator.
- Observe for soot or burn around the GSW and document its presence and distribution. Use a culture tube swab dampened with sterile water to swab around the area of the GSW prior to cleansing. This will collect any gunshot residue for use as evidence and determines the distance of the weapon from the victim. Store in the culture tube labeled for chain of custody and surrendered to the police.

- If a forensic expert is present, allow him or her to collect evidence from the wound prior to cleansing
- Do not cut through holes or tears in clothing as these may be necessary as evidence
  — Place clothing in separate paper bags as plastic destroys evidence and enhances mold growth
  — If wet or damp, hang to dry before bagging
  — Label per hospital policy for chain of custody and hand off to police or coroner
- Foreign body handling
  — Remove bullets with rubber tipped forceps to avoid marking the bullet
  — Place in a sterile specimen container, place loose gauze inside, seal, and label
- All evidence collected must be labeled and chain of custody maintained until turned over to legal authorities

Assessment

Skin wounds can be superficial, with or without loss of integrity of the skin surface. Skin wounds are caused by the impact of a blunt force to the skin or by a sharp object penetrating the skin surface. In trauma, wounds are described as blunt (MVC, falls, assault) or penetrating (GSW, stabbing, impalement). In forensic medicine, the medical examiner describes injuries as blunt (MVC, falls, assault, GSW) and sharp (stab, cut with a sharp object). In addition to identifying all skin injuries, any possible associated fractures should also be identified to rule out open fracture. These open fractures require orthopaedic management.

- Describe the length, depth, shape, presence of foreign body, and color
- Check pulses distal to the wound
- Check for active bleeding
  Skin injuries are described as

External Injuries

Contusion—breakage of small blood vessels within the soft tissue, resulting in "black and blue" mark from impact with a blunt object; skin intact; also called hematoma (if more consolidated) or ecchymosis; can occur at the edges of a sharp wound

Abrasions—loss of the outer epidermal layer of skin, leaving an open, weeping wound, painful; similar to a superficial partial thickness burn; may have scratches associated with it; demonstrates the direction of injury, eg, a skin roll at the edge shows the direction in which the abrasion ended; usually caused from "skidding" across roadways or other surfaces; tattooing may occur permanently imbedding debris into the skin; also described as "road rash"

Lacerations—open wound through the skin surfaces made by a blunt object impact to the skin, especially over bony prominences when the skin "splits"; can extend to or through muscle layers; bridging veins can be seen within deep lacerations; edges are ragged

Cut—open wound through the skin surface made by a sharp object; edges are clean; wound longer than deep; also referred to as "incision"

Stab—open wound through the skin made by a sharp object; edges are clean and may take on the shape of the object as well as the direction of entry; if imbedded to the hilt, the shape/design of the object will be present; deeper than long

Puncture wound—caused by a piercing object and may have imbedded foreign body; includes bites; human bites are contaminated with Gram-positive and Gram-negative bacteria

An avulsion is a complete tearing away of the skin from the structures below. It is usually described by size (eg, 4 cm × 4 cm or 16 cm^2). The wound requires surgical repair and may require grafting.

Degloving injuries are a complete tearing away of the skin from the underlying structures, including underlying structures such as subcutaneous tissue. On the hands and feet it appears as quite literally a "degloving" of the skin and other structures, leaving raw muscle and tendons behind. These injuries also require surgical repair.

Patterned injury and the pattern of injury are two distinct concepts that are important to wound documentation. A patterned injury leaves behind the shape, distinct markings, and size of the object used to inflict the injury. This can be a blunt or penetrating wound. Photos and/or tracings of the wound should be undertaken prior to any cleansing or surgical repair. A sizing object, such as a ruler or coin, must be in at least one photo.

The pattern of injury is a series of events leading up to the current injury. It may be multiple visits to the hospital for what appear to be benign injuries or complaints. It may be a series of wounds in various stages of healing on the present hospital visit. In either case, suspicion of abuse for both adults and children needs to be considered and documentation appropriate for such. In these cases the exigent evidence needs to be photographed for later use.

Impaled objects result in both a skin wound and possibly injury to deeper structures. The object should be stabilized, photographed, and not removed until determined by the surgeon.

Management

Emergent management of skin wounds focuses on stopping active bleeding. As discussed in Chapter 2, a component of the primary assessment of circulation is to halt any active bleeding. Scalp wounds are a primary source for this, especially in children. Pressure held on the wound is usually sufficient. In the patient with scalp wound, surgical clips along the edges of the wound or quick suturing may abate the bleeding. A wound should then be monitored for new onset or ongoing bleeding.

Wound cleansing

Wound cleansing occurs when the other life-threatening or limb-threatening injuries are managed.

- Abrasions should be cleansed with antibacterial soap and water or a polymer cleanser, which decreases discomfort
  - Pain management should be undertaken prior to cleansing as these wounds are very painful when touched
  - Deeper wounds may require several liters of irrigation if they are dirty
  - These abrasions as best managed by keeping them moist, usually with a antibacterial ointment applied after cleansing daily
  - Be sure to assess allergies in patients prior to applying antibacterial ointment as an allergy may exist
  - Full or partial thickness abrasions may require STSG
  - After the scabbing from the wounds is healed, aloe vera is useful to continue the skin healing process and keep the wound supple
- Solutions such as povidone-iodine diluted in NSS are useful for the initial cleansing but should not be repeated as they hinder cell healing. Use them only when initially removing bacteria and debris from the wounds.
  - Use a bulb syringe for irrigation preferably with isotonic saline if no debris is present
  - If debris is present, a 35 mL Luer-Lok syringe with a 19 g needle and splash shield will provide the pressure necessary to remove debris
  - Sharp debridement rapidly removes necrotic or devitalized tissue
- Local anesthetics such as lidocaine 0.5% to 2% have a rapid onset and allow for better cleansing and closure
- Clip hair around the wound but never the eyebrows
- High-risk wounds for infection include puncture wounds, particularly the foot, and bites, especially human

Closure

Closure occurs in wounds that are bleeding and those too deep to heal and that need reapproximation. Closure should occur within 6 to 8 hours. The face and scalp can tolerate repair up to 24 hours later. Face lacerations are usually closed to provide cosmetic healing. Very small sutures are used to decrease any possible defect after healing.

- Primary closure uses skin tapes, glues, staples, or sutures
  - Adequate tissue must be present
  - No tension when approximated
- Skin glues (octylcyanoacrylate) can be used only on areas without a lot of motion, low tension, and which will not frequently be wet
  - The hands are a poor choice for skin glue use as hands are involved in activity as well as frequently wet
  - Cleanse the area, dry, approximate, and apply the glue, hold for 30 to 40 seconds
  - Prevent the glue from entering the wound itself to prevent skin reaction
- Suturing can involve both the under layers of the skin and then the epidermis. The layering of sutures depends on the depth and extent of the wound
- Staples are useful in areas that are not of cosmetic significance (eg, scalp, torso, lower extremities)
  - Shorter time to wound closure
  - Less expensive
  - Rapid application
- Deep wounds should be taken to surgery for irrigation and repair. Puncture wounds and contaminated wounds are not closed because of potential for infection or retained foreign body
- Delayed primary closure for contaminated or ischemic wounds
  - Closure of puncture wounds and bites occurs as delayed primary intention. These can be closed within 3 to 5 days if no infection is present

Wound healing

Healing of skin injuries occurs via primary and secondary intention.

- Primary intent—wounds granulate on their own; may produce minor scarring; require only daily cleansing to prevent infection; ideal for small wounds
  — Usually heal within 14 to 28 days
  — Closure assists with the promotion of healing by primary intent
- Secondary intent—allowed to heal and granulate over time (eg, human bites)
  — Delayed closure
  — Necessary for wounds with infection, devitalized tissue, excessive debris
- Maintenance of oxygenation for cell function, collagen production, and angiogenesis
- Nutrients
  — Vitamins A, C, and zinc for tissue repair
  — Iron for collagen synthesis
  — Protein for cell growth

Deterrents to wound healing include

- Immunocompromised burn or trauma patient experiences cellular dysfunction
- Inflammation
  — Caused by devitalized tissue or foreign bodies
- Bacteria
  — Devitalized tissue provides an environment for growth
  — Release of OFRs and proteolytic enzymes prolong inflammation
- Further injury to the area of the wound
- Poor nutrition leads to decreased cell repair
  — Dehydration inhibits the delivery of nutrients
- Hypoxia or hypovolemia result in poor tissue oxygenation

- Application of antiseptic agents over a prolonged period
  — Kills bacteria but also destroys newly forming cells
  — Sodium hypochlorite (Dakin solution) and acetic acid are cytotoxic due to pH
  — Povidone-iodine, iodophor, hydrogen peroxide are cytotoxic to fibroblasts
  — Povidone-iodine is nephrotoxic if used over large surface area (Nayduch 1999)
  — Surfactant cleansers can also be cytotoxic

Daily care involves the promotion of healing and the prevention of injury and infection. The goal is promotion of granulation while controlling bacterial proliferation.

- Moist environment—accelerates epithelialization
  — When granulation tissue is present maintain a moist environment
- Cleansing
  — Remove inflammatory materials, devitalized tissue, debris
  — Irrigate with isotonic solutions, such as saline to remove debris in the initial cleansing
- Antibacterial agents
  — Use only in infected wounds
- Debridement
  — Application of enzymatic agents; inactivated in the presence of antiseptic agents
  — Mechanical—wet to dry dressings (wet with saline) changed 2 to 4 times daily
    - Useful for thick exudates or necrotic tissue
    - Nonselective, stripping granulation tissue, painful
    - Wetting dressings for removal negates the purpose
- Dressings
  — Prevent contamination and absorb drainage
  — Small wounds need daily cleansing and a thin film of antibiotic ointment and no dressing

— Occlusive provide moisture
— Never use occlusive dressings on an infected wound

 Critical Lifesavers

- **[Inhalation injury causes an] insidious onset of edema 24 to 48 hours, even up to 72 hours after injury; vigilant airway assessment is necessary to prevent crisis**
- **Timing for fluid resuscitation begins at the time of the burn, not at the time of patient arrival**
- **An additional maintenance IV that includes dextrose should be maintained during fluid resuscitation in children**
- **All evidence collected must be labeled and chain of custody maintained until turned over to legal authorities**
- **DO NOT apply soaks or ice [to burns] as it will increase the depth of the burn**

REFERENCES

American Burn Association. *Advanced Burn Life Support.* Chicago, IL: American Burn Association (ABA); 2007

American College of Surgeons. *Advanced Trauma Life Support* (ATLS). 7th ed. Chicago, IL: American College of Surgeons; 2004.

Auerbach P. *Wilderness Medicine.* 5th ed. St Louis, MO: Mosby; 2007.

Dyster-Aas J, Willebrand M, Wikehult B, et al. Major depression and posttraumatic stress disorder symptoms following severe burn injury in relation to lifetime psychiatric morbidity. *J Trauma.* 2008;64(5):1349-1356.

Emergency Nurses Association. *Trauma Nursing Core Curriculum* (TNCC). 6th ed. Chicago, IL: Emergency Nurses Association; 2007.

Ipaktchi K, Arbabi S. Advances in burn critical care. *Crit Care Med.* 2006;34(9):S239-S244.

Kramer G, Hoskins S, Copper N, et al. Emerging advances in burn resuscitation. *J Trauma.* 2007;62(6):S71-S72.

Lynch V. *Forensic Nursing*. St Louis, MO: Elsevier Mosby; 2006.

Murray CK. Infections in burns. *J Trauma*. 2007;62(6):S73.

Nayduch DA. Trauma wound management. *Nurs Clin North Am*. 1999;34(4):895-906.

Osborn K. Nursing burn injuries. *Nurs Manage*. 2003;34(5):49-56.

Thombs B, Singh V, Halonen J, et al. The effects of preexisting medical comorbidities on mortality and length of hospital stay in acute burn injury: evidence from a national sample of 31,338 adult patients. *Ann Surg*. 2007;245(4):629-634.

Thombs BD. Patient and injury characteristics, morality risk, and length of stay related to child abuse by burning: evidence from a national sample of 15802 pediatric admissions. 2008. *Ann Surg*. 247(3):519-523.

White CE, Renz EM. Advances in surgical care: management of severe burn injury. *Crit Care Med*. 2008;36(7):S318-S324.

Ziglar M, Bennett V, Nayduch D, et al. *The Electronic Library of Trauma Lectures*. Chicago, IL: Society of Trauma Nurses; 2004.

Chapter 11

TRAUMA IN WOMEN

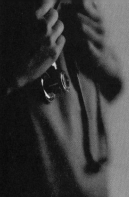

INTRODUCTION

Trauma statistics demonstrate that individuals involved are usually males, aged birth to 44 years. Trauma in women, however obviously occurs and with increasing frequency because women live longer than men and remain active both as they age and during pregnancy. Although the reproductive organs of women are relatively protected by the pelvis, there are times when the organs become vulnerable and need to be taken into consideration during resuscitation and management of the trauma patient.

ASSESSMENT

As with all trauma, assessing and managing airway, breathing, and circulation are the first priority. In addition, if the woman is pregnant, information regarding the fetus is also necessary. The primary focus of care is the mother and in turn the fetus will be provided the optimal environment. Other injuries can occur to women whether they are pregnant or not and are included below.

History

Begin with the history of the trauma event, including the use of safety equipment as well as proper use of those devices. Every trauma event is a teaching opportunity for safety. As with all patients, the past medical history is important to understanding of the total patient. In this situation the usual history should include the following specifics:

- Surgical history—hysterectomy? cesarean section? abortion?
  — Breast implants? Can potentially rupture from blunt or penetrating mechanisms or high altitude
- Last menstrual period (LMP)— >1 month prior consider possible pregnancy
  — Menopause? postmenopause?
- Obstetrical history
  — Premature births
  — Full-term births
  — Miscarriages
  — Abortion
  — Delivery history
- Current pregnancy—gestation, problems, medications, fetal movement, amniocentesis
  — Estimated date of confinement = LMP − 3 months + 7 days
- Medical history
  — Medication use to include contraceptives and hormone replacement therapy (estrogen) use both of which increase the risk for venous thromboembolism
  — Osteoporosis: prevalent in middle-aged and older women; decreases bone healing and increases the potential for fracture associated with minor mechanisms
    ▪ Diet history: calcium intake, vitamin D, sun exposure
  — Past medical history, particularly diabetes, hypertension, cardiac disease and hypothyroidism

Trauma Assessment

The principles of trauma assessment are unchanged in the pregnant trauma patient. The primary and secondary surveys need to focus on the mother with additional components for the fetus. It is essential to understand that the mother can lose 1200 to 1500 mL of blood without any signs of hypovolemia. Fetal heart tones may be the cue to impending maternal or fetal death before maternal changes in vital signs (ATLS 2008). Table 11-1 delineates the physiologic changes during pregnancy that should be taken into account during assessment.

- Initiate routine trauma evaluation of airway, breathing, circulation, and neurologic assessments (Chapter 2) in conjunction with appropriate actions to correct problems in these areas
- Expose the patient as usual for full examination
- Fetal heart tones (FHT)—as soon as possible with an obstetric Doppler, not a standard Doppler; heard at 20 weeks, seen on ultrasound (U/S) at 10 to 14 weeks; cardiotochodynamometer is useful for monitoring FHT and contractions >20 to 24 weeks
  — Listen/observe for 2 minutes
  — U/S every 4 to 6 hours
  — Normal 120 to 160 bpm
    ▪ Bradycardia <110 bpm
    ▪ Tachycardia >160 bpm
  — Check variability, decelerations
  — Be sure to differentiate between mother and fetal heart rate
  — Fetal distress indicates impending maternal and/or fetal decompensation; the only way to decrease fetal loss is early detection of fetal distress (Ikossi et al. 2005).
    ▪ Decreased movement
    ▪ Bradycardia or tachycardia, repetitive decelerations
    ▪ Beat to beat variability
- Secondary assessment
  — Contractions, tenderness, cramping, low back pain
    ▪ Contractions >6/hour may indicate labor
  — Fetal movement: palpable and mother's interpretation

Table 11-1   Physiologic Changes in Pregnancy

System	Alterations	Impact in Trauma
Respiratory	↑ minute ventilation ↑ tidal volume (TV) Elevated diaphragm: ↓, functional residual capacity ↑ O_2 consumption: ↑ risk of hypoxia	↓ PCO_2 30 to 34 mm Hg PCO_2 35 to 40 mm Hg indicates impending respiratory failure ↓ bicarbonate 18 to 22 mEq/L ↓ tolerance to hypoxia Requires O_2 supplementation
	Engorged upper airway	Risk of bleeding with placement of airway
Cardiovascular	↑ blood volume up to 50% by 34th week ↑ cardiac output after 10 weeks ↑ heart rate by 15 to 20 bpm ↓ peripheral vascular resistance (PVR) ↓ systolic BP by 0 to 15 mm Hg ↓ diastolic BP by 10 to 20 mm Hg second trimester	Uterine vasoconstriction during hemorrhage results in fetal hypoxia ↑ blood volume can mask 30% gradual blood loss or 10 to 15% acute loss 20% of cardiac output feeds the placenta in the third trimester
	Supine hypotensive syndrome: aortocaval compression (compression of IVC) ↑ temperature ECG changes: T wave flattening or inversion, Q waves	↓ venous return by 30% if supine

(Continued)

Table 11-1   Physiologic Changes in Pregnancy

System	Alterations	Impact in Trauma
Hematologic	↑ plasma volume, Hct 32-34%	Dilutional anemia
	↑ WBC: up to 20,000/mm^3	
	Hypercoagulability: ↑ fibrinogen and clotting factors	↑ risk of DIC and DVT
	Shorter PT and PTT with clotting times unchanged	
Gastrointestinal	↓ motility, relaxed gastroesophageal sphincter	Prone to vomiting and aspiration
	Upper intestine displaced into upper abdomen	
	Stretched abdominal wall	Masks abdominal assessment
	↑ stomach acidity from gastrin and progesterone released from the placenta	↓ rebound and guarding
Genitourinary	↑ compression of the bladder	↑ risk of injury
	Glycosuria	
	↑ glomerular filtration rate (GFR)	

(Continued)

Table 11-1   Physiologic Changes in Pregnancy (*Continued*)

System	Alterations	Impact in Trauma
Uterus	Does not autoregulate in response to blood loss	↑ uterine vascular resistance causes, ↓ fetal O_2
	Placenta is inelastic; sensitive to catecholamine stimulation	
	Intra-abdominal organ at 12 weeks	↑ risk of injury
	Descends in the last 2 weeks	
	Fetus: second trimester, cushioned by amniotic fluid; third trimester uterus thin and large	Third trimester pelvic fracture can result in fetal skull fracture
Musculoskeletal	Widened symphysis pubis 4-8 mm by 7 months	↓ risk of fracture
	Pelvic veins congested in third trimester	↑ risk of hemorrhage with pelvic fracture

— Perineum: check for blood, amniotic fluid (pH 7.5 represents ruptured membranes), prolapsed cord, crowning or fetal presentation (imminent delivery)

— Abdomen: shape; palpate uterus size, shape, tonicity, irritability; contusions

— Fundal height: not the definitive determination of gestational age, however in the emergent situation it provides a strong estimate (Figure 11-1)

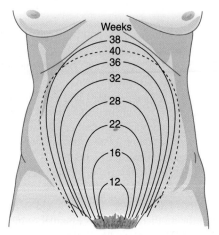

Figure 11-1   Fundal height. (Illustration by Maggie Reynard)

- ■ Symphysis pubis—12 weeks
- ■ Umbilicus—20 weeks
- ■ Costal margin—36 weeks
- ■ Increased fundal height may indicate intrauterine hemorrhage
— Pelvic examination: if able, assess for cervical effacement or dilation indicating labor
— Ultrasound (U/S): assesses obstetric (OB) issues and the focused abdominal sonogram for trauma (FAST), which can decrease the need for radiation exposure (Bochicchio et al. 2002). FAST assesses gestational age, fetal weight, heart rate, viability (>25 weeks, >750 g), placenta evaluation, and the maternal organs liver, spleen, heart, bladder. Diagnostic peritoneal lavage (DPL) can also be used to evaluate the abdomen for injury if it is done with the open technique and positioned above the fundus

— Labs
  - Beta HCG—pregnancy test positive as early as 1 to 2 weeks' gestation
  - Point of care testing may also be available for bedside determination of pregnancy
  - Kleihauer-Betke—determines fetal red blood [cell] count (RBC) in the maternal circulation from fetal hemorrhage through the placenta; Rh^- mother with an Rh^+ fetus will produce sensitization of the mother and requires Rh_o immune globulin within 72 hours
  - Fibrin split products—assess for potential disseminated intravascular coagulation (DIC)
— Radiographs are not delayed or withheld as the management of the mother's injuries is essential to maintaining a viable fetus (Meroz et al. 2007). It is important to do only essential films to diagnose injury, limiting overall exposure. Radiographs after 20 weeks' gestation are safe (Rosen and Barkin 1998)

DOCUMENTATION

Documentation should include, in addition to the routine trauma and forensic documentation

- OB history—list parity in this order: full, premature, aborted, currently alive
- Fetal heart tones
- Assessment of the abdomen
- Vaginal bleeding and perineal assessment
- Uterus fundal height, contractions and frequency, irritability, tone
- Fetal movement
- Photographic evidence of contusions, abrasions, or other injuries associated with domestic violence (follow the hospital permission policy)

MANAGEMENT

Vaginal and Perineal Injury

Overall, the vagina is well protected by the symphysis pubis. Injuries are most frequently caused by pelvic fractures that penetrate the vaginal wall. Any mechanism resulting in pelvic fracture in a woman should be evaluated for vaginal injury. Other mechanisms include straddle injury, jetski crashes, sexual assault. Injury can be masked by vaginal spasm. The expected vaginal bleeding may not be evident. In the patient with possible vaginal laceration associated with pelvic fracture, a speculum pelvic examination will be necessary. Surgical repair of the wound with irrigation and debridement should be expected. Diligent wound care of the open pelvic fracture should prevent osteomyelitis and wound infection.

Visual examination is essential, especially in cases of sexual assault. Look for lacerations, contusions, and/or abrasions to the introitus and anorectal areas. In the victim of sexual assault, a colposcope provides magnification for better injury identification. A sexual assault nurse examiner is a resource available to many emergency departments to perform the initial examination, interview, and evidence collection. Prepare for this evaluation by careful handling of the victim's clothing for evidence preservation.

Uterus and Ovaries

The uterus and ovaries are also rarely injured as they are well protected within the pelvis. However, these organs are susceptible to penetrating trauma even in the nonpregnant state. Gunshot wounds (GSW), stab wounds, impalement injuries are all examples of penetrating trauma. In these patients, any peritoneal signs (guarding, rebound, distention, rigidity) indicate abdominal injury. As with all GSW to the abdomen that cross the peritoneal wall, transport to the operating suite is expected for exploratory laparotomy. The priorities of laparotomy are to identify all injured organs and repair when possible. In regards to the uterus and ovaries, repair is the first choice, however some injuries cannot be repaired and require oophorectomy or hysterectomy. Typical surgical complications can occur with these injuries as with any abdominal injuries and include abscess, fistula, and sepsis.

Trauma in Pregnancy

The priority for management of trauma in pregnancy is the stabilization and management of the mother (Muench et al. 2004, Sisley et al. 1999, Hoyt and Selfridge 2007, Ziglar et al. 2004, ATLS 2008, ENA 2007). The fetus is completely dependent upon the mother. Initial stabilization is no different for the pregnant trauma patient with additional management needs. Priorities include

- Provide oxygen as there is a higher demand and potential fetal hypoxia without evidence of maternal decompensation
- Be careful of tubes placed via the upper airway (endotracheal, nasogastric) as they may result in hemorrhage from the engorged nasal passages and upper airway.
- After 16 to 20 weeks' gestation, tilt the backboard 30 degrees left to relieve pressure from the gravid uterus on the inferior vena cava (IVC)
  — Compression can result in significant hypotension from decreased venous return
  — During operative procedures and throughout hospital care, the supine position should be avoided in these patients
  — If the patient is undergoing an abdominal procedure, the uterus may need to be manually displaced to the left
- Avoid vasopressors that further decrease uterine blood flow and increase fetal hypoxia
- Obtain OB consult to assist during resuscitation, including an OB nurse to provide uterine and FHT monitoring and assist with delivery if imminent

- Consider hyperventilation if the PCO_2 is >35 to 40 mm Hg
- Rapid management of any of the obstetric situations presented below to decrease both maternal and fetal death

SPECIAL SITUATIONS

Preeclampsia and Eclampsia

Eclampsia is not commonly associated with trauma mechanisms. However, the predisposing event to the trauma may be the result of preeclampsia or eclampsia. Recognition of these events will enable rapid management of the complication of pregnancy.

- Preeclampsia—occurs in 5% to 7% of pregnancies (Ziglar et al. 2004) and can progress to eclampsia if undiagnosed or untreated
- Eclampsia—the life-threatening result of untreated preeclampsia. Eclampsia is life threatening to both the mother and fetus. It can also mimic head injury in the trauma patient and should be ruled out as the cause of coma and hypertension.

Signs and Symptoms of Preeclampsia

Acute hypertension
Proteinuria
Peripheral edema

Signs and Symptoms of Eclampsia
Proteinuria with peripheral edema
Hypertension
Grand mal seizures
Hyperreflexia
Coma

Premature Labor and Ruptured Membranes

Premature labor is the most common complication after trauma (Hoyt and Selfridge 2007, ENA 2007). Contractions should be monitored for frequency and intensity. The occasional contraction will usually resolve within a few hours. History should include any previous experience and treatment of preterm labor with this or other pregnancies. The presence of vaginal discharge may indicate ruptured membranes. In this situation, evaluation for prolapsed cord or fetal presentation is essential.

Signs and Symptoms of Premature Labor

Frequent contractions >6/hour or every 10 minutes
Back pain
Clear or bloody vaginal drainage (pH 7.5 = amniotic fluid)
Pelvic pressure
Cervical dilation or effacement
Can be precipitated by dehydration

Management

- If membranes are not ruptured and the trauma patient is stable, uterine contraction inhibitors may be administered
- Note that the use of tocolytics to inhibit contractions, such as magnesium sulfate, decrease deep tendon reflexes affecting the neurologic examination
- If prolapsed cord is present, cover with saline-soaked gauze and prevent pressure on the cord
  — Place the patient in Trendelenburg position if able from a trauma perspective
  — If the fetus is presenting, lift the presenting part off the cord
- A sterile speculum is necessary if a pelvic examination is to be done and ruptured membranes are present

- Labor may be allowed to continue if the mother is stable, or cesarean section may be performed if maternal instability is present

Abruptio Placenta

Abruptio placenta is the most common cause of fetal death after injury with maternal survival (Metz and Abbott 2006, Mattox et al. 2005, Hoyt and Selfridge 2007, ENA 2007). It can occur in up to 40% to 50% of major trauma (Ziglar et al. 2004). Abruptio placenta is the premature separation of the placenta from the uterus in part or total. This results in disruption of the fetal circulation causing fetal hypoxia and death. There may be no external signs and the mother may demonstrate normal vital signs. Abruption can occur up to 48 hours after injury (ENA 2007). A complete abruption is usually evident within 6 hours (Ziglar et al. 2004). Signs and symptoms are not always evident. Vaginal bleeding occurs ~70% of the time with no bleeding if the abruption is partial (ATLS 2008).

Signs and Symptoms of Abruptio Placenta

Vaginal bleeding
Abdominal tenderness
Uterine contractions and/or premature labor
Tetany or irritable uterus
Pain, cramping
Ultrasound evidence of the abruption
Fetal distress—altered FHT, decreased or no fetal movement
Maternal hemorrhage and/or shock
Increased fundal height

Management

If the mother is without additional injury and is hemodynamically stable, the abruption can be managed in labor and delivery with the OB team. However if the mother is critically injured or has other injuries, she will usually be managed by the trauma service with an OB consult and assistance in the ICU or hospital bed.

- Extensive abruption can result in coagulopathy progressing to DIC through depletion of fibrinogen
- Uterine evacuation is emergent in this situation to reverse the coagulopathy and salvage the mother
- If the fetus is of a viable gestation, survival may occur if the evacuation is immediate
- Replacement of clotting factors and platelets is also necessary

Ruptured Uterus

A ruptured uterus occurs <1% of the time with an almost 100% fetal mortality (Hoyt and Selfridge 2007). A history of a previous cesarean section increases the possibility of ruptured uterus. Unfortunately, a ruptured uterus usually also results in a hysterectomy.

Signs and Symptoms of Ruptured Uterus

Tender, rigid abdomen with guarding
Palpable fetus separate from the uterus itself
Abnormal fetal position
No palpable fundus
Pain may or may not be present
Vaginal bleeding possible, hemorrhage, shock
No FHT

Management

An immediate cesarean section is required to control hemorrhage, save the mother and attempt to save the fetus. An associated bladder rupture may also have occurred as the bladder is an intra-abdominal organ when the uterus is large and experiences the same kinetic energy transfer as the uterus.

Maternal Arrest

When maternal death occurs, cesarean section within 5 minutes of the death may be successful (ATLS 2004, ENA 2007). Gestation of 26 to 28 weeks is also part of the success of the procedure. Cardiopulmonary resuscitation (CPR) must be continued throughout the delivery as well as correction of metabolic acidosis that is usually present. CPR may need to be performed slightly above the midsternum or with open cardiac massage as the best option. If the patient is defibrillated, the fetal monitor must be removed prior to the actual defibrillation. It is rare for the mother to improve even after cesarean section. Survival of the fetus will be dependent upon the gestational age, length of maternal arrest prior to delivery, length of hypoxia to the fetus prior to the death of the mother, and injuries to the fetus itself.

In the case of fetal death, the fetus must be delivered if disseminated intravascular coagulopathy (DIC) is present. If not, the mother may be allowed to proceed to labor and delivery over the normal course of events.

Domestic Violence

Although commonly associated with women, and increased during pregnancy, domestic violence can occur with men, children, and the elderly and therefore should be considered when taking the history of injury for all patients. Domestic or intimate partner violence is defined as an ongoing pattern of coercive control which includes physical and/or sexual assault or similar threats. For women >18 years, 75% of the acts of violence against women are committed by their cohabitating partner, husband, exhusband, or date/boyfriend. The partner can be of the same or opposite sex (Ziglar et al. 2004). Approximately 4.8 million domestic violence assaults and rapes occur each year. In 2004, >1500 deaths occurred directly related to intimate partner violence with 75% of those women. (CDC 2006)

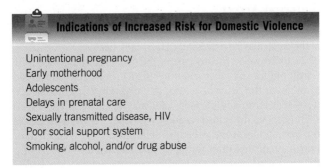

Indications of Increased Risk for Domestic Violence

Unintentional pregnancy
Early motherhood
Adolescents
Delays in prenatal care
Sexually transmitted disease, HIV
Poor social support system
Smoking, alcohol, and/or drug abuse

Coercive control includes physical or sexual abuse, threatening behaviors, and/or psychological and emotional abuse. The control and power over the individual is dependent upon intimidation. The victim fears retaliation by the perpetrator. Definitions of types of coercive control include

- Sexual abuse—includes any unwanted touching, fondling, sexual actions that are inclusive of sexual intercourse but it is not a requirement. These include any coercion into the sexual act against the will of the victim
- Psychological and emotional abuse—includes humiliation or embarrassment in public, controlling activity especially outside the home, controlling relationships with friends and family, isolation from friends and family, controlling financial and other resources, withholding information, destroying personal possessions, threatening a pet or child, using or threatening with weapons

The cycle of violence often starts as psychological abuse which is often dismissed by the victim as stress or unintentional. The violence continues and can accelerate or escalate to physical abuse, even to the point of homicide. Throughout the cycle, the abusive phases are usually tempered by kindness, tenderness, or gifts. During these times, the victim forgives the perpetrator or makes excuses for the behavior. Then the violence occurs again, and again. As trauma staff, identification of the cycle is part of holistic care.

The interview should be conducted with

- Direct questions with focused listening
- Observation of the patient, interactions, and comments
- Documentation in the patient's own words, diagrams of injuries, photographs with consent
- Without the partner in attendance
- Private environment

Hospitals are required to ask all patients about their perception of safety at home, with their partner or family, and elsewhere within their lives. Screening and observations should include

- Past medical history—frequent emergency or clinic visits, chronic pelvic pain, headaches, vaginitis, depression or suicide attempts/ideation, anxiety, irritable bowel syndrome, substance abuse, childhood abuse or living in an abusive household as a child
- History of the injury that is not consistent with the actual physical injuries; downplaying the injury event, for example, "just a fall"
- Multiple injuries in various stages of healing
- Redness from slapping-type mechanisms
- Weight loss
- Self-abuse
- Frequently misses work
- Low self-esteem
- Partner—oversolicitous, will not leave the patient alone, answers questions for the patient, hostile or demanding, monitors all verbal and nonverbal responses of the patient, possessive

- Psychological—anxious, flat affect, dissociation, startle response, overcompliant, distrustful

The caregiver should provide a safe environment where the victim can express her feelings and describe her circumstances without fear of retaliation. The victim is hoping for someone to reach out to her and will often respond positively to information, time, and repeated support. The victim usually stays in the situation for the children, hopes that the perpetrator will change or get through the stress, feels powerless, and/or is afraid of offending the partner by acknowledging the abuse.

Domestic violence increases with pregnancy as noted above. Symptoms include less weight gain than expected during pregnancy, increased anemia, infection, bleeding, depression, and suicide. Use of smoking and alcohol may also increase or begin if domestic violence is present. Domestic violence is not limited to a specific culture, economic group, or community. There are specific questions that can be asked to assess the home situation. From 65% to 70% detection is possible if asked without the partner (ATLS 2008). An index of suspicion is needed to identify these patients and later provide for a safe home situation.

POSTRESUSCITATION MANAGEMENT AND REHABILITATION

- The risk of deep venous thrombosis (DVT) is five times higher in the pregnant trauma patient due to the hypercoagulable state, increased fibrinogen, factor VII, VIII, IX and decreased plasminogen activator
  - DVT prophylaxis is required in these patients as early as implementation can be initiated
  - Use of contraception or hormone replacement prior to arrival increases DVT risk
- Pregnant trauma patients also have decreased calcium, magnesium, creatinine, and blood urea nitrogen (BUN)
  - Take these into consideration when evaluating lab work and in providing nutrition for the mother

- After delivery, the uterus requires routine postpartum care with the guidance of an OB nurse and includes
  — Every 15 minute massage of the uterus for the first hour, and then every hour for the next 4 hours
  — Monitoring for increased height, bogginess, or increased bleeding is essential and must be reported to OB for evaluation of continued uterine bleeding
- Temperature and vaginal drainage needs monitoring for infection in the postpartum period as well
  — The mother is postpartum whether or not she is critical and potential infections of breast milk as well as the uterus or incision must be included in infection evaluations
- Other routine postpartum care such as infant care, breast-feeding, and bonding should be provided to the extent that the mother can participate in these events
- When the mother is critical, care should be taken to assure that the father spends time with the newborn
  — It is difficult to split the family time between the critical patient and the newborn
- In the case of fetal and/or maternal death, grief management should be provided to the family as with any loss
  — This should be provided for the mother as well when she is capable of participating in the counseling process
- Other injuries to the female genitalia and reproductive organs are managed as with an abdominal injury
  — Open pelvic fractures require diligent wound care for prevention of infection
  — Prevent DVT, pneumonia, and other complications of immobility and postoperative care

The care of the pregnant trauma patient involves the complete resuscitation of the mother in every effort to provide for both patients through her stabilization. The only opportunity for fetal survival is maternal survival. Overall, most pregnant trauma patients are not seriously injured and require only monitoring by the OB service for stability of the fetus and prevention of preterm labor.

Critical Lifesavers

- **The principles of trauma assessment are unchanged in the pregnant trauma patient**
- **Fetal distress indicates impending maternal and/or fetal decompensation**
- **The priority for management of trauma in pregnancy is the stabilization and management of the mother**
- **When maternal death occurs, cesarean section within 5 minutes of the death may be successful**
- **Increased blood volume can mask 30% gradual blood loss or 10% to 15% acute loss**

REFERENCES

American College of Surgeons. *Advanced Trauma Life Support* (ATLS). 7th ed. Chicago, IL: American College of Surgeons; 2004.

American College of Surgeons. *Advanced Trauma Life Support* (ATLS). 8th ed. Chicago, IL: American College of Surgeons; 2008.

Bochicchio GV, Haan J, Scalea TM. Surgeon performed focused assessment with sonography for trauma as an early screening tool for pregnancy after trauma. *J Trauma.* 2002;52(6):1125-1128.

Centers for Disease Control and Prevention (CDC). Understanding intimate partner violence. Available at://http:www.cdc.gov/injury. Accessed March 08, 2008.

Emergency Nurses Association (ENA). *Trauma Nursing Core Curriculum.* 6th ed. Chicago, IL: Emergency Nurses Association; 2007.

Hoyt KS, Selfridge TJ. *Emergency Nursing Core Curriculum.* 6th ed. St Louis, MO: Saunders; 2007.

Ikossi DG, Lazar AA, Morabito D, et al. Profile of mothers at risk: an analysis of injury and pregnancy loss in 1195 trauma patients. *J Am Coll Surg.* 2005;200(1):49-56.

Mattox KL, Goetzi L. Trauma in pregnancy. *Crit Care Med.* 2005;33 (10 supp):S385-S389.

Meroz Y, Elchalal V, Ginosar Y. Initial trauma management in advanced pregnancy. *Anesthesiol Clin.* 2007;25(1):117-129.

Metz TD, Abbott JT. Uterine trauma in pregnancy after MVCs with airbag deployment: a 30 case series. *J Trauma.* 2006;61(3):658-661.

Muench MV, Baschat AA, Dorio PJ, et al. Successful pregnancy outcome after splenic artery embolization for blunt maternal trauma. *J Trauma.* 2004;56(5):1146-1148.

Rosen P, Barkin RM. *Emergency Medicine: Concepts and Clinical Practice.* 4th ed. St Louis, MO: Mosby Year Book; 1998.

Sisley A, Jacobs LM, Poole G, et al. Violence in America: a public health crisis—domestic violence. *J Trauma.* 1999;46(6):1105-1113.

Ziglar M, Bennett V, Nayduch D, et al. *The Electronic Library of Trauma Lectures.* Chicago, IL: Society of Trauma Nurses; 2004.

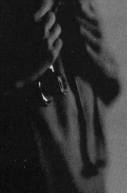

Chapter 12

SPECIALTY POPULATIONS

INTRODUCTION

There are specific groups who arrive as trauma patients and require special attention. The principles of resuscitation remain the same for all types of trauma patients. However pediatrics, geriatrics, and obese patients have unique physiology and anatomy issues, which need to be taken into account. In addition, substance abuse patients experience the effects of alcohol and/or drugs during resuscitation and through rehabilitation.

PEDIATRICS

Assessment

The assessment approach to the child follows the same approach as in Chapter 2. However, the assessment of a child is driven by anatomical and physiological differences at each age. The changes in the anatomy of the child and the ability to participate in the assessment are outlined in this section.

History

Children at various stages of development have different abilities to participate in the taking of their history. In addition to obtaining medical history there is also the history of the event itself. Table 12-1 describes the development and approach to children by age group. When obtaining the history be attentive to inconsistencies in the history, time from injury to arrival,

Table 12-1 Age-Specific Development

Age	Development	Approach
Infant 0 to 3 months	Parental contact essential; poor head control, obligate nose breather, helpless in water; learning trust	Parents present Comforts child Relieves parental distress
3 to 6 months	Rolls over; hand to mouth	Do not leave alone, hold infant Eye contact is threatening
6 to 12 months	Crawls; stands, cruises Fears separation and the unknown	Still need parents present to comfort child; stranger anxiety
Toddler 1 to 3 years	Walks, climbs, runs; limited language; short memory; tests reality Autonomy Fears separation, strangers, and especially loss of "special object" Concrete thinkers	Parents present Keep security blanket/ object with the child Keep child in motion/occupied Restrain gently by human contact when possible Reassuring tone of voice
Preschool 3 to 6 years	Constant motion; curious; clever; imagination, magic Increased verbal skills but limited comprehension "I'll do" Fears separation, punishment, loss of control, and body integrity	Parents present "Play" to accomplish assessment and treatment; be honest; examine painful area last Slow, nonthreatening approach with simple words for child and family "OK" to cry Clean and cover wounds

(Continued)

Table 12-1 Age-Specific Development (Continued)

Age	Development	Approach
School-age 6 to 12 years	Explores, creates, increased communication skills; growth spurts Modesty Increased importance of peers Needs some control; wants to cooperate Fears separation, punishment, pain, loss of body integrity, body image, and death	Parental contact Explain actions, will help if asked "Play" to accomplish assessment and treatments; be honest Protect modesty by avoiding overexposure Examine painful area last Reassure; include child in conversation; obtain medical and event history from child Respect complaints of pain
Adolescents 12 to 16 years	Good historian; responds to peer pressure Magical thinker, dreamer Modesty Often dramatic, overreacts, or hysterical Fears separation from peers and parents; pain; disability; disfigurement; death	Parental and peer contact Explain actions; provide information about condition; be honest Offer choices, privacy Recognize tendency to overreact; use calm tone; reassure as fear leads to overreaction Obtain medical and event history from teenager Use care provider of same sex when possible

multiple emergency visits, and inappropriate parent/guardian behavior as indicators that abuse may have occurred.

Trauma assessment

Physical alterations in children affect the likelihood of certain injuries as well as protection from injury. Trauma assessment and management priorities are airway, breathing, and circulation. Immediate use of a length-based resuscitation tape will assist with determining approximate patient length and weight. The tape also provides approximate tube sizes and medication dosages. Anatomical differences include

- Airway
  - Obligate nose breather until 6 months; then deep abdominal breather
  - Large tongue obstructs airway until 5 years
  - Hyperextension or flexion of neck obstructs airway
  - Larynx anterior and cephalad; floppy epiglottis
  - Short trachea
  - Cricoid most narrow part of airway until 9 years
- Breathing
  - Chest wall is thin; breath sounds can be reflected to the opposite side
  - Compliant chest: rib fractures are a sign of severe force and injury (rare injury)
  - Grunting, nasal flaring, retractions are signs of respiratory distress
  - Increased metabolic rate causes increased oxygen consumption
  - Hypoxia results in bradycardia; most common terminal pathway
- Circulation
  - Palpate brachial pulses on infants
  - More tolerant of blood loss; compensation through increased heart rate (HR) and peripheral vascular resistance up to 30% blood loss

- — May be no change in blood pressure (BP) up to 50% blood loss; uncompensated shock
- — Indications of blood loss—delayed capillary refill, cool extremities, weaker peripheral than central pulses, mottling
- — Blood volume 80 mL/kg
- Neurologic exam
  - — Large occiput causes flexion of the neck when supine (see Chapter 5, positioning on the backboard)
  - — Anterior fontanel closes age 9 to 18 months
  - — Posterior fontanel closes age 2 months
  - — Open fontanels more tolerant of intracranial pressure
  - — Upgoing Babinski until 2 years
  - — Able to fixate on objects at 4 months
  - — Seizure after injury more common, but self-limiting
  - — Thin skull prone to fracture; large subarachnoid space
  - — Preverbal: difficult to explain/express headache, nausea, blurred vision, dizziness
  - — Weak neck with a large, heavy head; flat facets
  - — Interspinous ligament laxity; spinal cord injury without evidence of radiographic abnormality (SCIWORA) most common <8 years
  - — Pseudosubluxation of C2 on C3
- Exposure
  - — No shivering response <3 months
  - — Large body surface area causes rapid heat loss and hypothermia; results in metabolic acidosis, hypoglycemia, apnea, coagulopathy, respiratory depression
  - — Glycogen stores rapidly depleted
- Secondary survey
- Head and neck
  - — Increased vagal response from hypoxia, laryngoscope during intubation

— Increased distance between the dens and C1 normal variant
— Cervical ligamentous laxity can result in SCIWORA (Chapter 5)
• Chest and abdomen
  — Pulmonary contusion is common
  — Swallowed air can occur with crying or bag-valve-mask ventilation
  — Gastric distention decreases diaphragm excursion
  — Lap-belt sign on the abdomen may indicate abdominal injury or lumbar spine Chance fracture
  — Handlebar injuries can result in duodenal hematoma; may develop up to 24 hours later
  — Spleen, most common solid organ injured
  — Kidneys are mobile; liver is anterior
  — Bladder is an abdominal organ
  — Abdominal muscle wall is less developed
• Extremities
  — Elasticity of bones results in less facial and long-bone fractures
• Triage

Pediatric triage requirements differ from adult requirements. Use adult triage criteria with these additional pediatric criteria
  — Any peripheral symptom of poor perfusion, assume bleeding
  — Respiratory rate (RR) >60 breaths/minute
  — RR <20 when <6 years; <15 when <15 years
  — HR >200 or <60 beats per minute (bpm)
  — Neurologic changes such as lethargy, drowsiness, low Glasgow Coma Score (GCS)
  — Assisted respirations, intubation
  — Falls <20 feet or two times the height of the child may cause significant injury
  — Any "ill-looking" child after trauma suspect internal injury or hemorrhage

Documentation

Documentation principles remain the same as for adults. Children must have a weight in kilograms documented or document the "color" from the length-based resuscitation tape. If a pediatrician or pediatric surgeon respond to the trauma activation, arrival times of the surgeon as well as rest of the team should be documented. If the facility is not capable of managing pediatric trauma, the communication regarding transfer, method of transfer, and transfer time should be documented as well. In the patient with a burn, be sure to use the age-appropriate burn diagram (Chapter 10, Figure 10-1).

Management

Airway, breathing, circulation

Be aware of the following when managing the pediatric trauma patient:

- Airway—loss of airway is the leading cause of arrest
  - Use chin-lift method for opening the airway; use jaw-thrust method only as a secondary attempt
  - Use the sniffing position with the external auditory canal parallel to the backboard
  - Maintain the head in a neutral position, requiring the placement of a folded towel beneath the torso to elevate the chest and provide straight alignment with the occiput up to 8 years (Chapter 5)
  - Do not rotate oral airways; place them into the mouth directly
  - Avoid nasal tubes especially in obligate nose breathers; may cause injury to the pharynx; also difficult to place because of the angle of the pharynx; may increase intracranial pressure
  - Little finger of the child is the size needed for an endotracheal tube (ETT); or use the length-based resuscitation tape

— Uncuffed ETT for child <8 years; monitor the tube as it can move even though the cricoid is naturally holding the tube in place; sizes 2.5 to 5.5 mm

— Airway occlusion can occur rapidly from burn edema, tongue, or foreign body

— Shallow respirations are a sign of impending arrest

— Immobilize neck in size appropriate cervical collar; can use cardiopulmonary resuscitation (CPR) board as backboard for small children; a papoose can be used if <5 years

• Breathing

— Tidal volume 6 to 8 mL/kg

— Count respirations for 1 full minute because of irregular breathing patterns in children

— Monitor breath sounds bilaterally as the sound is reflected onto the opposite side

— Hypoxia is the most common cause of arrest and secondary brain injury

— Monitor pressure when ventilating children, especially with bag valve mask to prevent lung injury and gastric distention

• Circulation

— Monitor capillary refill, skin color, and peripheral pulses; BP changes are late signs

— Urine output should be monitored along with frequent vital signs (Table 12-2)

— Do not assume that a normal BP means the child is stable; normal BP = 80 mm Hg + 2 × age (years)

— BP lower limit = 70 mm Hg + 2 × age (years)

— All fluids must be warmed to prevent hypothermia

— Place 2 peripheral IV; if unable to obtain IV within two tries, place intraosseous catheter (IO) in the distal femur, proximal or distal tibia (Figure 12-1)

— IO is done with downward pressure angling away from the growth plate. Aspirate bone marrow to confirm placement;

Table 12-2   Normal Pediatric Vital Signs

Age	Blood Pressure Systolic	Pulse	Respirations	Urine Output
Newborn	60-90 mm Hg	120-160 bpm	60/minute	2 mL/kg
1 year	65-95 mm Hg	80-140 bpm	25/minute	2 mL/kg
3 years	70-100 mm Hg	80-120 bpm	20/minute	1.5 mL/kg
5 years	70-100 mm Hg	70-115 bpm	20/minute	1.5 mL/kg
7 years	70-100 mm Hg	70-115 bpm	25/minute	1.5 mL/kg
10 years	90-120 mm Hg	70-115 bpm	30-35/minute	1.5 mL/kg
15 years	102-140 mm Hg	70-90 bpm	18/minute	1 mL/kg until no growth then 0.5 mL/kg as per adult

anchor firmly. Begin infusion immediately to prevent clotting. Infusions may include IV fluids, antibiotics, anticonvulsants, atropine, epinephrine, mannitol, sodium bicarbonate

— Do not place IO in a broken tibia or femur, or in children with osteogenesis imperfecta

— Warm IV normal saline solution (NSS) or lactated ringer (LR) at 20 mL/kg; can be repeated twice (takes up to 60 mL/kg to replace a 25% blood loss)

— Transient or nonresponder to crystalloids requires warm packed red blood cells at 10 mL/kg

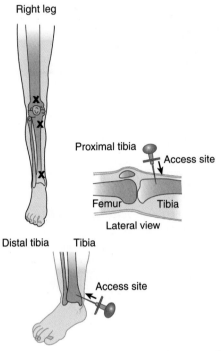

Figure 12-1   Intraosseous catheter placement. (Courtesy of Professor Mike South, Royal Children's Hospital, Melbourne Australia.)

— <15 kg weight, use a straight catheter for the bladder

— Hypovolemia and hypoxia will result in secondary brain injury and overall poor outcome; rapidly identify hemorrhage, including scalp lacerations

— Tachycardia may identify hemorrhage, stress, pain, fear

Neurologic and secondary surveys

• Deficit

— For infants and toddlers, use the pediatric GCS to document neurologic response to stimuli (Table 12-3); the GCS is an assessment of head injury, not spine injury

Table 12-3   Pediatric Glasgow Coma Scale

Assessments	Score
Eye opening	
Spontaneous	4
To speech	3
To pain	2
None	1
Verbal response	
Coos, babbles	5
Irritable cry, consolable	4
Cry to pain, unconsolable	3
Moan to pain	2
None	1
Motor response	
Normal, spontaneous	6
Withdraw to touch	5
Withdraw to pain	4
Decorticate posturing	3
Decerebrate posturing	2
None	1
TOTAL Pediatric GCS	3 to 15

— GCS <9 or a GCS motor score of 1 or 2 should be evaluated by a neurosurgeon
— Assess fontanels up to age 18 months; bulging fontanels indicate increased intracranial pressure
— Ondansetron (Zofran) should be administered for nausea as it is less sedating than promethazine (Phenergan)
  ▪ Promethazine also results in tissue necrosis if extravasation occurs or with peripheral IV administration
— For spinal cord injury, the use of high-dose methylprednisolone has not been studied in children <13 years
— Seizures immediately after the event are not usually associated with a positive head CT; seizures >20 minutes after

injury have a greater correlation with intracranial injury and associated seizures later

- Exposure
  - Warm room, fluids, blankets or blanket warmer to prevent hypothermia
  - Cover child for modesty as well; cover wounds
  - Scalp lacerations can result in serious hemorrhage; evaluate for scalp laceration and close or apply pressure dressing as early as possible
  - Cover burn wounds to decrease evaporative loss
- Secondary survey
  - Place nasogastric or orogastric tube to decrease gastric distention
  - If a diagnostic peritoneal lavage (DPL) is performed, use LR (prevent cramping associated with NSS) 10 mL/kg; positive findings are the same as for adults (Chapter 8)
  - Missed abdominal injury can result in rapid acidosis; examine the abdomen when the child is calm to determine rigidity
  - Most solid organ abdominal injuries are managed nonoperatively; when these injuries require operative treatment, the majority are emergent
  - Fractures may present close to the growth plate (physis); greenstick fractures are incomplete fractures with angulation or cortical splinters (Chapter 9, Table 9-3)
  - If the child is not moving or refusing to use an extremity, examine for fracture/dislocation

Special Situations

Head injury

Mild traumatic brain injury (TBI) is a GCS of 13 to15. There may be a brief loss of consciousness (<30 minutes) with amnesia for <24 hours with normal computed tomography (CT) scan of the head and neurologic exam (Cook et al. 2006).

Symptoms Post-TBI

Physical changes:
Headache, dizziness
Fatigue
Nausea/vomiting
Sensitivity to noise and/or light
Blurred vision, diplopia
Sleep disturbances

Cognitive changes:
Decreased attention, impaired concentration
Short term memory deficits or delayed processing of information

Behavioral changes:
Irritability, emotional lability
Depression, anxiety

These should resolve within 3 months of onset. If a preexisting head injury has occurred or premorbid learning or behavioral disorder, the child is likely to experience inattention, hyperactivity, and exacerbated behavioral issues.

Children in sports should not return to play until all symptoms are resolved. Second impact syndrome occurs when a child returns to play too soon after a TBI and can result in vasospasm, cerebral edema, increased intracranial pressure, hemorrhage, and even death. Children should be evaluated by neuropsychology ~4 weeks after injury to determine deficits and return to school. Ibuprofen should be given <3 times per week to avoid rebound headache.

In children with a GCS <13, focal neurologic deficits or scalp hematoma in infants should receive a head CT. In children <2 years, a scalp hematoma is associated with a positive head CT for brain injury in 93% of the cases (Cook et al. 2006). According to the Brain Trauma Foundation guidelines, a child with a GCS <8 needs an intracranial pressure (ICP) monitor (Adelson et al. 2003).

- For increased ICP, sedatives and analgesics should be given (Adelson et al. 2003)
- Repeat head CT are necessary to monitor changes in the brain as well as identify any hematoma that may require surgery
- If a ventriculostomy is present, cerebrospinal fluid (CSF) can be drained to lower ICP
- Neuromuscular blockade is the next step in the process for persistent increased ICP
- If serum osmolarity is <320 mOsm/kg, mannitol may be administered and if the osmolarity is <360 mOsm/kg, hypertonic saline (3%) may be administered as well
- If the elevated ICP persists, mild hyperventilation (PCO_2 30-35 mm Hg) may be added to the regimen

  Refractory ICP at this point requires more intensive therapy.

- Check the ventriculostomy to determine it is not obstructed or clotted
- Decompressive craniectomy may be considered if cerebral edema is evident on the CT
  — Decompressive craniectomy provides room for the brain to continue to swell without the constraints of the skull
  — The child will need a helmet to protect the head after he or she is stable and for the rehabilitation process until the bone flap is replaced
- If the electroencephalogram (EEG) is active, barbiturate coma induction may be considered
- Hypothermia to 32°C to 34°C is considered if there is evidence of ischemia on the head CT (Chapter 4)

Child abuse

Abuse is defined as a failure to act or an act committed by a caregiver that results in injury (physical or emotional), sexual abuse or exploitation, placing the child at risk or death (Ziglar et al. 2004). The injuries are intentional. The children who suffer abuse most often are <3 years. Common symptoms are

Suspected Child Abuse Symptoms

Inconsistent history of the event
History of the event that keeps changing
Patterned injuries (reflect the object used, Figure 12-2)
Multiple injuries of various stages of healing, including
    fractures, bruises, abrasions
Caregiver states child is clumsy or frequently injures self
Poor nutrition and hygiene
Mechanism is inconsistent with developmental stage of child
Withdrawn or acting out behavior
Delayed arrival for treatment
Repeated injuries treated at different emergency departments
    or clinics
Inappropriate parental/guardian behavior; unusual interaction
    between the child and parents/guardian

Child abuse or suspected child abuse must be reported to the authorities following the protocol in the individual facilities and local government requirements. Common injuries include cigarette burns, fractures, subdural hematoma(s), retinal hemorrhages, ruptured solid organs without severe blunt abdominal mechanisms, bites, burns with demarcation. Approximately 6% to 20% of abuse cases involve immersion burns that are found on bilateral hands and/or legs in a stocking-glove distribution. The burns have a sparing of the tissue folds and no splash burn which is indicative of the child being held in the scalding water. Of abuse deaths, 50% were previously victims of unreported or uninvestigated abuse. Full body x-rays are usually taken to evaluate for fractures and dislocations. Retinal exams are done by ophthalmology. Head CT scans are done to evaluate for head injury and skull fractures.

Postresuscitation Management and Rehabilitation

Most children respond well and heal quickly after injury. In the case of minor TBI, there may be transient neurologic sequelae

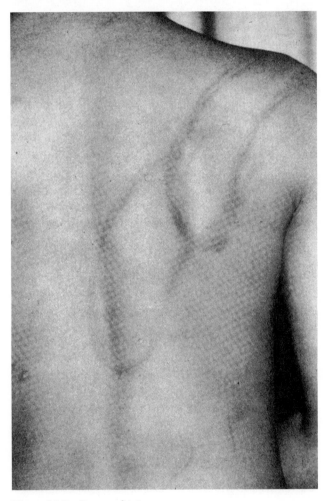

Figure 12-2 Patterned injury.

in function, behavior, or cognitive areas. However, there can be a delay in symptoms for up to 2 years (Cook et al. 2006). TBI children need ongoing evaluation for their response to neurologic injury. Severe TBI in children <3 years of age have a worse outcome than older children. Children overall have a better outcome than adults after TBI.

Orthopaedic injury may have long-term effects related to bone growth and extremity-length discrepancies if the fracture involved the physis (growth plate). Severe trauma results in 60% of children with personality changes up to 1 year after injury. Up to 50% of injured children may have cognitive and physical handicaps, including learning disabilities. After motor vehicle collisions (MVC), up to 25% of children demonstrate posttraumatic stress disorder (PTSD). It is clear that children require follow-up for both the physical injuries as well as the emotional response to injury for up to at least a year after the event.

GERIATRICS

There is an increasing geriatric population across the world. In the United States, 41.6% of all emergency visits are patients >65 years. Geriatric individuals comprise only 15% of the population but use >33% of trauma health-care resources (ATLS 2004, Wright and Schurr 2001). Associated diseases exist on >81% of the geriatric trauma patients (Yilmaz et al. 2006).

Assessment

As with children, the elderly have anatomic and physiologic differences from the general population. These differences alter their potential for injury as well as the actual injuries they experience. The assessment and management of the elderly trauma patient is, as always, the same as described in Chapter 2 with the following important additions.

History

Comorbidities or past medical history and a medication list are essential components of the history of an elderly trauma patient.

Both seriously affect outcome as well as assessment and management of the injury.

- Asthma and chronic obstructive pulmonary disease (COPD) can result both in hypoxia and hypercarbia, requiring management of chest injury and comorbidities with bronchodilators or early mechanical ventilation
  — COPD patients are dependent upon oxygen, not carbon dioxide levels, to stimulate respiration. This must be taken into account when applying typical oxygen therapy on arrival.
- Left ventricular heart failure may require inotropic agents although right ventricular heart failure requires a fluid challenge for hypotension
- Dementia, stroke, diabetes mellitus, and epilepsy can result in altered level of consciousness, requiring an evaluation for head injury as well as the medical issues
- Rheumatoid arthritis and degenerative disc/bone diseases can lead to difficulties with neck movement and spinal cord injuries as well
- Chronic renal failure requires careful fluid balance and medication administration

Some of the most significant medications are anticoagulants, which will result in uncontrolled bleeding. Early identification of their use is essential to initiate the proper reversal agent, eg, warfarin (Coumadin), and administer clotting factors or platelets in an attempt to mitigate the antiplatelet effects of the other agents, eg, clopidogrel (Plavix) and aspirin. In addition early identification of any areas of bleeding and rapid management of these areas is necessary to prevent hemorrhage. The principles of resuscitation and rapid injury identification must remain the focus of the initial assessment.

Trauma assessment

Changes occur in the body as it ages that result in less ability to compensate for injuries. Each of the changes has an impact on either assessment or the long-term healing after the injury has occurred. Table 12-4 describes these changes. With the anatomic

Table 12-4 Changes with Aging

Alterations	Effects
Airway-Breathing	
↓ airway/lung compliance	↑ airway resistance
↓ glycogen stores	Exhaustion; arrest with rapid RR
↓ surface area for gas exchange	Hypoxia-hypercarbia
Chronic colonization of *Haemophilus*	↑ risk of infection
Cervical osteoarthritis or degenerative diseases; Cervical stenosis	Difficulty with intubation; ↑ incidence of central or anterior cord syndromes, cervical fracture
COPD—loss of hypercapnia drive for breathing	Careful oxygen administration
Cardiac	
↓ vital capacity	Inability to tolerate supine position
↓ ability to generate increased HR with hypotension; ↓ response to catecholamines; also caused by beta-blockers	Normal HR despite hypotension; continued decompensation;
Normal increased BP	Normal BP may actually be hypotension
Presence of anticoagulants or NSAID use	Ineffective platelets; require reversal; rapid identification of hemorrhage
Maximum HR that can be generated = (220 minus age)	
Neurologic	
↓ cerebral blood flow	↓ level of consciousness
Cerebral atrophy, ↑ intracranial space	↑ space for hemorrhage before signs and symptoms of head injury; ↑ movement of the brain; Stretching of bridging veins in subdural space causing hemorrhage
Musculoskeletal/Integument	
↓ muscle mass, dermis, and subcutaneous fat	Hypothermia; loss of balance and strength

(Continued)

Table 12-4 Changes with Aging (Continued)

Alterations	Effects
↓ ability to vasodilate or vasoconstrict with calcium channel blockers in response to temperature; ↓ ability to sweat	Hypothermia or hyperthermia due to inability to thermoregulate
↓ thirst mechanism	Dehydration before patient is aware they are thirsty
Osteoporosis from ↓ activity, estrogen, calcium consumption or absorption	↑ risk of fracture with minor mechanisms; ↓ healing
Renal	
↓ renal excretion	Medications requiring renal clearance may remain longer in the blood; nephrotoxic medications, eg, aminoglycosides, diuretics, and contrast may severely affect renal function
↓ ability to concentrate urine	Urine output not reliable predictor of fluid status
↓ sodium absorption and potassium excretion	Hyponatremia; hyperkalemia; monitor electrolytes
Diuretic use	Hypokalemia
Gastrointestinal	
↓ peristalsis and motility	Malnutrition
↓ absorption of nutrients; ↓ metabolic rate	Malnutrition; ileus
Other	
↑ incidence of retinal detachment	Consider this with blindness or ocular pain even with a minor mechanism
↓ visual acuity	Safety issues with rehabilitation
↓ ability to hear high-pitched frequencies	Affects ability to hear questions and instructions
Friable nasopharynx	Bleeding with nasal tube placement
Pancreatitis, hypothyroidism	Hypothermia prone
↓ Immunity, febrile response, WBC response, steroid use	↑ risk of infection without clinical evidence of ↑ WBC or fever

and physiologic changes in the elderly, >70 years, should be included as a criteria for triage and trauma team activation decreasing mortality by ~20% and disability by ~4% (Demetriades 2002).

Management

The management of geriatric trauma remains the same as for all ages, airway, breathing, circulation, and neurologic evaluation. Aggressive resuscitation and injury identification is necessary to provide the optimal setting for survival and successful rehabilitation. The leading causes of mortality and morbidity are failure to recognize injury, errors in management, and a failure of the patient's physiologic reserve. Special situations with respect to the elderly patient include

- Monitor for hypoxia; unrecognized hypoxia is unrecoverable
- Base deficit <−5 indicates severe injuries, unrecognized injury, and/or continued shock
- Acknowledge and reverse anticoagulation
- Maintain hemoglobin >10 g/dL; maximizes oxygen-carrying capacity
- Early invasive monitoring such as Swan-Ganz lines provide vital information regarding the cardiovascular response to injury and resuscitation
- Chest injury, particularly rib fractures are associated with increased mortality
  - Pain control, epidural may be most effective
  - Pulmonary toilet, incentive spirometry
- Cervical spinal cord injury, primarily central cord injury, occurs with hyperextension from falls or MVC when the vehicle is rear-ended
- Clinical predictors of cervical injury may be present in <50% of the time (Schraq et al. 2008)
- Early head CT to evaluate for subdural hematoma (SDH)
  - SDH are three times more likely in elderly patients (ATLS 2008, Ziglar et al. 2004)

- Supplement nutrition as baseline malnutrition may exist, as well as malabsorption and decreased healing and immunity
- Nonoperative management of organ or bony injury may have higher risks than operative management
- Anticipate intensive care unit (ICU) admission to provide close monitoring for cardiovascular response to injury
- Common fractures include proximal femur, hip component of the femur, proximal humerus, and distal radius/ulna

Special Situations

Burns

Burns in the elderly pose a significant problem. In addition to the normal changes in aging and responses to injury, the geriatric patient has a thinner dermis and less subcutaneous tissue. As a result, the burn will have more depth. The skin growth is slower as well as less vitamin D production, resulting in longer healing time. There is also an increased risk of inhalation injury caused by decreased ciliary action. The healing time for inhalation injury is also increased.

Elder abuse

Like children, elders are susceptible to abusive situations with an inability to manipulate the situation for safety. Abuse is defined as willful infliction of injury or intimidation or confinement against the person's will or punishment or deprivation. Abuse is not necessarily physical. The caregiver may withhold medications, food, money, or hygiene. Coercion to sign papers, release property or finances without consent is also abusive. Abuse can include emotional and physical abuse as seen frequently in children.

As with any abusive situation, any question of abuse needs to be reported. History of the event that changes or is inconsistent with injuries should raise awareness for abuse. Patients with poor hygiene, malnutrition, hypothermia should also be considered potential abuse cases and caregivers should be evaluated.

Postresuscitation Management and Rehabilitation

Managing cardiovascular and respiratory issue rapidly is the primary way to a successful outcome in the elderly. Acute respiratory distress syndrome (ARDS) is the leading cause of death for the elderly within the first 24 hours after injury (Ziglar et al. 2004). Prevention of complications and prevention of a compromised state leads to less mortality and morbidity. The patient's premorbid activity level will determine the likelihood of return to home. Early mobilization is the key to prevention of complications and improved healing. Functional decline in the hospital is one of the leading causes of late hospital mortality. A favorable functional outcome of up to 4 years after injury is not uncommon. The goal for all rehabilitative efforts is return to previous level of function with minimal deficits. Many geriatric trauma patients find recovery best in short-term placement in a skilled nursing facility to receive therapy in a safe environment. The long-term goal for these patients is return to independent or previous level of function.

Any discussion of outcome in the geriatric trauma patient must include end-of-life decisions. The need to have advanced directives in the event that the patient cannot coordinate his or her own plan of care is essential and best if prepared prior to any injury event. A living will and do not resuscitate (DNR) status should be identified early on so that the patient's wishes are met. Patients have the right to self-determination. Care needs to be provided with the patient's best interests in mind, not the interests of the family. Final decisions should be based upon the determination of benefits that outweigh adverse outcomes.

OBESITY

Obesity is defined as a body mass index >30 kg/m². The average male has ~18% body fat and the female, 25%. Up to 61% of Americans are overweight or obese and ~300,000 deaths annually are associated with obesity. Overweight individuals are at increased risk for hypertension, stroke, diabetes mellitus type II, myocardial infarction, asthma, sleep apnea, thromboembolism, and cholelithiasis. There is also increased risk of certain cancers specifically, endometrial, breast, and colon. There are genetic, social, and cultural factors affecting obesity.

Assessment

Multiple physiologic and anatomic changes alter the obese patient's response to injury. These include

- Abdominal fat inhibits the excursion of the diaphragm reducing functional residual capacity
  — Causes atelectasis and increased risk of pneumonia
- Decreased lung compliance
- Increased work of breathing to expand the diaphragm
- Increased risk of heart failure
- Increased cardiac output due to the increased blood volume to the adipose tissue
- Malnutrition is common with low protein stores

Trauma assessment

As usual, airway, breathing, and circulation take priority in trauma assessment. Identification of injuries may be difficult because of weight restrictions on CT and magnetic resonance imaging (MRI) scanners, inability to penetrate with radiation for clear plain films, and the ineffectiveness of the abdominal ultrasound (U/S). Palpation of the abdomen may also result in an apparently benign abdomen because of the depth of palpation required to effect a response. It may also be difficult to assess abdominal rigidity for the same reason. It may be hard to hear breath sounds with the decreased excursion of the diaphragm. Pulses are often difficult to palpate under the adipose tissue. Skin folds can hide external injury as well as fractures.

Management

When managing the obese patient, there are specifics that can be anticipated before the patient arrives, as well as special attention throughout the patient's stay.

- Prehospital
  - Extrication is difficult and more likely because of entrapment
  - Special lifts are available to assist with removing patients from the ambulance or vehicle and into the hospital
  - Immobilization devices may not fit or may be rendered ineffective
  - Transport stretchers have a weight limit; lifting an obese patient also places the crew at risk
- Resuscitation
  - Venipuncture poses difficulties with identification of the vein and placement of the catheter
  - Diagnostic peritoneal lavage must be performed as an open procedure to ensure access to the abdominal cavity
  - Blood volume should be calculated on the patient's ideal body weight and not the actual current weight of the patient
- Equipment
  - Larger BP cuffs
  - Extra-wide wheelchairs
  - Larger stable beds, preferably that convert to sitting to enhance pulmonary toilet
  - Cervical collars require extensions; patient may also have a very short neck
  - CT scanners capable of handling certain weights can only be found in veterinary schools which requires transport of the patient; the patient must be stable to transport
  - Operative tables typically handle weights up to 450 pounds; some can handle up to 1000 pounds.
- Critical care
  - Invasive monitoring of the critical obese patient is necessary to obtain an accurate assessment of hemodynamic status
  - Oxygenation decreases as body mass index increases
    - Chronic under-ventilation of lower lung alveoli
  - Increased risk of pneumonia; pneumonia increases risk of respiratory failure

— Ventilation
- First choice is noninvasive ventilation
- Fatty neck makes intubation difficult
- Early tracheostomy decreases ventilator days
- Prone to respiratory muscle fatigue
- Risk for gastric reflux and aspiration; elevate the head of the bed or use reverse Trendelenburg position

— Pharmacokinetics
- Malnutrition decreases drug binding, causing increased free-circulating drug levels
- Hydrophilic medications have a partial distribution in adipose tissue; includes antibiotics; therapeutic levels should be monitored
- Lipophilic medications are rapidly absorbed into adipose tissue and are then slowly released, resulting in delayed awakening from pain medications and anxiolytics; use pain and sedation scales to monitor response

— Medication administration
- Subcutaneous injections have decreased uptake due to decreased blood supply causing delayed onset of action and unpredictable duration
- Intramuscular injections may never reach muscle
- Cutaneous patches have a delayed onset of action with erratic and unpredictable effect because of decreased cutaneous perfusion

Postresuscitation Management and Rehabilitation

Prevention of complications is essential. The obese patient is already at increased risk for complications; therefore extra care must be taken to prevent them.

- Thromboembolic events are prevented with early mobilization and the use of low molecular weight heparin (LMWH) at an increased dosage (Frezza and Chiriva-Internat 2005).

Weight-based heparin dosing is another option for prevention of deep vein thrombosis (DVT) and hence pulmonary emboli (PE). Inferior vena cava filters also prevent DVT from becoming PE.

- Decubiti can be prevented through the usual means of turning and early mobilization. Special mattresses can also assist with decreasing pressure points, however these are limited for the larger beds required for obese patients. Skin folds should be assessed for breakdown and assure the folds are dry after bathing. The patient is at risk for necrotizing infection if these folds breakdown and become infected.

- Renal failure is an increased risk in obese patients especially with preexisting dehydration. Close monitoring of hemodynamics is essential.

- Obese patients are also at risk for myocardial infarction, respiratory failure, sepsis, wound complications such as delayed healing and infection, organ failure, and surgical sudden death. Prevention of pneumonia through mobilization and pulmonary toilet is part of the daily routine for all patients and particularly with the obese patient.

SUBSTANCE ABUSE

Trauma patients frequently arrive under the influence of alcohol or drugs. The presence of these substances alters the patient's response to injury as well as their response to stimuli. In some cases the response is accelerated or exaggerated and in others the patient may appear sleepy to comatose. An awareness of the effects of the substances on the body and psyche will assist the provider in determining injury from influence of drugs or alcohol.

Assessment

Assessment for trauma remains the same as for all trauma patients (Chapter 2). It is essential however to identify injury first as well as substances that may be affecting the patient's response. Both need evaluation and management.

History

Abuse is defined as a mild dependence upon a substance. There is episodic or short-term use of the substance or combination of substances. Dependence, however, is use over a long duration in which tolerance is demonstrated or withdrawal when the substance is removed, such as after trauma. A patient's history of drug and alcohol use should be part of the review of systems. The length of use, amount, and substance should be documented.

Management

Management is first and foremost about the injuries present and the treatment of the injuries. However, management of trauma includes the fact that substance abuse seriously affects a patient's level of consciousness. There is also an increased potential for aspiration from vomiting. Precautions such as a gastric tube for decompression of the stomach will decrease aspiration. When possible, elevation of the head of the bed will also decrease aspiration.

The presence of substances can also change patient behaviors such as

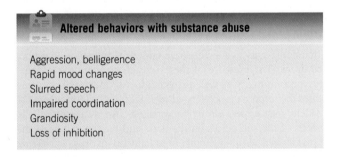

Altered behaviors with substance abuse

Aggression, belligerence
Rapid mood changes
Slurred speech
Impaired coordination
Grandiosity
Loss of inhibition

Caregivers must ensure both patient and staff safety. Restraint may be necessary. Benzodiazepines, an antianxiety agent, can be used for sedation. Sedation also prevents exhaustion and promotes rest during this phase of recovery. Patients who are substance dependent are also usually malnourished, especially thiamine deficiency. A means of decreasing withdrawal effects is to provide the "banana bag," intravenous vitamins (including thiamine) and nutrition. Approaching the patient in a calm and firm manner also assists with helping the patient remain calm and as reality-based as possible. Symptoms of acute withdrawal include uncontrollable fear, anxiety, hallucinations, tremors, incontinence, and agitation. The patient tends to be very talkative and preoccupied, making it difficult to focus on rehabilitation of injury. A quiet nonthreatening environment decreases input, calming the patient.

Other effects of alcohol include coagulopathy from liver damage and can result in significant head injury from a simple fall mechanism. Hepatic failure and hypoglycemia also occur with long-term alcohol abuse.

Specific drugs affect the body in different ways. There are classes of drugs that are commonly abused. These include stimulants, depressants, opioids, amphetamines, inhalants, and hallucinogens. Some patients mix these drugs together to experience both the "up" and then "down" effect. Unfortunately, the drugs do not always respond as expected, may not be cut purely and the effects of the "base" can be toxic as well, or tolerance exists, requiring higher and higher doses to achieve the same "experience."

The following is a brief description of each drug type and its effects:

Stimulants

- Includes cocaine which can be inhaled (snorted), smoked (free-basing), intravenous, or even mixed with heroin
- Toxicology screen, especially on autopsy, may demonstrate benzoylecgonine, a cocaine metabolite

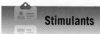
Stimulants

CNS stimulant; causes seizures; increased energy, agitation, aggression, hypervigilance
Increase heart rate, blood pressure, temperature
Ventricular dysrhythmias

(Continued)

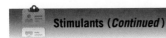

Stimulants (*Continued*)

Euphoria followed by anxiety, insomnia, sadness
Hallucinations and delusions
Extreme paranoia
Short-lived symptoms

- Management
  — Airway, breathing support
  — Seizure management and prevention of injury
  — Lidocaine and defibrillator available in case of ventricular dysrhythmias
  — Evacuate stomach if taken by mouth
  — Manage hyperthermia

Amphetamines (stimulant/hallucinogen)

- Includes 3,4-methylenedioxymethamphetamine (MDMA, ecstasy), 3,4-methylenedioxy-N-ethylamphetamine (MDEA), amphetamine, dextroamphetamine
  — "Ice," "rocks," "crystal meth" are smoked
  — MDMA is both a hallucinogen and a stimulant

Amphetamines

Tachypnea
Palpitations, tachycardia, hypertension
Seizure, coma
Anxiety, fearful, hostility, paranoia
Diaphoresis, mydriasis, hyperthermia, rhabdomyolysis
Repetitive behavior, irritability, insomnia, agitation
Nausea, vomiting, anorexia
Hallucinations—visual and auditory
Hyperactivity, rapid speech, euphoria, hyperalertness, decreased inhibition

- Management
  - Airway, breathing support
  - Gastrointestinal (GI) evacuation if oral overdose; use activated charcoal
  - Place in a calm, cool, quiet environment; cool patient if hyperthermia is present
  - Small doses of diazepam or haloperidol decrease hyperactivity
  - Manage hypertension or ventricular dysrhythmias
  - Manage sympathetic stimulation with beta-blockers

Hallucinogens

- Includes lysergic acid diethylamide (LSD), phencyclidine HCl (PCP), mescaline, cannabinoids (marijuana), ketamine (special K)

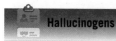

Hallucinogens

Nystagmus, confusion, borderline panic, incoherence
Hypertension, mild
Hyperthermia, renal failure
Hyperactivity, combative, delirium, mania, self-injury,
   aggressiveness—lasting 6 to 12 hrs
Withdrawn
Hallucinations
Flashbacks may occur weeks to months after using the drug

- Management
  - Airway, breathing support
  - Attempt to communicate with the patient helping to overcome fears, connect to reality
  - Reassure patient that the fears and hallucinations are temporary; keep eyes open
  - Place in a calm, quiet, dim environment; keep patient safe

— Administer diazepam or other benzodiazepine to calm hyperactivity
— Evaluate for any self-inflicted injury caused by acting on the hallucinations
— Monitor and manage seizures
— Monitor for hypertensive crisis
— If PCP was used—maintain calm, quiet environment and protect from harm; do not leave patient alone or unobserved; symptoms can exacerbate

Depressants

• Include pentobarbital, gamma-hydroxybutyrate (liquid ecstasy), secobarbital

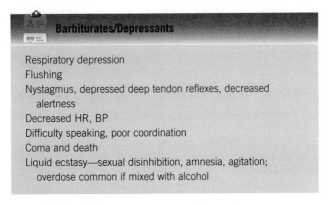

Barbiturates/Depressants

Respiratory depression
Flushing
Nystagmus, depressed deep tendon reflexes, decreased alertness
Decreased HR, BP
Difficulty speaking, poor coordination
Coma and death
Liquid ecstasy—sexual disinhibition, amnesia, agitation; overdose common if mixed with alcohol

• Management
— Airway, breathing support including intubation if necessary
— Respiratory depression most common cause of death
— IV fluids to support hemodynamic instability
— Evacuate stomach; use activated charcoal
— Hemodialysis may be required in severe intoxication
— Prevent injury as the patient emerges from an overdose
— Reverse benzodiazepines with flumazenil (Romazicon)

Opioids/narcotics

- Include heroin, opium/paregoric, morphine, codeine and the semisynthetic derivatives, fentanyl

Opioids/Narcotics

Respiratory depression, respiratory arrest
Pinpoint pupils
Decreased BP
Stupor, coma, seizures
Check for skin abscesses or needle marks—check hidden
   places (eg, between toes)

- Management
  — Airway, breathing support
  — IV fluids to maintain hemodynamic stability; may need glucose administration if hypoglycemic
  — Administer reversal agent naloxone hydrochloride IV or IM; may need to repeat in cases of heroin use as duration of action of naloxone is shorter than that of heroin
  — Observe for pulmonary edema
  — Hemodialysis may be indicated for overdose; oral ingestion may be treated with activated charcoal

Inhalants

- Include amyl nitrate, propane, freon, trichloromethylene, toluene (metallic paint spray), gasoline

Inhalants

Respiratory depression
Vasodilation, nose bleeds
Dizziness, imbalance similar to alcohol

(Continued)

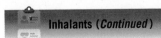

Inhalants (*Continued*)

Aplastic anemia
Renal, hepatic, and cardiac toxicity may be evident
Euphoria, altered level of consciousness, headache

- Management
    — Airway, breathing support may include intubation
    — Manage cardiac dysrhythmias and hypotension
    — If amyl nitrate is combined with MDMA and sildenafil, monitor for profound hypotension

Postresuscitation Management and Rehabilitation

With the incidence of substance abuse and its direct effect on trauma, confronting the patient about the abuse must be done. Intervention at this point greatly decreases the risk of recidivism. One of the ways to assess the patient's degree of dependence is the CAGE questionnaire (Ewing 1984). There are four simple questions. If the answers are positive, a substance abuse referral is next.

CAGE Questionnaire

Have you ever felt you needed to cut back on your drinking?
Have people annoyed you by criticizing your drinking?
Have you ever felt guilty about drinking?
Have you ever felt you needed a drink as an "eye-opener" in the morning to steady your nerves or get rid of a hangover?

The American College of Surgeons recognizes the importance of addressing substance abuse by requiring trauma centers to perform a screening, brief intervention, and referral (SBIR) for all patients with positive drug and alcohol screens (Sise et al. 2005, American College of Surgeons 2006). The purpose of the screen and provision of a brief intervention provides clinical benefit as well as decreases the risk of recurrence in a population where recidivism runs high (Gentilello 2005). The difficulty with the trauma population is the follow through with referral. During the brief intervention up to 85% of individuals state an intention to address the substance abuse issue. However, only 29% are found to have an absolute willingness, and none accessed resources after discharge (Yonas et al. 2005). Gentilello (2007) demonstrated that the brief alcohol intervention resulted in decreased consumption and a 47% decrease in readmission.

In addition to initiating substance abuse referrals and interventions, managing the patient's new "abstinence" cannot be ignored. Withdrawal prevention starts at admission. Pain management can be very difficult as some patients have a high tolerance caused by the drugs and alcohol they use daily. A consult to the pain management service assists with this issue. Patients with substance abuse issues have two health problems after trauma—healing the injuries and dealing with their dependence.

 Critical Lifesavers

- Large tongue (in children) obstructs airway until 5 years
- Rib fractures (in children) are a sign of severe force and injury
- Most common errors (in pediatric trauma) are lack of airway maintenance, fluid management in head injury, and unrecognized internal hemorrhage
- Glasgow coma scale is an assessment of head injury, not spine injury
- Hypoxia is the leading cause of arrest in children
- Large body surface area (in children) causes rapid heat loss and hypothermia
- Chest injury, particularly rib fractures (in the elderly) are associated with increased mortality

REFERENCES

Adelson PD, Bratton SL, Carney NA, et al. Guidelines for the acute medical management of severe traumatic brain injury in infants, children, and adolescents. *Pediatr Crit Care Med.* 2003; 4(3 Suppl): S72-S75.

American College of Surgeons. *Advanced Trauma Life Support* (ATLS). 7th ed. Chicago, IL: American College of Surgeons; 2004.

American College of Surgeons. *Advanced Trauma Life Support* (ATLS). 8th ed. Chicago, IL: American College of Surgeons; 2008.

American College of Surgeons Committee on Trauma. *Resources for Optimal Care of the Injured Patient 2006.* Chicago, IL: American College of Surgeons; 2006.

Cook RS, Schweer L, Shebesta LF, et al. Mild traumatic brain injury in children: just another bump on the head? *J Trauma.* 2006;13(2):58-65.

Demetriades D, Karaiskakis M, Velmahos G, et al. Effect on outcome of early intensive management of geriatric patients. *Br J Surg.* 2002;89(10):1319-1322.

Ewing, JA. Detecting alcoholism: the CAGE questionnaire. *JAMA* 1984; 252(14):1905-1907.

Frezza EE, Chiriva-Internat M. Venous thrombo-embolism in morbid obesity and trauma. *Minerva Chir.* 2005;60(5):391-399.

Gentilello L. Confronting the obstacles for alcohol problems in trauma centers. *J Trauma.* 2005;59(3):S137-S143.

Gentilello LM. Alcohol and injury: American College of Surgery Committee on Trauma requirements for trauma center intervention. *J Trauma.* 2007;62(6):S44-S45.

Schraq SP, Toedter LJ, McQuay N. Cervical spine fractures in geriatric blunt trauma patients with low energy mechanisms: are clinical predictors adequate? *Am J Surg.* 2008;195(2):170-173.

Sise M, Sise CB, Kelley D, et al. Implementing screening, brief intervention, and referral for alcohol and drug use: the trauma service perspective. *J Trauma.* 2005;59(3):S112-S118.

South M. Intraosseous Access. Available at: http://www.rch.org. au/clinicalguide/cpg.cfm?doc_id=9747. Accessed May 25, 2008.

Wright AS, Schurr MJ. Geriatric trauma: review and recommendations. *WMJ.* 2001;100(2):57-59.

Yilmaz S, Karcioglu O, Sener S. The impact of associated diseases on the etiology, course, and mortality in geriatric trauma patients. *Eur J Emerg Med.* 2006;13(5):295-298.

Yonas M, Baker D, Cornwell E, et al. Readiness to change and the role of inpatient counseling for alcohol/substance abusing youth with major trauma. *J Trauma.* 2005;59(2):464-467.

Ziglar M, Bennett V, Nayduch D, et al. *The Electronic Library of Trauma Lectures.* Chicago, IL: Society of Trauma Nurses; 2004.

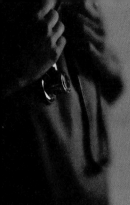

Chapter 13
CRITICAL CARE

INTRODUCTION

Resuscitation is the initial challenge for the trauma center. Trauma deaths, however occur in one of three phases, at the scene, during resuscitation, or later from complications. The patients with the greatest potential for complications are those requiring critical care. The patient is struggling with healing the injuries. Energy is also expended in preventing complications which could change the patient's long-term outcome. A review of common complications and means of prevention follows.

ACUTE RESPIRATORY DISTRESS SYNDROME (ARDS)

Lung injury can present from the trauma itself or be acquired from the inflammatory response associated with multiple injuries. The inflammatory response that drives acute lung injury (ALI) begins with edema and protein leak into the interstitial space and alveoli. A loss of surfactant and collapse of terminal bronchioles further exacerbates the hypoxemia and increases dead space. The lung becomes "stiff" and difficult to ventilate without high pressures. The progression into acute respiratory distress syndrome (ARDS) results in prolonged ventilation requirements, and can progress to multiple organ failure and death.

ALI has an acute onset of pulmonary infiltrates that are not associated with congestive heart failure. The PaO_2/FiO_2 ratio is ≤ 300.

With progression to ARDS the PaO_2/FiO_2 ratio drops to 200. Mortality from this syndrome relates to the patient's response to positive end expiratory pressure (PEEP), presence of multiple organ failure, degree of recruitable lung, and the presence of refractory hypoxemia (Derdak 2007).

Signs and Symptoms of ARDS

Hyperventilation, rales/crackles
Low $PaCO_2$ initially with progression to hypercapnea
Gradual increase in respiratory insufficiency
Progression to persistent low PaO_2 despite increased FiO_2
Pulmonary edema: frothy sputum, tachypnea, hypotension
Chest x-ray (CXR): bilateral infiltrates, ground glass appearance
Hypoxemia PaO_2 <50 mm Hg on FiO_2 60%
Absence of cardiogenic pulmonary edema

Prevention and Prophylaxis

Prevention of ARDS focuses on respiratory and circulatory management. Fluid volume resuscitation needs to be appropriate but not excessive. Monitoring base deficit and lactate can provide guidance for resuscitation and recognition of normovolemia. The more resuscitation is prolonged, the more likely complications will occur. In addition, pulmonary toilet is always a high priority for intensive care unit (ICU) patients. Close pulmonary monitoring may provide early warnings of hypoxia, hypercapnea, tachypnea, and pulmonary infiltrates.

Management

Early identification of ALI is essential to the prevention of full ARDS. Treatment of the underlying cause of ARDS is the first priority. The goal is prevention of further alveolar damage.

- Types of ventilation
  - Controlled mechanical ventilation (CMV) is a preset number of breaths per minute at a preset tidal volume
  - Assist-control ventilation (A/C) provides a preset number of breaths per minute at a preset tidal volume, however between these breaths the patient can trigger a spontaneous breath to which the ventilator responds (assists) with the preset tidal volume; tidal volume is guaranteed for all breaths, ventilator and patient initiated
  - Intermittent mandatory ventilation provides a preset number of breaths per minute at a preset tidal volume, however between these breaths the patient may initiate spontaneous breaths of variable volume and patient dependent
- Ventilator management
  - Lung protective strategies need to be implemented early to decrease morbidity
  - Maintain tidal volume ≤6 mL/kg based upon the patient's predicted body weight (Derdak 2007, Dellinger et al. 2008)
  - Consider using lower tidal volumes early in patient management to avoid ventilator associated lung injury
  - High-frequency oscillatory ventilation can be provided up to 15 Hz, minimizes tidal volume; use the highest frequency that will allow clearance of CO_2 (Fessler et al. 2008, Derdak 2007)
    - Useful for refractory hypoxemia, respiratory acidosis, high peak airway pressures
  - Airway pressure release and high frequency percussive ventilation are other methods of ventilation useful for ALI and ARDS
    - Pressure control ventilation determines the airway pressure based upon inspiratory flow pressure
    - Volume is variable
    - Dependent upon lung complicance, inspiratory time, and airway resistance

— Maintain $PaCO_2$ ~40 mm Hg and PaO_2 >70 to 80 mm Hg
— Minimize FiO_2 to prevent oxygen toxicity
— Peak airway pressures should be maintained <30 cm H_2O by decreasing tidal volume
— Inverse inspiratory:expiratory (I:E) ratio ventilation increases inspiratory times and allowing for higher lung volume resulting in intrinsic PEEP
  ■ PEEP maintains open alveoli on expiration, preventing full collapse
  ■ High levels of PEEP can result in barotrauma
— Consider permissive hypercapnea to assist with minimizing plateau (peak) pressures and tidal volume
— Nitrous oxide may be administered to prevent oxygen toxicity
— Maintain head of bed ≥30 degrees if not contraindicated
— Weaning protocols should include
  ■ Spontaneous breathing trials
  ■ Patient should be arousable, demonstrate hemodynamic stability, low ventilator pressure requirements, and require an FiO_2 that can be delivered safely via face mask or nasal cannula
• Prone positioning
— Useful for both ALI and ARDS by recruitment of otherwise dependent alveoli
— Has demonstrated decreased pneumonia and ARDS by increasing the PaO_2/FiO_2 ratio to >300 (Voggenreiter et al. 2005)
— Proning can be accomplished with a prone pillow/device designed for this use
— Challenges to nursing care include monitoring lines and tubes during the proning process to prevent dislodgment
• Aggressive pulmonary toilet to remove secretions and prevent pooling
— May include bronchoscopy

- Surfactant may be administered to assist with keeping alveoli from collapse
- Corticosteroids are not helpful and do not prevent mortality
- Early tracheostomy
  — No demonstrated decrease in mortality, however decreases total ventilator days and ICU days in any ventilated ICU patient
  — Consider tracheostomy for a ICU patient who will likely remain ventilated for >7 days (Holevar et al. 2006)
  — Patients who benefit from early tracheostomy include (Goettler et al. 2006)
    - Glasgow coma scale (GCS) = 3 at 24 hours after admission with age >70 years
    - Age >55 years
    - Severe abdominal, chest, and extremity injuries (AIS = 5) and >60 years
    - Craniotomy patients >50 years; increased intracranial pressure (ICP) and >40 years
    - Bilateral pulmonary contusions with >8 rib fractures
    - Paralysis and >40 years
- Aggressive maintenance of hematocrit within normal levels
- Aggressive maintenance of cardiac output

VENTILATOR-ASSOCIATED PNEUMONIA (VAP)

Many trauma patients have already aspirated at the scene or from vomiting during resuscitation. In these situations, the lungs are already seeded with bacteria ripe for proliferation. Other sources of bacteria include the oral cavity and the sinuses. The presence of the endotracheal tube provides a route for transmission of bacteria into the lungs. The inflammatory response present in the trauma patient promotes the development of ALI and is predictive of pneumonia as well. The pooling of secretions can result in microaspiration as the patient has a decreased gag reflex resulting in the pooling in the subglottic space. The head-injured or previously ventilated patient may have silent aspiration thus a swallow study is beneficial for evaluation of swallow prior to oral feedings. The diet should then be modified to a texture that the patient can swallow safely such as thickened liquids. VAP increases the risk of mortality as well as ICU and ventilator length of stay.

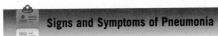

Signs and Symptoms of Pneumonia

Rhonchi present in the lung fields
Hypoxia, poor ventilation
Fever, increased white blood cell count (WBC)
CXR: pulmonary infiltrates
Culture positive for bacteria, fungus

Prevention and Prophylaxis

Prevention of pneumonia is a basic routine for nursing and respiratory staff. All patients should receive pneumonia prevention and that does not include prophylactic antibiotics.

- Wash hands before and after patient care and particularly between patients
- Wash hands before any actions relating to the ventilator and endotracheal tube
- Centers for Disease Control and Prevention (CDC) guidelines for VAP (VAP bundle) prevention include (Cason et al. 2007, Tolentino-DelosReyes et al. 2007)
  — Increasing the head of the bed where possible to 30 to 45 degrees

— Wear gloves when handling respiratory secretions or equipment
— Subglottic suctioning before removal of the endotracheal tube or deflating the cuff to eliminate pooled secretions
— Change the ventilator circuit at every 48 hours
— Provide oral hygiene to clean and decontaminate the mouth with or without antiseptic

- Other recommendations include (Tollentino-DelosReyes et al. 2007)

  — Check nasogastric residuals every 4 to 6 hours when providing tube feeds
    - Hold feeds for an hour if the total residual is >1.5 times the amount instilled per hour or >150 mL
  — Minimizing rings and washing hands with an alcohol-based solution decreases the presence of *Staphylococcus aureus,* Gram-negative bacilli, and *Candida*
  — Minimize endotracheal suctioning to when needed and not on a routine every 2 hour schedule
    - Do not instill saline into the endotracheal tube prior to suctioning
  — Turn the patient every 2 hours or use a kinetic therapy bed if spine precautions must be maintained
    - Provide chest physical therapy, coughing and deep breathing, and use of the incentive spirometer to increase lung volume preventing alveolar collapse (atelectasis) and trapping of secretions
    - If the patient can mobilize, increasing ambulation also increases deep breathing and prevention of atelectasis
  — Bronchoscopy is a useful adjunct to clear deep secretions, provide cultures, and open collapsed airways; also allows for visualization of the airways
    - Blind bronchial-alveolar lavage may be used to obtain specimens for quantitative culture
    - Cultures with $<10^5$ colony forming units are not diagnostic for VAP (Brown et al. 2001)

— Use of H_2 blockers and proton pump inhibitors (PPI) decrease gastric pH

  ▪ Gastric acidic pH may prevent enteric bacteria from migrating to the lungs

Management

Management of VAP or other pneumonia includes intense pulmonary care and treatment of the infection. The goal of prevention was to keep the airways open so that bacterial or fungal growth would not occur. In the presence of VAP, the goal now is to treat the infection and minimize lung injury and progression towards ARDS or sepsis.

- Culture secretions first; send for culture, sensitivity, and Gram stain
- Provide a broad-based antibiotic regimen only until the cultures return and then immediately adjust the regimen to sensitivities of the specific organism
- In the patient with methcillin-resistant *Staphylococcus aureus* (MRSA), vancomycin or ciprofloxacin is usually the medication of choice
  — These antibiotics should not be used arbitrarily as vancomycin-resistant *Enterococcus* may also proliferate
- Aggressive pulmonary toilet is essential to moving secretions out of the lung, decreasing the culture medium available for bacterial or fungal growth
  — Chest physiotherapy
  — Manage ventilation to prevent ALI or ARDS
  — If unventilated, cough and deep breathe along with incentive spirometry
  — Kinetic therapy bed or frequent turning to avoid pooling
- Treat fever with the antipyretic of choice specific to the patient
- Follow the prophylaxis of pneumonia criteria from CDC as the behaviors listed above will continue to protect the lungs even during an infectious process (Cason et al. 2007)

- Careful washing of hands to prevent transmission of the bacteria to other patients
  — MRSA isolation precautions should be observed to prevent cross-contamination
  — Evidence of MRSA must be eradicated from the patient prior to transfer to a rehabilitation or skilled nursing facility to prevent introduction of the bacterium into these populations

SYSTEMIC INFLAMMATORY RESPONSE SYNDROME (SIRS)/SEPSIS

Again, the inflammatory mediators present after trauma can induce a full body response to the injuries similar to ALI but widespread. SIRS is the evidence of the inflammatory process at work without evidence of a source of infection. The only real difference in presentation between sepsis and SIRS is the presence of infection and progress toward multiple organ failure evident in sepsis. It is also possible that bacteria can be present in the bloodstream without resulting in the septic response. This requires treatment for the bacteremia. A positive blood culture may also come from improper site preparation prior to drawing the culture. This would be a contaminant only, not bacteremia or sepsis.

From the arrival of the patient, complete resuscitation preferably within the first 24 hours is the goal to prevent complications. Monitoring base deficit and lactate levels assists with identifying the resuscitated patient. Microcirculatory alterations occur during the SIRS/sepsis processes resulting in multisystem organ failure. Prevention of these alterations is the goal of therapy.

A frequent source of sepsis is the presence of a central line, either venous, percutaneously introduced central catheter (PICC), or arterial lines. Peripheral intravenous lines can also be the source if placed without aseptic technique or a dressing contamination. Line sepsis results from direct entry of bacteria to the bloodstream. All line dressing changes should be through aseptic/sterile technique as well as during placement of the lines.

Signs and Symptoms of SIRS/Sepsis

Fever >38°C or hypothermia <36°C

Increased WBC >12,000/mm³ or decreased <4000/mm³ with >10% bands

Decreased systemic vascular resistance (SVR), arterial hypotension, increased cardiac output with widened pulse pressure

Poor perfusion, increased lactate

Tachycardia, tachypnea

Positive fluid balance

Culture blood and lines prior to antibiotic administration; check presence of organism

Signs of cellulitis or infection including abdominal abscess or any tube/line site (IV, chest, intracranial drain)

Signs of organ dysfunction: acute lung injury, renal failure, altered mental status, altered liver function tests

Prevention and Prophylaxis

Prevention of sepsis is routine nursing care. In some patients, contamination may already be present in a dirty wound from the field. However, the majority of cases of sepsis are hospital acquired. Sepsis increases the risk of mortality as well as length of ICU stay.

- Use sterile technique when placing central and peripheral lines
- Use aseptic technique when changing dressings on all central lines and wound care
- Decontamination of wounds on arrival to prevent wound infections and cellulitis, which can progress to sepsis
  — Monitor incisions and wounds for infection
  — Culture dirty wounds on initial irrigation to identify infectious sources

- Maintain normovolemia and oxygenation to prevent SIRS and sepsis (Dellinger et al. 2008)
  — Monitor and treat base deficit and lactate and normalize as quickly as possible (see Chapter 2)
  — Maintain
    - Central venous pressure (CVP) 8 to 12 mm Hg
    - Mean arterial pressure (MAP) >65 mm Hg
    - Urine output >0.5 mL/kg/hour
    - Mixed venous oxygen saturation >65%
  — Continue fluid resuscitation including packed red blood cells (PRBC) to maintain hematocrit >30%
- Early recognition of the presence of SIRS and sepsis to initiate immediate treatment and halt the progression of the inflammation and coagulopathy associated with sepsis
  — Swan-Ganz cardiac output and SVR monitoring
  — Monitor C-reactive protein, arterial blood gases, and oxygen saturations

Management

After sepsis is identified, treatment involves supporting the organs though the process and treating the infection at the source (Dellinger et al. 2008). It is imperative that lines are removed and replaced in a new site to prevent further contamination from the old sites.

- Obtain blood and other cultures prior to administration of antibiotics
- Site control of the source
  — May require computed tomography (CT) scan to identify abdominal, thoracic, or cerebral sources
  — Identify source of infection within 6 hours of onset
  — Consider percutaneous drainage of abscesses and culture
  — Remove lines that may be infected
- Initiate IV antibiotics as early as possible after culture
  — Broad-spectrum antibiotics initially until culture sensitivities are returned

— Treatment usually lasts 7 to 10 days unless the source of infection cannot be drained

- Do not administer antimicrobials if there is no positive culture result
- Provide fluid resuscitation
  — Maintain CVP
  — Fluid resuscitate as needed to prevent sepsis-induced tissue hypoperfusion, which will result in organ failure
  — Avoid over resuscitation resulting in pulmonary edema or congestive heart failure; monitor
  — Maintain mean arterial pressure >65 mm Hg
    ■ Administer vasopressors as needed such as norepinephrine or dopamine
    ■ Epinephrine, phenylephrine, and vasopressin are alternative vasopressors but should not be administered as initial treatment
    ■ Ensure that the trauma patient does not have any sites of ongoing hemorrhage
  — Inotropes
    ■ Dobutamine may be useful in patients with myocardial dysfunction
  — IV hydrocortisone may be helpful in septic shock refractory to fluid resuscitation and vasopressors
  — Recombinant human activated protein C should be considered in patients with sepsis-induced organ failure/dysfunction at high risk for death
    ■ Decreases mortality
    ■ Bleeding is a common side effect and must be taken into consideration for the trauma patient
    ■ Mechanism of action is unknown
    ■ Improves severe sepsis by repairing the microvascular alterations thus increasing the percentage of perfused capillaries within 4 hours and may also provide a more rapid clearance of increased lactate (DeBacker et al. 2006)

— Blood products
  ▪ Maintain hemoglobin (Hgb) minimum of 7 to 9 g/dL or preferably higher in the trauma patient
  ▪ For the treatment of sepsis, do not use fresh frozen plasma (FFP) in the trauma patient, however, FFP may be warranted for reasons other than sepsis
  ▪ Maintain platelets as needed
  ▪ Restricted transfusion practices may alter protocols to transfuse for Hgb < 7 g/dL as opposed to 7 to 9 g/dL mentioned above
    ○ Lower transfusion triggers reduce septic mortality
— Sedation
  ▪ Follow appropriate hospital-based protocols for sedation and analgesia in patients who are mechanically ventilated
  ▪ If neuromuscular blockade is necessary, monitor with train of four to ensure appropriate blockade
— Glycemic control
  ▪ See later discussion on Hyperglycemic Management
— Management of any associated organ failure may require temporary dialysis or renal replacement therapy until the failure resolves
— Prevent other complications associated with the critical care patient while experiencing sepsis

THROMBOEMBOLIC EVENTS

A complication that can occur with the trauma patient is a venous thromboembolism (VTE). This complication occurs from prolonged immobility in conjunction with the coagulopathy that accompanies trauma. Head and spinal cord injured patients are particularly at risk. In addition, patients experiencing shock, obesity, and age >40 years are at risk for deep vein thrombosis/pulmonary emboli (DVT/PE). The predisposing factors to thrombus for trauma patients are described in Virchow's triad of venous stasis, hypercoagulability, and vascular damage

(Ziglar et al. 2004). Prevention is required for all trauma patients and particularly critical care trauma patients. The incidence of DVT and PE are low as long as prophylaxis is in place.

DVT usually occur in the lower extremities, but with the increased use of PICC lines, upper extremity DVT are more prevalent. Superficial venous thromboses may also be detected upon screening but do not require treatment unless they move within the deep vein system. A PE occurs when the thrombus from the deep veins becomes mobile and traverses the right ventricle entering the pulmonary system. A PE is life-threatening as it obstructs portions of the lung allowing ventilation but without any perfusion from the obstructed artery. The absolute life-threatening situation is when the embolus enters the bifurcation of the pulmonary artery obstructing both the right and left circulation (saddle embolus).

Signs and Symptoms of Deep Vein Thrombosis

Pain with passive stretch (Homan sign)
Venous obstruction
Redness, warmth, swelling
Tachycardia, fever

Signs and Symptoms of Pulmonary Embolism

Feeling of impending doom ("I'm going to die")
Sudden onset hypoxia, pale, diaphoretic, cyanosis (late)
Substernal chest pain, hypotension, tachycardia
Tachypnea, shallow respirations
Shortness of breath, acute dyspnea
New onset murmur
Altered level of consciousness
Low-grade fever
Anterior T-wave inversion and/or ventricular strain
Cardiopulmonary arrest

Prevention and Prophylaxis

From admission, DVT prevention must be part of the initial order set for trauma patients both in the ICU and out. Surveillance for DVT is another component of prevention so that early detection can allow for treatment before PE occurs. Therefore, DVT prevention is also PE prevention.

- Maintain mobility, active range of motion (ROM) where possible
  — Ambulation 3 to 4 times each day for ~20 minutes each (McQuillan et al. 2009)
  — Prevent dependent positioning when out of bed
  — Frequent position changes, active ROM, isometric exercises while on bedrest
- External devices
  — Sequential compression device (SCD) should be placed on all trauma patients in critical care and any immobile patients on the units
  — Foot pumps are a viable alternative to the SCD when a lower extremity fracture prevents placement of SCDs (Rogers et al. 2002)
  — Use in conjunction with anticoagulation in high-risk patients
- Anticoagulation
  — Can be initiated when the risk for bleeding is lower
  — At risk for bleeding patients include
    ▪ Operative cases
    ▪ Solid organ injuries
    ▪ Head injury with hemorrhage or hematoma present
  — Low molecular weight heparin (LMWH) as per protocol
    ▪ Do not use LMWH in the presence of an epidural catheter
  — Low dose subcutaneous unfractionated heparin as per protocol
    ▪ There is insufficient evidence to use low dose heparin alone for prophylaxis in trauma patients (Rogers et al. 2002)

— Warfarin

  ■ Useful if long-term anticoagulation is needed after discharge (immobility)

  ■ May convert subcutaneous heparin or LMWH to warfarin prior to discharge to manipulate the INR to the appropriate level

  ■ Maintain both LMWH and warfarin during conversion until INR approaches the desired level and before establishing maintenance warfarin doses

• Surveillance

— Venous duplex studies should be performed within the first 72 hours

  ■ Repeat every 5 to 7 days (Fitzpatrick et al. 2006)

  ■ Identifies up to 86% of DVT (Adams et al. 2008)

— Include upper extremities especially when a PICC line is in place

• Inferior vena cava filter (IVC-F) placement

— Prevents the thrombus from reaching the pulmonary system

— Particularly important in the patient who is immobile, however cannot receive anticoagulation

— Removable IVC-F are the most commonly used filters

  ■ Retrievable avoids chronic sequelae

  ■ Follow-up with patients after discharge can be difficult, leaving some IVC-F as permanent due to

    ○ Lack of revisit for removal

    ○ Clot within the filter

  ■ Should be MRI compatible

— Prophylactic placement for (Cherry et al. 2008)

  ■ Spinal cord injuries

  ■ Head injuries with GCS <8

  ■ Complex pelvic fractures with or without long-bone fractures

  ■ Multiple long-bone fractures

- High grade liver or spleen injury
- Nonoperative cases in whom anticoagulation cannot be started within 72 hours
- Patients with hemorrhage on full anticoagulation
— Monitor for sequelae of IVC-F
  - Caudal movement occurs in up to 18% of IVC-F (Adair et al. 2008)
  - Movement may be affected by vigorous pulmonary toilet and quad cough procedure (Kinney et al. 1996), however these should not be avoided for fear of IVC-F migration
  - Filter fracture can occur
  - Filter tilt can occur; when >14 degrees a PE can occur from clot bypassing the IVC-F
  - Penetration of the inferior vena cava requires removal and repair

Management

Management of DVT and PE require immediate treatment. In the case of DVT the treatment is focused on prevention of movement of the thrombus. For PE, removal or decreasing the size of the clot to restore perfusion is the goal of management.

- DVT
  — Bedrest
  — Management with unfractionated heparin or LMWH followed by oral anticoagulation for up to 3 months
  — Duplex monitoring for resolution of DVT and/or movement
  — Placement of IVC-F to prevent thrombus from becoming an embolus
- PE
  — Most patients do not demonstrate the classic symptoms but more commonly acute dyspnea and tachypnea (Shaughnessy 2007)

- Rare symptoms include hemoptysis, cough, pleural friction rub
— Manage airway and oxygenation immediately
  - Place airway as needed and administer oxygen
  - Mechanical ventilation with endotracheal tube placement
  - Monitor ABG
— Provide fluid resuscitation and/or vasopressors
— Early identification of PE may prevent serious sequelae such as cardio-vascular collapse
  - Helical CT-A of the chest has replaced most ventilation-perfusion ($\dot{V}/\dot{Q}$) scans as the means of diagnosis for PE
  - $\dot{V}/\dot{Q}$ scans demonstrate high probability of PE when >2 segments of lung perfusion defects are present
  - Pulmonary angiogram is another means of diagnosis of PE
— Administer anticoagulation with heparin IV or LMWH (Shaughnessy 2007)
  - Contraindication to anticoagulation includes patients who received operation in the previous 10 days
  - LMWH is effective for DVT and small PE
  - Heparin does not dissolve the clot, but prevents further development
  - Convert to warfarin with an overlap of 4 days
  - Maintain on warfarin for 3 to 6 months with a goal INR 2 to 2.5
— May consider thrombolytics in some patients, although it is difficult to administer these in trauma patients
  - Approved for PE treatment include urokinase, streptokinase, and alteplase
  - Dissolves the clot
— Operative management may be required, particularly with saddle emboli
  - Surgical embolectomy

- Catheter embolectomy
- Placement of an IVC-F if lower extremity DVT is present
• Reversal of anticoagulation
  — In the rare occasion of bleeding associated with DVT prophylaxis or PE treatment, preparation for reversal is essential
    - Warfarin reversal requires oral or intravenous (IV) vitamin K administration to an INR range of 2 to 3
    - Reversal of unfractionated heparin is accomplished with protamine
    - Anaphylaxis is possible with vitamin K administration
    - FFP may be administered, involves volume and the waiting period for thawing; may not achieve complete reversal
    - Recombinant factor VIIa (rFVIIa) can decrease INR within 10 to 15 minutes for warfarin reversal (Coursin 2007)

Heparin-Induced Thrombocytopenia

Although not common, heparin-induced thrombocytopenia (HIT) is a serious side effect of heparin administration. This includes unfractionated heparin, heparin, and LMWH. The risk for HIT has increased with the widespread use of heparin and is more commonly associated with unfractionated heparin than with LMWH. HIT risk can be decreased with careful use of heparin-coated catheters and with flushing of lines with saline instead of heparinized saline.

HIT-1 occurs within 2 to 3 days of administration and is usually self-limiting and resolves despite continued heparin administration. The occurrence of HIT-1 is up to 15% of cases exposed to heparin. It is nonimmune mediated. HIT-2 is immune mediated and occurs in only 2% to 3% of patients. It is however more severe and can result in embolic complications. HIT-2 may not occur for 5 to 14 days or more after exposure to heparin. The syndrome is evidenced by a drop in platelets of up to 30% to 50%. A percentage change in platelets may be more appropriate in the trauma patient who has a higher platelet count in the initial post-trauma period. HIT-2 may occur in <5 days if the patient has recently been exposed to heparin prior to the current administration. In addition the syndrome can present more than a week after stopping heparin administration.

HIT-2 management includes

- Identify arterial or venous thromboses
- Immediately stop the heparin
- If previous exposure to heparin, HIT-2 presents with rapid onset and anaphylactic-like reaction with hypotension, shortness of breath, cardiovascular collapse, and even death
- Replace anticoagulation with nonheparin anticoagulants (direct thrombin inhibitors)
  — Argatroban
    ▪ Monitor activated partial thromboplastin time (aPTT) and maintain at 1.5 to 3 times control (AACN 2006)
    ▪ Metabolized in the liver
  — Lepirudin
    ▪ Monitor aPTT and maintain 1.5 to 2.5 times control
    ▪ Metabolized in the kidney
    ▪ May increase risk of bleeding
  — Manage with direct thrombin inhibitors for 5 to 7 days before converting to warfarin with an overlap of 4 to 5 days and attainment of INR >2 (Cooney 2006)
  — Warfarin inhibits protein C, causing a procoagulable state in these patients
- Anticoagulation must be maintained as clotting during HIT-2 can progress to loss of limb, stroke, or myocardial infarction (MI)
  — Skin necrosis may occur at the injection site
  — Up to 20% experience amputation
- There is a 50% occurrence of DVT and 25% occurrence of PE (Cooney 2006)
- Rule out disseminated intravascular coagulation, hemodialysis, hypercoagulability, and multisystem organ dysfunction as the cause of thrombocytopenia

ADRENAL CORTICAL INSUFFICIENCY

There has been intense study into critically ill patients and the relationship of severity of illness and adrenal insufficiency. It is believed that a degree of corticosteroid resistance exists. This resistance leads to an exaggerated proinflammatory response. Evidence of resistance is demonstrated by refractory hypotension to fluids and vasopressors in which there is no ongoing bleeding. There is no documentation that shows trauma patients benefit from the use of corticosteroids for adrenal insufficiency. In practice, critical care medicine physicians apply the principles of managing adrenal insufficiency in trauma patients who are not responding well to treatment. Research in the trauma population will drive future practice in this regard.

- Test random total cortisol <210 micrograms/dL
  - Cosyntropin stimulation tests identify adrenal insufficiency
- Treat with (Marik et al. 2008)
  - Glucocorticoids (hydrocortisone) for vasopressor dependent septic shock in the presence of ARDS
    - In ARDS corticosteroids may decrease fibrosis, improving lung compliance
  - Methylprednisolone may be used for severe early ARDS
  - Glucocorticoids must be weaned when completing treatment
  - Overall dosing should be based upon the stress experienced and administered at low doses over a short period to decrease risks
  - Dexamethasone is not appropriate treatment for adrenal cortical insufficiency
  - There is some question that patients who receive etomidate for RSI may experience adrenal insufficiency more often than those who do not
- Risks of steroid administration include
  - Immunosuppression and increased risk of infection
  - Hyperglycemia
  - Hypertension

HYPERGLYCEMIC MANAGEMENT

Recently glucose control has become a central component of critical care management, including the trauma patient. Hyperglycemia, defined for the general critical care patient as >200 mg/dL, has been associated with increased mortality and increased rates of infection. The stress of trauma and critical illness causes increased hepatic glucose production, decreased glucose uptake. These changes cause hyperglycemia and the resultant infectious complications and longer lengths of stay and ventilation.

- For the trauma patient
  — Admission glucose levels >200 mg/dL have demonstrated 40% mortality
  — Admission glucose levels between 141 to 200 mg/dL are associated with 20% mortality
  — Mortality drops to 3.3% when initial glucose levels are <140 mg/dL
  — The authors postulate that maintaining glucose levels <140 mg/dL is sufficient for trauma patients and do not identify a higher infection rate with glucose up to 140 mg/dL (Wahl et al. 2008, Scheuren et al. 2006, Laird et al. 2004)
- Blood glucose levels on admission correlate closely with lactate levels and outcome (Duane et al. 2008)
- Worsening, consistently high, and variable glucose levels are predictive of poor outcome

Management

Management begins when the patient arrives to ICU.

- Diligent blood glucose monitoring should occur every 1 to 2 hours
- Insulin drip protocols should adjust to the blood glucose for tight glycemic control
  — On average the duration of insulin therapy is ~6.5 days
  — A low percentage of patients experience hypoglycemia

- Glycemic management is a component of the ventilator-associated pneumonia bundle
- ICU protocols or computer-driven protocols have been developed that can be used to guide glucose measurement and insulin infusion

STRESS ULCER

The stress experienced by the trauma and/or burn patient is the highest of the critically ill patients. Prevention of stress ulcers is also a part of the initial trauma orders for all critical trauma patients. Stress ulcers can progress to hemorrhage and perforation. Both of these complications are serious and especially for trauma patients in whom an additional source of hemorrhage is devastating.

Prevention and Prophylaxis

Prevention of gastric stress ulcers is straightforward and routine.

- Should be used in patients with
    — Mechanical ventilation
    — Head injury
    — Burns
    — Coagulopathy
    — Multisystem trauma
    — Sepsis
    — Renal failure
    — A trauma patient on high-dose steroids
    — Delayed feeds
- Administer H_2 blockers, cytoprotective agents, or PPIs per protocol
    — No difference between the medications in preventing stress ulcer (Guillamondegui et al. 2008)
    — Avoid aluminum-containing medications in patients on dialysis

— Prophylax the patients until off mechanical ventilation and until able to take enteral feedings (Guillamondegui et al. 2008)
- Monitor gastric pH to maintain within normal
- Provide feeds to prevent excess acid damage to the stomach lining
  — Preferably oral feedings when possible
  — When providing duodenal or jejunal tube feeds, ensure that H_2 blockers or PPI for stomach protection are administered
  — Some evidence exists that decreased stomach acid results in migration of bacteria into the airway and increased incidence of pneumonia
- Manage stressors
  — Decrease stressors through maintenance of airway, control of hemorrhage
  — Promote rest, calm environment
  — Identify and treat complications

SKIN BREAKDOWN

Skin breakdown from pressure is a preventable complication during illness. Skin breakdown occurs when the pressure applied exceeds capillary closure pressure. Pressure begins with the placement of the spine backboard for spine protection. In addition to the board, rigid cervical collars and extrication collars can also initiate skin breakdown from the scene. Early identification of pressure points and efforts to remove them are essential to patient care.

Prevention and Prophylaxis

Prevention begins on the arrival of the patient and continues until all sources of pressure are removed including the cervical collar. If the collar is to be worn after discharge, the potential for breakdown continues.

- Upon secondary survey, the backboard should be removed upon turning and examination of the back
  — Maintain spinal precautions through logrolling until injury is ruled out
- Clear the cervical spine and remove the cervical collar to prevent breakdown on the pressure points of the chin, occiput, ears, mandible, clavicles (Swartz 2000)
  — If cervical spine injury exists, change the cervical collar as early as possible to a low-pressure collar (eg, Aspen or Miami-J)
  — When using the low-pressure collars, change the pads daily, washing and drying the used pads for reuse
  — Provide hygiene to the neck under the collar and dry prior to replacing the collar
    - Maintain in-line immobilization while the collar is off for neck cleansing
    - Ensure pads are dry when reapplying the following day
- Patients with immobility because of critical illness, fractures, spinal cord injury, head injury need strict observation and management of the skin
  — Frequent turning every 2 hours to avoid prolonged pressure
  — Diligently check skin every 2 hours
  — Do not allow skin to remain wet; do not apply powder
    - Clumps and causes excoriation
  — Use of low air loss beds
  — Massage areas of pressure, bony prominences
  — Prevent sliding against sheets by positioning the patient appropriately
  — Redness (stage I decubiti) can occur within 2 hours of pressure
  — Act when the skin demonstrates a stage I alteration; do not wait for open skin injury to make interventions
- Skin alterations
  — If redness begins, apply skin barrier cream to protect the area

— In areas of moisture or soiling, skin barrier cream is also useful to prevent breakdown from excoriation

— Stages

  ▪ Stage I decubiti involve erythema, warmth, inflammation

  ▪ Stage II decubiti involve as above with the addition of loss of the outer layer of skin

  ▪ Stage III decubiti involve as above with the inclusion of subcutaneous tissue disruption, and/or death of the tissue

  ▪ Stage IV decubiti continue to proceed to the level of muscle and bone with necrosis and/or dry gangrene

— Monitor sites around drains and fistulae to prevent skin contact with body fluids

Management

Management of skin breakdown is a specialty in and of itself. Briefly interventions include

• Continuing preventative activities which will stop the decubitus from deepening

• Early consultation with the enterostomal therapy/wound care nurse for optimal management and healing of the skin breakdown

— Consultation should begin prior to the development of skin open wounds

• Multiple specialty wound care products exist for varying depths of ulceration

— Choice of product is dependent upon the state of the patient as well as the optimal product for the specific wound and wound site

— If the wound develops to a stage IV full-depth ulceration, surgical coverage with a flap and/or skin graft may be the final management option

— Before surgery can be successful, pressure to the site must be prevented and the skin bed demonstrates healthy granulation tissue to accept the flap/graft

SPECIAL SITUATION

End-of-Life Decisions

The goal of critical care management is to save the life of the patient as well as provide for optimal functional outcome. There are, however, times when the actions are futile, or by the choice of the patient and family, the goal is redirected to easing into an end-of-life decision. Many patients already have an advanced directive refusing futile care or long-term ventilation, feedings, cardiopulmonary resuscitation, and more. When these directives are not in place, the decisions may need to be made by family based upon their interpretation of the patient's desires. In the case of brain death (discussed in Chapter 4), decisions regarding organ donation need to be made.

Interventions that assist with this difficult time for the family include (VanHorn 2007)

- Family involvement in decision-making from the early admission
- Discussions with the family daily to keep them abreast of the progress of the patient
- Making end-of-life decisions
  — Pain control for the patient to provide comfort
  — Do not prolong the dying process
  — Allow the family and/or patient some control over decisions and patient management
  — Maintain a strong, open, honest relationship with the family
  — Provide comfort care interventions; include chaplain and palliative care consults
- Provide counseling opportunities to the ICU staff

POSTRESUSCITATION MANAGEMENT AND REHABILITATION

Rehabilitation in the ICU

Despite the critical aspect of the patients in the ICU, rehabilitation cannot be ignored or postponed. Early physiatry consultation is essential to design a rehabilitation plan to start in ICU and progress as the patient heals. Turning, positioning, prevention of skin breakdown, nutrition, maintenance of bowel and bladder function are all components of the rehabilitation program that can be initiated in the ICU from admission. Range of motion (ROM) can be performed by the nurse or physical therapist. Occupational therapy can place splints to prevent contractures and maintain function. Speech therapy can initiate cognitive evaluation and swallow studies in the non-ventilated head injury patients. Moving the patient out of bed to the chair also promotes stimulation of the patient and prevents complications, such as skin breakdown and pneumonia. Even in its simplest forms, rehabilitation activities should begin on arrival and be adapted to the capabilities, stability, and specific needs of the patient.

 Critical Lifesavers

- **Lung protective strategies need to be implemented early to decrease morbidity**
- **Blind bronchial-alveolar lavage may be used to obtain specimens for quantitative culture**
- **Lower transfusion triggers reduce septic mortality**
- **Maintain LMWH and warfarin during conversion until INR approaches the desired level and before establishing maintenance warfarin doses**
- **Despite the critical aspect of the patients in the ICU, rehabilitation cannot be ignored or postponed**

REFERENCES

Adair JD, Harvey KP, Mahmood A. Inferior vena cava filter migration to the right ventricle with destruction of the tricuspid valve: a case report. *J Trauma.* 2008;64(2):509-511.

Adams R, Hamrick M, Berenguer C, et al. Four years of aggressive prophylaxis and screening protocol for venous thromboembolism in a large trauma population. *J Trauma.* 2008;65(2):300-308.

American Association of Critical Care Nurses (AACN). Implications, management, and prevention of heparin-induced thrombocytopenia in the critical care setting. *AACN News.* 2006;November, S3-S13.

Brown DL, Hungness ES, Campbell RS, et al. Ventilator associated pneumonia in the surgical intensive care unit. *J Trauma.* 2001;51: 1207-1215.

Cason CL, Tyner T, Saunders S, et al. Nurses' implementation of guidelines for ventilator-associated pneumonia from the centers for disease control and prevention. *Am J Crit Care.* 2007;16(1): 28-36.

Cherry RA, Nichols PA, Snavely TM, et al. Prophylactic inferior vena cava filters: do they make a difference in trauma patients. *J Trauma.* 2008;65(3):544-548.

Cooney MF. Heparin-induced thrombocytopenia: advances in diagnosis and treatment. *Crit Care Nurse.* 2006;26(6):30-36.

Coursin DB. *Sepsis, Glycemic Control, and Antithrombotics in Critical Care.* Des Plaines, IL: SCCM; 2007.

DeBacker D, Verdant C, Chierego M, et al. Effects of drotrecogin alpha activated on microcirculatory alterations in patients with severe sepsis. *Crit Care Med.* 2006;34(7):1918-1924.

Dellinger RP, Levy MM, Carlet JM, et al. Surviving sepsis campaign: international guidelines for management of severe sepsis and septic shock. *Intensive Care Med.* 2008;34(1):17-60.

Derdak S. Acute respiratory distress syndrome in trauma patients. *J Trauma.* 2007;62(2):S58.

Duane TM, Ivatury RR, Dechert T, et al. Blood glucose levels at 24 hours after trauma fails to predict outcomes. *J Trauma* 2008;64(5):1184-1187.

Fessler HE, Hager DN, Brower RG. Feasibility of very high frequency ventilation in adults with acute rsespiratory distress syndrome. *Crit Care Med.* 2008;36(4):1043-1048.

Fitzpatrick MK, Reilly P, Stavropoulos SW. The use of retrievable inferior vena cava filters in trauma: implications for the trauma team. *J Trauma Nurs.* 2006;13(2):45-51.

Goettler C, Fugo J, Bard M, et al. Predicting the need for early tracheostomy: a multifactorial analysis of 992 intubated trauma patients. *J Trauma.* 2006;60(5):991-996.

Guillamondegui OD, Gunter OL, Bonadies JA, et al. Practice management guidelines for stress ulcer prophylaxis. 2008. Available at: http://www.east.org. Accessed November 11, 2008.

Holevar M, Dunham JCM, Clancy TV, et al. Practice management guidelines for the timing of tracheostomy. 2006. Available at: http://www.east.org. Accessed November 11, 2008.

Kinney T, Rose S, Valjo K, et al. Does cervical spinal cord injury induce a higher incidence of complications after prophylactic Greenfield inferior vena cava filter usage? *J Vasc Interv Radiol.* 1996;7(6):907-915.

Laird AM, Miller PR, Kilgo PD, et al. Relationship of early hyperglycemia to mortality in trauma patients. *J Trauma.* 2004;56(5): 1058-1062.

Marik P, Pastores S, Annane D, et al. Recommendations for the diagnosis and management of corticosteroid insufficiency in critically ill adult patients: consensus statements from an international task force by the American College of Critical Care Medicine. *Crit Care Med.* 2008;36(6):1937-1949.

McQuillan KA, Flynn Makic MB, Whalen E. *Trauma Nursing from Resuscitation through Rehabilitation.* 4th ed. Philadelphia, PA: Saunders Elsevier; 2009.

Rogers FB, Cipolle MD, Velmahos G, et al. Practice management guidelines for the management of venous thromboembolism in trauma patients. *J Trauma.* 2002;53(1):142-164.

Scheuren L, Baetz B, Cawley MJ, et al. Pharmacist designed and nursing-driven insulin infusion protocol to achieve and maintain glycemic control in critical care patients. *J Trauma Nurs.* 2006;13(3):140-145.

Shaughnessy K. Massive pulmonary embolism. *Crit Care Nurs.* 2007;27(1):39-50.

Swartz C. Resuscitation considerations to prevent pressure ulcers in trauma patients. 2000. *Int J Trauma Nurs.* 6(1):16-18.

Tolentino-DelosReyes AF, Ruppert SD, Shiao SY. Evidence-based practice: use of the ventilator bundle to prevent ventilator-associated pneumonia. *Am J Crit Care.* 2007;16(1):20-27.

VanHorn JM. A case study of right ventricular rupture in an elderly victim of MVC: incorporating end of life care into trauma nursing. *J Trauma Nurs.* 2007;14(3):136-143.

Voggenreiter G, Aufmkolk M, Stiletto RJ, et al. Prone positioning improves oxygenation in post-traumatic lung injury—a prospective randomized trial. *J Trauma.* 2005;59(2):333-343.

Wahl WL, Taddonio M, Maggio PM, et al. Mean glucose values predict trauma patient mortality. 2008. *J Trauma.* 2008;65(1):42-48.

Ziglar M, Bennett V, Nayduch D, et al. *The Electronic Library of Trauma Lectures.* Chicago, IL: Society of Trauma Nurses; 2004.

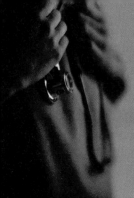

Chapter 14

ENVIRONMENTAL INJURY

INTRODUCTION

Trauma occurs in many different settings. Because of this, the trauma practitioner must include the effects of exposure and environment in the assessment and management of the trauma patient. Each of these unique situations affects the outcome of the patient and requires specific interventions to optimize that outcome.

HYPOTHERMIA

Risks

Exposure to both heat and cold results in physiologic alterations that affect the outcome of trauma patients. Hypothermia is more common than hyperthermia as injury lends itself toward loss of heat or loss of the ability to maintain body temperature. Each year in the United States, there are approximately 650 deaths from hypothermia (Jurkovich 2007). Areas of moderate temperature, especially those with rapid changes in night temperatures, are the source of the majority of hypothermia deaths. Summer season has only 10% less deaths from hypothermia than the winter season (Neno 2005). Excess exposure and/or an inability to generate body heat increases risk. For example, people at risk are the elderly and very young because of less body fat, hypothyroid disease, medications, spinal cord injury, alcohol, mental illness, immobilization, and shock/trauma.

In the patient with blunt trauma, core temperature <32°C without vital signs is lethal at almost 100% (Jurkovich 2007, Sicoutris 2001). Immersion in cold water increases temperature loss by 32 times normal. Wind and wet clothing also increase temperature loss. The lethal triad for the trauma patient is hypothermia, coagulopathy, and acidosis (Sicoutris 2001). Hypothermia itself exacerbates the acidosis and coagulopathies that may already be present after injury. Clotting is a temperature dependent process. Thus as body temperature decreases, clotting activity is impaired in a dose-response fashion.

Assessment

The body regulates temperature continuously with the goal of a constant internal environment. The ability to recognize changes in temperature, "feeling cold," is one of the first defense mechanisms of the body. As the body ages, it loses this sense of cold. This behavioral thermoregulation triggers the need to add clothing, a blanket, or perhaps increase the ambient temperature. Covering the head can decrease 60% radiant heat loss.

The hypothalamus is in control of thermoregulation. As temperature decreases, the body's typical responses include

- Vasoconstriction shunting blood to the core
- Piloerection to trap air for insulation
- Shivering increases heat production by up to 4 times normal
- Initial hypermetabolism later decreases by 10% for each 1°C loss

As temperature continues to fall, the body is unable to maintain thermoregulation attempts. Figure 14-1 demonstrates the changes in body responses as temperature drops.

Temperature loss occurs through

- Radiation: 55% to 65% loss
- Conduction: contact with the body surface; increases 5% with wet clothing and 25% with immersion
- Convection: air currents/wind
- Evaporation: 2% to 9% loss through inspired air; overall 20% to 27% loss through skin and lungs

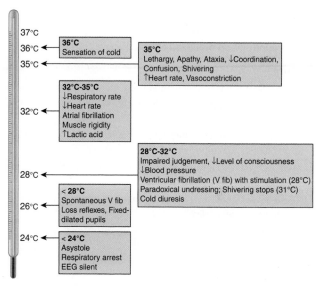

Figure 14-1   Effects of hypothermia.

Types and classification

Types of hypothermia include

- Primary unintentional: excessive cold stress usually from exposure or immersion
- Secondary unintentional: abnormal thermoregulation even with mild exposure (high risk groups)
- Chronic: inability to generate heat (altered autoregulation caused by continuous exposure)

  Hypothermia is then classified as

- Mild: 32°C to 35°C (trauma 34°C to 36°C)
- Moderate: 28°C to 32°C (trauma 32°C to 34°C)
- Severe: <28°C (trauma <32°C)

Because of the severe effects of hypothermia on trauma patients, it has been proposed that the scale for hypothermia classification should be altered as noted above (Jurkovich 2007).

History

The history of the trauma event should include the duration of exposure to the elements—temperature, humidity, wind chill, rain/dry.

- If the event includes water, such as boating incidents, MVC into water or upside down in water, swimming
  - If known, the temperature of the water and the outdoor temperature is also helpful
  - Survival decreases proportionately as the temperature of the water decreases
- Age of the patient should be taken into consideration as increased age causes decreased shivering, decreased metabolic rate and vasoconstriction, and decreased perception of the cold.
- Other factors to include are use of
  - Cannabinoids, phenothiazines, antidepressants, and alcohol
  - History of hypothyroid disease
  - Malnutrition
- Note the onset of spinal cord injury along with degree of exposure as spinal cord injured patients are poikilothermic, unable to regulate temperature.

Trauma assessment

Temperature assessment is included in the initial set of vital signs and must be a core measurement. Core measurements include tympanic, bladder, esophageal, and rectal temperature access methods. If the temperature demonstrates mild hypothermia or more severe, continuous core monitoring should be established. Bladder temperature via the Foley catheter is one of the easiest to secure as a Foley catheter is in place for fluid monitoring as well. Note that if magnetic resonance imaging (MRI) is anticipated, a temperature Foley has a ferrous thermistor tip that is not MRI compatible. A rectal probe can also be used and is more feasible in the intensive care unit (ICU) where the patient is not being moved as often as in the ED.

Alterations in the normal assessment can be seen as temperature decreases and can result in misinterpretation of information unless taken in the context of hypothermia (Table 14-1). An organized electrical cardiac rhythm without palpable pulses should be considered "alive" until warmed. End points of resuscitation include potassium >10 mEq/L, pH <6.5, and severe coagulopathy.

Management

In addition to rewarming, the hypothermic trauma patient needs the following
- Oxygen—corrects hypoxia
  - Administer warmed and humidified
  - Intubation necessary for altered level of consciousness or instability
- IV fluids—manage hypovolemia and cold diuresis
  - Administer rapidly and warmed to 42°C to 44°C
  - A Foley should be placed to monitor urine output and core temperature
  - Avoid lactated ringers as the liver will not metabolize lactate well when hypothermic
- Monitor for cardiac dysrhythmias
  - Gently move the patient to prevent initiating a dysrhythmia from an irritable myocardium
  - Defibrillation and cardiac medications are ineffective with core temperatures <28°C
    - Bretyllium tosylate was recommended for core temp <30°C
    - However, bretyllium is no longer manufactured or available (Edelstein et al. 2007)

Table 14-1   Alterations with Hypothermia

Oxygen consumption/delivery	↑ oxygen consumption ↑ minute ventilation Anaerobic metabolism Acidosis Impaired oxygen delivery: ↑ affinity for hemoglobin (left shift of oxyhemoglobin curve)
Cerebral blood flow	↓ by 6% for each 1°C drop
Cold diuresis	Vasoconstriction shunts blood to the core ↑ urine output Relative hypovolemia ↓ antidiuretic hormone
Coagulation	Labs use standard temperature of 37°C—labs may appear normal Cold platelets morphologic change affecting ability to adhere (even mild hypothermia) Coagulation path slowed in proportion to hypothermia
Hyperglycemia	Inhibition of insulin release ↑ resistance to insulin
Shivering	↑ oxygen consumption Ceases at 32°C resulting in muscle rigidity and passive heat loss
Electrolyte imbalance	Hyperkalemia Hyponatremia

- Dopamine has some action
- For ventricular fibrillation, attempt defibrillation immediately
  - If unsuccessful, hold all defibrillation and antiarrhythmics until warmed to 30ºC (Edelstein et al. 2007)
  - If remains in ventricular fibrillation when >30ºC, use amiodarone
— Widened QRS, prolonged PR interval, J wave (Osborn wave) at the junction of QRS and ST segments
— Organized electrical activity without pulses, do not initiate cardiopulmonary resuscitation (CPR); CPR can initiate ventricular fibrillation

Passive external rewarming—mild hypothermia

- Ensure hydration
- Avoid caffeine

Passive External Rewarming

Remove wet clothing
Cover with prewarmed blankets
Cover head
Dry skin by patting to prevent moving cold blood to core by rubbing
Cover with laminate reflective blanket, especially during transport

Active external rewarming—moderate hypothermia; faster than passive external rewarming

- Incorporate passive external rewarming measures in addition to active external rewarming
- Warm at rate of 0.5ºC to 1ºC per hour
  - Warming too rapidly increases oxygen consumption and myocardial demand as well as vasodilation; these result in decompensation

- Core temperature afterdrop—core temperature decreases after cold peripheral blood circulates into the core as peripheral vasodilation occurs
- Rewarming Shock—drop in blood pressure (BP) caused by peripheral vasodilation during warming

Active External Rewarming

Forced-air blanket warmers
Overbed radiant heaters 70 cm above the patient
Immersion into 40°C bath

Active core rewarming—severe hypothermia
- Warm up to 3°C per hour
- Warm humidified air provides very slow rewarming due to the low quantity of heat transferred
- Body cavity rewarming limited by the volume of fluid necessary
  — As the body warms, the dwell time required increases
- Continuous arteriovenous rewarming (CAVR) provides rapid rewarming without the need of a perfusionist or heparin;
  — CPR can be performed during rewarming
  — Rate of rewarming is dependent upon BP driving the system
  — Requires a BP >80 mm Hg; weight >40.9 kg
- Continuous venovenous rewarming (CVVR) provides rapid rewarming through the use of a roller pump
  — Independent of BP
  — At a temperature of 40°C rewarming can occur at 1°C per hour
- Hemodialysis requires hemodynamic stability and systemic heparinization
- Cardiopulmonary bypass for unstable patients/arrest
  — Requires perfusionist and heparinization
  — Warm at a rate of 1°C to 2°C every 2 to 3 minutes

— Oxygenate and perfuse simultaneously

— Relative contraindication for trauma patients with the potential for bleeding

Active Core Rewarming

Blood warmer—40°C to 44°C, rapid infuser
Humidified, warm ventilation 40°C to 45°C
Warm lavage abdomen 40°C to 45°C instilled at 6 L/hour
Hemodialysis
Cardiopulmonary bypass
CAVR
CVVR

SUBMERSION AND IMMERSION

Risks

Injuries involving water are complicated by the presence of water in the lungs, water temperature, and duration of exposure. Immersion is considered exposure to water without the head going below the surface. Submersion is the total body going below the surface.

There are more than 8,000 drownings each year in the United States and is the second leading cause of unintentional injury in children. Small children can drown in as little as 2 in of water and do not require submersion. Most of these drowning occur in pools, fish ponds, buckets, and while bathing. Near-drowning is submersion, followed by 24 hours of survival. Drowning is submersion followed by death from asphyxia. Risk factors include alcohol, an inability to swim, loss of consciousness or spinal cord injury, hypothermia, and exhaustion.

Assessment

The outcome of submersion is dependent upon many factors. Water temperature is critical. Water cools the body 32 times faster than air. Survival in water at 0°C is <1 hour. Water at 15°C produces survival up to ~6 hours. At that time, the victim is hypothermic and will no longer be able to attempt to stay above the surface. There is a survival advantage when the patient is hypothermic prior to hypoxia because of the decrease in metabolic rate. With aspiration of cold water, core cooling continues. Movement or struggling in the water increases heat loss so that swimming and treading water decreases survival time.

The primary issue in drowning is anoxia. The victim initially gasps after initial immersion and then hyperventilates. Aspiration can occur with the initial gasp. Fatigue and muscle cooling can impair the victim's ability to swim. Once submerged, exhausted, or unconscious, the victim takes a terminal breath aspirating the water and then the water enters the airways passively. Few people have a "dive reflex" that decreases heart rate, closes the airway (laryngospasm), and shunts blood to the brain. The dive reflex may be more prevalent in children, which gives them a survival advantage. These are patients with a dry drowning as the reflex protects against aspiration of water at least temporarily.

History

When taking the history of trauma events that include water, the following information should be collected

- Type of water—fresh versus salt
- Amount of water aspirated—if it can be determined; patient can aspirate up to 2 L of fluid into the lungs
- Temperature of the water involved
- Duration of exposure to the water for temperature alterations and degree of fatigue

Obtain all of the components of the trauma event, eg, motor vehicle collision (MVC), fall/dive, struck in the process of entering the water or once in the water.

Trauma assessment

The primary and secondary surveys of the trauma patient should include issues with hypothermia as well as submersion. Additional factors include

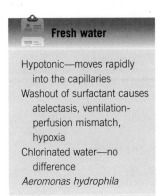

Fresh water

Hypotonic—moves rapidly
into the capillaries
Washout of surfactant causes
atelectasis, ventilation-
perfusion mismatch,
hypoxia
Chlorinated water—no
difference
Aeromonas hydrophila

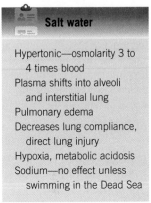

Salt water

Hypertonic—osmolarity 3 to
4 times blood
Plasma shifts into alveoli
and interstitial lung
Pulmonary edema
Decreases lung compliance,
direct lung injury
Hypoxia, metabolic acidosis
Sodium—no effect unless
swimming in the Dead Sea

Other airway issues include the aspiration of mud or sand in addition to water. Include the assessment and management associated with hypothermia discussed earlier in this chapter.

After submersion the patient may be essentially asymptomatic with some shortness of breath and mild hypoxia.

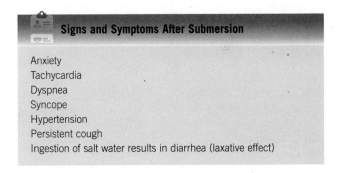

Signs and Symptoms After Submersion

Anxiety
Tachycardia
Dyspnea
Syncope
Hypertension
Persistent cough
Ingestion of salt water results in diarrhea (laxative effect)

Management

The primary goal of managing the near-drowning patient is controlling hypoxia. As this is the same goal for trauma patients, the focus remains the same with some critical care management specific to water aspiration. Asymptomatic patients should receive oxygen at 8 to 10 L/minute and observation for ~4 to 6 hours. Check for hypothermia and rest the patient to prevent rapid flow of cold peripheral blood back to the core. Symptomatic patients need the following.

- Initiate CPR in the field as rapidly as possible; warm the patient
  — Follow the principles of hypothermia management
- Airway management and oxygen administration
- Place a nasogastric (N/G) tube to prevent vomiting/aspiration of gastric contents
- Pulse oximetry monitoring
  — Maintain PO_2 >90 mm Hg and PCO_2 < 45 mm Hg
- Pulmonary toilet, bronchoscopy
- Diuresis
- Sodium bicarbonate—impairs oxygen delivery
  — Administer half the expected dose only after arterial blood gas monitoring
  — Causes paradoxical increase in lactate production
  — Increases CO_2 production and acidosis
- Mechanical ventilation with positive end-expiratory pressure (PEEP)
  — Moves interstitial water into the capillaries
  — Increases lung volume preventing atelectasis
  — Increases diameter of airways
  — Increases alveolar ventilation and improves ventilation-perfusion ratio
- Warm and dry
- Manage persistent arrhythmias following Advanced Cardiac Life Support recommendations (AHA 2006)
  — Monitor core temperature to avoid hypothermic effects on rhythm

- Support BP with vasoactive drips if needed (dopamine, dobutamine)
  - Insert Swan-Ganz catheter for full cardiac monitoring
- Protect cervical spine, especially if a diving mechanism or struck by boat/object

Common management errors include administration of steroids and antibiotics without positive cultures. End points of resuscitation include severe unsurvivable injury and/or normothermia without vital signs.

HIGH ALTITUDE EXPOSURE

Risks

Injury can happen anywhere, anytime. There are temperature and water risks as well as risks associated with altitude. Recreational activities such as skiing, snowboarding, hiking, and more occur at altitude and injuries resulting from these activities are also treated at altitude. Many of the injured do not reside at altitude, therefore may have a degree of altitude sickness as well as injury.

Most people do not experience any effects of altitude until above 7000 feet. However, high altitude is considered anywhere above 4900 feet, where decreased exercise performance is already evident. At altitudes above 11,000 feet, PaO_2 is <60 mm Hg and oxygen saturations drop <90% (Auerbach et al. 2007). Altitude illness occurs at >8500 feet in 25% of patients and above 10,000 feet in 42% of patients (Rodway et al. 2003).

Assessment

Altitude sickness is classified into three groups. Each is progressively worse than the others. Acute mountain sickness (AMS) ranges from mild to severe before progressing to high-altitude pulmonary edema (HAPE) and/or high-altitude cerebral edema (HACE).

- AMS
  - Self-limiting with resolution by day 5; maximal symptoms day 2 to 3

AMS

Dyspnea with exertion
Headache
Dizziness, poor sleep, feels "hungover"
Nausea and vomiting
Loss of appetite
Irritable

- HAPE
  — Majority of deaths are caused by HAPE
  — Usually begins at night within 3 days after arrival
  — At least 50% will have experienced AMS; <20% have HACE in addition to HAPE (Rodway et al. 2003)

HAPE

Dyspnea at rest, cough, weakness, fatigue
Chest tightness and congestion
Decreased exercise performance/endurance
Rales, wheezes, tachypnea
Central cyanosis
Pulmonary hypertension, noncardiogenic
Tachycardia

- HACE
  — Hypoxemia results in cerebral herniation and brain death
  — Occurs from 12 hours to 3 days after arrival
  — Check for hypothermia as the cause of symptoms
  — Cranial nerve palsies are rare

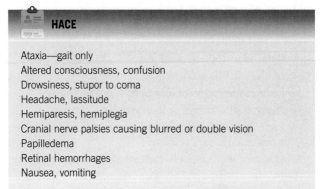

HACE

Ataxia—gait only
Altered consciousness, confusion
Drowsiness, stupor to coma
Headache, lassitude
Hemiparesis, hemiplegia
Cranial nerve palsies causing blurred or double vision
Papilledema
Retinal hemorrhages
Nausea, vomiting

History

When taking the history of injury, include the altitude at which the injury occurred and whether the patient is a resident of that altitude or is a visitor. It is also helpful to know how long the patient has been at altitude and if any symptoms were present prior to the injury. As with submersion, temperature may also be a factor in the overall patient presentation, especially if any prolonged exposure occurred. Other factors to include in the history are resting altitude and the rate of ascent to that altitude.

Trauma assessment

Trauma can mimic many of the symptoms of altitude sickness, and these symptoms can mimic trauma, particularly head injury, abdominal injury, and especially trauma complicated by hypothermia. Identify injury as well as altitude sickness symptoms.

Management

Altitude sickness management requires descent from altitude. The final altitude for descent is dependent on the severity of the illness. Management for AMS includes

- Minimization of activity to allow the body to acclimatize up to 3 days

- Oxygen administration, low flow, 2 L/minute
- Descent if any neurologic symptoms or no response to rest and oxygenation
  — Descend to 1500 to 3000 feet
- Acetazolamide BID accelerates acclimatization
  — Reduces resorption of bicarbonate and sodium
  — Avoid in sulfa allergy or increased liver enzymes
  — Begin 24 hours prior to arrival at altitude and continue for a minimum 3 days at altitude
- Avoid respiratory depressants such as sedation or sleep-inducing agents
- Administer analgesics and antiemetics as needed
  — Ibuprofen, aspirin, or acetaminophen for headache
- Dexamethasone may mitigate symptoms, but symptoms will recur when the drug is stopped
- Consider *Ginkgo Biloba* BID to mitigate symptoms (Auerbach et al. 2003)
  — May be more effective with acetazolamide
- In severe AMS or if descent is impossible
  — Portable hyperbaric chamber used to simulate 6000 to 7000 feet

  HAPE must be managed rapidly to control hypoxia with

- Descent to 2000 feet
- Oxygen administration for 48 to 72 hours
- Minimize activity to prevent increased oxygen consumption
- Consider the situation severe if oxygen saturations do not improve to >90% within 5 minutes of initiating oxygen therapy (Rodway et al. 2003)
- Consider nifedipine if unable to descend or no oxygen is available
  — Decreases pulmonary artery pressure by 30%

  HACE, like the above, must be managed rapidly as the hypoxia promotes vasogenic edema, increased intracranial pressure, and herniation. Management includes

* Descent to ≤2000 feet; or use of the hyperbaric chamber
* Oxygen administration
* Dexamethasone IV, IM or PO if the patient is able

The key to managing altitude sickness is removal of the patient from the situation through descent and if unable, provide oxygen or hyperbaric treatment to manage symptoms. Acclimatization is essential when making the ascent such as sleeping at lower altitudes, slower ascent, minimizing activity in the initial days. Other means of preventing altitude sickness include hydration and avoidance of caffeine and alcohol. However, patients injured at altitude may not have acclimatized and come for treatment with both trauma and altitude issues.

 Critical Lifesavers

* Immersion in cold water increases temperature loss by 32 times normal
* Covering the head can decrease 60% radiant heat loss
* Warm at rate of 0.5°C to 1°C per hour
* Primary goal of managing the near-drowning patient is controlling hypoxia
* Key to managing altitude sickness is removal of the patient from the situation through descent

REFERENCES

American Heart Association (AHA). *Advanced Cardiac Life Support Professional Provider Manual.* Dallas, TX: AHA; 2006.

Auerbach P. *Wilderness Medicine.* 5th ed. St Louis, MO: Mosby; 2007.

Auerbach P, Donner HJ, Weiss EA. *Field Guide to Wilderness Medicine.* 2nd ed. St Louis, MO: Mosby; 2003.

Edelstein JA, Li J, Silverberg MA, et al. Hypothermia. 2007. Available at: http://www.emedicine.com/emerg/Topic279.htm. Accessed December 17, 2008.

Jurkovich GJ. Environmental cold-induced injury. *Surg Clin North Am.* 2007;87(1):247-267.

Neno R. Hypothermia: assessment, treatment, and prevention. *Nurs Stand.* 2005;19(20):47-52,54,56.

Rodway GW, Hoffman LA, Sanders MH. High-altitude-related disorders-Part 1: pathophysiology, differential diagnosis, and treatment. *Heart Lung.* 2003;32(6):353-359.

Sicoutris C. Management of hypothermia in the trauma patient. *J Trauma Nurs.* 2001;8(1):5-12.

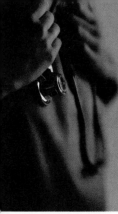

Chapter 15

MASS CASUALTY INCIDENTS

INTRODUCTION

There is always the possibility of a disaster happening close to home. There is no place that is immune to the potential..For some it is natural events, such as flooding or tsunami, tornadoes, hurricanes, earthquakes, forest fires, and volcanic eruptions. It could be small scale, such as a bus rollover or van filled with unrestrained passengers. In some parts of the world, it is disaster on a large scale with terrorist events or natural disasters where housing is poorly constructed or there are no resources to help. The world has been affected by disasters since the beginning of time. Terrorist-type events have been recorded since the 6th century BC when bioterrorism was used in warfare.

In any situation, the hospital and the trauma center must be prepared for a mass casualty situation. Any mass casualty situation is defined as an incident in which the number of casualties exceed the resources of the facility and/or region. It is essential for the facility to prepare with the community to manage any type of mass casualty incident (MCI), which could occur at any time and in any place.

INCIDENTS

There are many types of MCI events, including the use of weapons of mass destruction (WMD). These weapons are used with the intention of causing massive destruction, injury, and death. MCI events can occur individually but preparedness must include the potential for these to occur simultaneously. It is not unknown for terrorists to set off an incendiary blast device with a chemical or biologic weapon inside. Types of events include

- Natural—earthquakes, floods, volcanic eruptions, tornadoes, hurricanes, tsunami, and any other event that is the result of earth-made destruction. These may occur in one geographic area and have an impact on other regions of the globe
- Local—building, bridge or stadium collapse, fire, bus rollover, and any other local event. In addition to the stress of the situation and the number of casualties, some of them, as in natural disasters, may also be family and friends of the caregivers
- Chemical—vesicants, blood, and nerve agents. Chemicals are widely dispersed during a blast with the intention of widespread morbidity and mortality. Victims of the dispersion move from the site and spread the chemical on their clothes and skin to an even broader population resulting in contamination of caregivers and others not even present at the original event.
- Biological—infectious or debilitating biologic weapons dispersed into a population. Biologic agents such as smallpox were used in warfare to debilitate an army
- Terrorism—the systematic use of violence in attempts to coerce people toward an end—religious, political, or other. Terrorists empower their members to act on behalf of the group, thereby disengaging the person from the act and justifying the behavior to achieve the end.
- Radiation—external irradiation, contamination, incorporation. Nuclear radiation release is possible through "dirty bombs" that are easily concealable simple devices. This, like chemical and biological weapons, can result in widespread injury from the movement of victims with contaminated skin and clothing.
- Blast—multiphasic injury patterns after an explosive event that may or may not include secondary devices, eg, shrapnel, biological or chemical weapons, and more.

Disasters occur to varying degrees dependent upon their geographic location, number of victims involved, and the resources

needed. They are classified into three levels based upon the anticipated response needed.

- Level I—local response sufficient. Emergency response personnel
  and equipment can contain and manage the scene and aftermath
- Level II—regional response is sufficient. Emergency response
  from both the local and regional community resources are
  sufficient to manage both the scene and aftermath.
- Level III—both local and regional resources are over-
  whelmed. Emergency response assistance from state and federal agencies is needed. It is essential that a community plan
  for maintenance in isolation for up to 5 days before federal
  assistance may be available

PREVENTION AND PREPAREDNESS

Preparedness for disaster is more than a plan in a book. Facilities
as well as communities need to plan together and practice together
for readiness and action, not just preparedness. The plans must be
integrated as well as meet the requirements of the Department of
Homeland Security. State and local agencies include State Bureau
of Investigation (SBI), Centers for Disease Control and Prevention
(CDC), American Red Cross, and other local resources. The Office
of Emergency Management coordinates state disaster relief and
coordinates emergency personnel, provides leadership, and support staff at the state level. An awareness of the potential for MCI
and the use of weapons of mass destruction is important in every
community and hospital.

Federal Agencies

Federal agencies start with the Department of Homeland Security
created in 2001. The Federal Emergency Management Agency
directs the National Incident Management System (NIMS). Every
hospital disaster plan must incorporate the components of NIMS.
The plan provides consistency across the nation and between
communities. Other components of the federal response include
Urban Search and Rescue Teams and the National Disaster Medical

System (NDMS). NDMS includes Disaster Medical Assistance Teams, Veterinary Medical Assistance Teams, Disaster Mortuary Response Teams, and National Medical Response Teams for Weapons of Mass Destruction.

The federal government also determines the potential security threat level for the country. These levels are (DHS 2008)

- Red: severe; high possibility of a security threat that is site specific and should include lockdown for security, opening the Emergency Operations Center (EOC) and Incident Command Center (ICS)

- Orange: high; high risk of attack without site specific information that should include increasing security measures and anticipation of activating the EOC and ICS

- Yellow: elevated; moderate risk of security threat with no designated site and should include increased awareness and monitoring

- Blue: guarded; general security awareness, preparedness, and readiness without any definitive threat and should include practice drills and preparedness

- Green: low; no identified risk of attack but should include continued preparedness and practice drills

Local Hospital

The hospital emergency operations plan includes not only facility resources but an integration with the community, other nearby hospitals, emergency medical services, and volunteer organizations in the area. A Hazard Vulnerability Analysis is conducted for the region surrounding the facility and includes

- All real and potential threats both natural and manmade
  - Recognition of these vulnerabilities assist with the plan and needs assessment for drills, stockpiles of equipment and/or medications, security, and training
- Mutual aid agreements are designed with agencies that are beyond the vulnerabilities identified so that there are resources outside of the potential disaster region

- The hospital ICS is integrated with the emergency medical system to coordinate incoming information (Nicholson 2006)
  — The incident commander oversees all functions of the hospital during the disaster, coordinates many subofficers who manage security, supplies, staff, operations, and logistics
  — Coordination with mutual aid as well as state and federal resources all stem from the ICS

Overall the emergency operations plan that is activated is simple, flexible, and includes (Waugh 2007)

- Activation response
- Communications—internal and external
- Patient care coordination for movement into and out of the facility, as well as walking wounded
- Security
- Resource identification—external and internal, mutual aid
- People management—"flow"
- Data management—with and without electricity
- Demobilization—deactivation
- Debriefing and critique
- Practice drills
- MCI management—including morgue management
- Education and training

A very important liaison within the people management component is the person in charge of media control. There is a designated public information officer to provide information to the media as the spokesperson for the hospital whose intention is to protect privacy as well as prevent incorrect information being offered to the media. Media should not be allowed access to the patient care areas.

ASSESSMENT

During an MCI, triage is similar but not identical to emergency department triage. Emergency triage usually involves resuscitation, emergent, urgent, nonurgent, and minor categories. Resources are allocated to the patients who are critically ill. At the time of an MCI, triage is rapid and the focus is on patients with potentially survivable injuries and careful allocation of resources. Resources must be provided to the greatest number of people who will benefit the most from those resources. The first person to triage at the scene "labels" the patient according to a four-level system (Garner 2003).

MCI Triage Categories

Red—Immediate: life-threatening but survivable, eg, sucking chest wounds, pneumothorax, airway obstruction, open fracture, abdomen or chest injuries, second degree and third degree burns up to 40%

Yellow—Delayed: significant but can survive while waiting for medical care, eg, intact airway, abdominal injury without hypotension, fractures, eye injury

Green—Minor: minor injury that can wait hours to days for treatment, eg, minor wounds, sprains, psychological disturbances

Black—Expectant-Deceased: extensive injury without likelihood of survival, eg, severe head injury, high spinal cord injury, multisystem injury, burns >60%, fixed and dilated pupils, death

The second person at the scene initiates immediate lifesaving behaviors such as intubation and initiates transport. Patients are continually reassessed and can change triage category with improvement or deterioration. According to the START triage protocol (Newport Beach Fire 2008) the

- Initial triage person checks first for respirations and repositions the airway for improvement

- Respirations alone may precipitate "immediate" category triage
- Perfusion is checked next by assessing for radial pulse, capillary refill, and control of bleeding and may again precipitate and "immediate" category
- The final rapid check is mental status
  — Ability to follow commands with positive radial pulse and respirations places the patient in the "delayed" category
  — All walking wounded (if still at the scene) are "minor"
  — No respirations even with repositioning of the airway are "deceased"

For pediatric specific guidelines, see the JumpSTART triage protocol (Romig 1995) (Figure 15-1). JumpSTART should be used with any patient who looks like a child. There are no specific age guidelines. In a written communication with Lou Romig, MD (May 2008), once a child looks like a young adult, approximately 15 to 17 years, the START triage algorithm is applied. For small children and infants who cannot walk, the JumpSTART algorithm should be applied. Children meeting yellow criteria should be assessed for external injury such as large surface area burns, amputations, avulsions, abdominal distention, penetrating injuries, and possible airway burn. If any of these or other serious injuries are present, the child remains as a yellow. In the absence of significant injury, the child may be determined to be green (even though their normal is that they cannot walk).

The walking wounded present a specific problem, as they may start arriving at the hospital before it is ready to receive patients and possibly before a lockdown to filter all incoming through one triage entry point. The idea that there is a "safe zone" for hazardous situations where decontamination has already occurred and all personnel and people are safe for treatment and transport is a good idea, but unlikely due to the self-triage that occurs at the scene. It is impossible to contain a hazard (Phelps 2006). Self-evacuation usually precedes the arrival of emergency medical personnel from 2 to 5 minutes. This makes the hospital part of the scene itself.

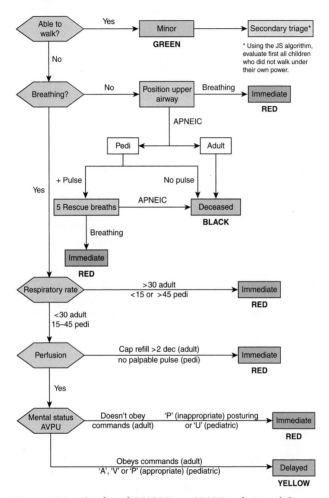

Figure 15-1 Combined START/JumpSTART pediatric-adult triage algorithm; RED = Immediate, YELLOW = Delayed, GREEN = Minor, BLACK = Expectant or Deceased. (With permission, from Lou E. Romig MD, FAAP, FACEP.)

Personal Protection Equipment

Personal protection equipment (PPE) is necessary at any level of activity with the victims of an event (Currance 1999). There are various levels of PPE, which depend upon the agent or suspicion of an agent present at the scene and through the hospital phases of care. PPE are intended to protect the staff from any chemical, biological, radiation, or other hazards present. PPE are effective only if worn prior to patient contact. There are four levels of protection

- Level A—highest level of PPE, including self-contained breathing apparatus and provides respiratory, skin, eye, and mucous membrane protection. It is vapor-tight with both gloves and boots
- Level B—provides the highest respiratory protection as with level A with a chemically resistant suit that is not vapor-tight, which decreases its skin and eye protection
- Level C—uses an air-purified respirator to cleanse the air in addition to a chemically resistant suit with boots, gloves, and a splash hood
- Level D—least protective level of PPE includes a typical uniform with the usual universal precautions of gloves, gown, mask with splash shield, and booties
- Dust particle masks decrease breathing in debris that may be on the victims clothing
- At the scene, other protective gear includes steel-toed shoes, hard hat

History

Increased awareness of the community and any changes can assist the facility in being ready for an MCI or any disaster-like event. Clusters of patients with an unusual illness presentation, increased number of people with flu-like symptoms, or any increase in a disease pattern in a community should be noticed and reported to the local health department or CDC office. When taking a patient history include the date, time and place of the event, when did signs and symptoms occur, recent travel or contact with others who are ill. Assistance regarding suspicious findings can be found through hospital infectious disease, material safety data sheets or the chem-trac database available at www.improchem.co.za, CDC, and the local poison control center. Any known exposure to an agent needs to be documented and determined if PPE are needed as rapidly as possible to contain the agent.

Trauma Assessment

After the patients arrive from the scene in their various assigned triage categories, the hospital re-triages them to ensure that the choice of category remains appropriate. In addition, a trauma resuscitation assessment is done for the usual airway, breathing, circulation, and neurologic review (Chapter 2). This is followed by a rapid secondary assessment and determination of care needs. Rapid life-saving interventions, eg, intubation, chest tubes, closed reductions of fractures, are instituted and the patient taken to the operating suite, intensive care, or floor as their needs dictate. Only patients with survivable, manageable injuries are taken to the operating room or intensive care units as the resources to manage a severe injury are not available.

DOCUMENTATION

Documentation is brief but complete. The initial triage person at the scene identifies the triage category but does not complete the triage tag. It is simply placed on the patient. The next in line for triage completes the rest of the tag. On arrival to the hospital, the brief history and assessment are documented. The facility must be prepared for the need to document on paper if they are currently using computer documentation. Documentation is done of the history of the event, patient involvement, signs and symptoms, onset, vital signs, and the usual emergency notes.

MANAGEMENT

Decontamination is usually provided first at the scene to decrease cross-contamination beyond the "hot zone." As stated previously, walking wounded frequently leave the scene before the arrival of assistance and before decontamination can be accomplished at the scene. Hospitals must provide an area for decontamination as well. In general decontamination starts with the

- Removal of clothing and jewelry followed by a rinse with water
  — Should remove the majority of contamination in most cases
- Second step is a thorough soap and water scrub followed by another rinse with water
- Waste water must be contained to prevent contamination of water tables and sewer systems
- Staff should be trained in decontamination procedures

Trauma management is otherwise the same standard of care discussed in Chapter 2. For specific situations such as chemical, biologic, and radiation exposures, the management is discussed below and may involve infectious disease, isolation, decontamination, and other services.

Natural Events

Natural disasters may be remote situations with little human involvement or may result in an MCI. A natural disaster results in loss of electricity, mobile and cell phones, and potable water.

- Electrocution is a common injury caused by downed power lines or power lines in contact with water
- Building collapse and excessive exposure to the elements are other effects of a natural disaster, resulting in injuries in addition to the original series of injured from the event itself
  — Victims trapped >2 to 6 hours have a decreased chance of survival because of untreated injuries and exposure

There are typically three waves of patients.

- First-wave patients are the initial walking wounded with minor injuries
- Second-wave and third-wave patients are triaged from the scene by emergency services and are usually the severely injured "immediate" category patients

- Finally, patients sustaining injuries from rescue and clean-up efforts can arrive for days to weeks later
  - Contaminated food and water may provide another source of victims as safe food is in limited supply especially in the initial stages
  - Exposure and other environmental injuries, eg, bites or venomous animal exposure may also result in injuries
  - Some of the typical waterborne and insect-borne agents that may present to the emergency department after a natural disaster include *Escherichia coli,* typhus, *Salmonella, Shigella,* malaria, tularemia, and *Leptospirosis*

Other naturally occurring disasters that may not seem such at the initial patient contact, are outbreaks of infectious diseases. Examples are influenza, bird flu, and the severe acute respiratory syndrome (SARS). A pandemic of influenza, especially H5NI Influenza A (avian flu) has been likened to a weapon of mass disruption where the citizens themselves become the weapon. Mortality in Southeast Asia for this strain of flu has been up to 50% of those <40 years. (Grigg et al. 2006). Vaccines provide for a degree of prevention. Retroviral administration can provide recovery if administered within the first 48 hours of symptom onset.

Blast Incidents

There are a multitude of possible blast scenarios. Bombings occur in both military and civilian arenas. Because of this, understanding the methods and likely injuries assist with planning for victims. Explosives can be packaged in various ways. Fertilizer made with ammonium nitrate can also be used as the explosive agent. A "dirty bomb" includes radioactive material within the bomb. The bomb serves as the means of dispersion of the radiation. Weapons used in terrorist attacks are more often improvised explosive devices (IED).

To increase the impact, a bomb can have the addition of nails, other shrapnel, and/or chemical or biological contaminants. The addition of shrapnel increases wounding when the victims are hit.

This is referred to as a secondary device. Other secondary devices include the collapse of the building or other structure.

A high-order explosive, such as dynamite or nitroglycerin has a supersonic overpressurization wave that results in serious internal injuries. Low-order explosives like the Molotov cocktail have a subsonic overpressurization wave. The patient injuries are dependent upon the presence of this wave. The pressure wave occurs when the liquid explosive rapidly converts to gas, expands, and compresses the surrounding air. The effects are most severe in enclosed spaces, amplifying the pressure wave. Superheated air flow is also associated with a blast and is called a blast wind and is not the pressure wave itself. Another important aspect to remember is that a terrorist may be one of the incoming patients and may still be a walking armed IED.

As with any mass casualty situation, there is a large number of walking wounded and on average ~20% of the total victims have severe injury (CDC 2008). The majority of fatal injuries are to the head (50-75%) however the majority of actual head injuries are not fatal or even severe. Almost any injury can be seen in blast incidents due to the blast itself, secondary injuries, and being struck by objects set in motion by the explosion. The blast has four categories of injury (Table 15-1). Common injuries include blast lung, tympanic membrane rupture, abdominal, and head injuries. Delayed deaths may be due to undetected abdominal injury from devascularized or perforated bowel or lung injury.

In the situation of blast injuries, pulmonary contusion is most common in children and may not be clinically apparent on arrival. It should be suspected with any signs of external chest injury. A chest radiograph is essential.

Blast lung injury

Blast lung is part of the primary blast injury. As the wave passes through the air-filled lungs, hemorrhage and tearing occur. Ventilation-perfusion mismatch results and it is possible for an air embolus to develop.

Table 15-1   Blast Injury Classification

Blast	Effect
Primary	Caused by actual over-pressurization wave **Spalling**: injury from the wave passing through the body; each tissue responds differently due to varying tissue densities **Implosion**: injury from expanding gases within hollow organs causing rupture **Shear:** injury from movement of different tissue densities against each other **Irreversible work:** possibly causes injury as the wave exceeds tensile strength of the tissue
Secondary	Injury from the debris within the bomb and objects set in motion by the explosion
Tertiary	Injury from being lifted, thrown, and dropped during the blast
Quaternary	Any other injury including long term effects, exacerbation of co-morbidities, and any complications of the previous blast effect
Quinary	Proposes that a hyper-inflammatory state develops in those closest to the blast or is the result of toxins from within the bomb (Kluger et al. 2006)

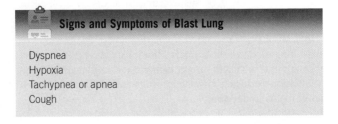

Signs and Symptoms of Blast Lung

Dyspnea
Hypoxia
Tachypnea or apnea
Cough

Chest pain
Pneumothorax or hemopneumothorax
Wheezing
Hemodynamic instability
Hemoptysis
Pulmonary edema

Management of blast lung includes the use of

- Oxygenation, continuous positive airway pressure (CPAP), and intubation with mechanical ventilation, especially in the event of respiratory distress, pulmonary edema, and hemoptysis
  — Independent lung ventilation may be necessary if there is significant hemoptysis or air leaks
  — Place a chest tube for pneumothorax or hemopneumothorax to decompress the lung.
- Fluid volume overload should be avoided to prevent pulmonary edema, yet enough fluid must be administered to maintain perfusion
- If an air embolism develops, position the patient in the prone to partial left lateral position and transport with 100% oxygen to the closest hyperbaric chamber for compression
- Can develop acute respiratory distress syndrome (ARDS) from the blast lung injury

Tympanic membrane rupture

Another primary blast injury is tympanic membrane (TM) rupture. The TM is the body's pressure transducer and responds to the pressure wave from the blast. As such, the TM is the most commonly injured organ of the body in a blast. Symptomatic patients usually have a large rupture. If the victim was in an enclosed space at the time of the explosion, there is an increased incidence of TM rupture. Ossicular disruption and foreign bodies in the auditory canal can also occur.

Signs and Symptoms of Tympanic Membrane Rupture

Hearing loss
Dizziness
Pain
Tinnitus
Otorrhea

Management of TM rupture is simple in most cases, as they heal spontaneously. Residual effects may include the need for hearing aids (~5% of patients) or mild high-frequency hearing loss (Ritenour et al. 2008).

Abdominal and head injuries

Abdominal and head injuries are common primary blast injuries. These are managed as any head or abdominal trauma patient would be. Abdominal injuries may not present for days after the event. Postconcussive syndrome is common as well as posttraumatic stress disorder (PTSD). Burns may be present caused by the explosion and fire resulting from the ignition of the bomb. Secondary and tertiary blast injuries are identified and treated as any trauma patient. Quaternary injuries include complications, such as acute respiratory distress syndrome, asthma and chronic obstructive pulmonary disorder (COPD) exacerbation. Injuries rarely occur in isolation. The usual trauma assessment and management is performed to prevent missed injuries and complications.

Biological Agents

Covert methods of causing widespread damage are not new to the terrorist or warfare. Biological weapons are one of the methods to disable a large part of a population. It takes more manpower to care for ill or injured victims than for the dead. Biological, chemical, and radiation weapons can be added to other methods of warfare and attack. Biological weapons result in both morbidity and mortality. With walking wounded and the general mobility of people, a disease can be spread over a large area quickly. In addition, the presentation of many biological weapons resembles common illnesses like influenza.

Biological weapons can be dispersed through droplet vaporization, foods, or direct contact. If a vector is used it can be animal, insect, or human. Rapid recognition of the agent is essential to assure appropriate PPE, decontamination if needed, isolation, vaccination, antidotes, and/or medication administration.

Ebola hemorrhagic fever

Ebola hemorrhagic fever virus (Ebola HF) is one of the most aggressive viruses in the filoviridae family. It is highly contagious and virulent with a biosafety level 4. There is ~50% to 90% mortality rate with this contagion. Ebola HF has sporadic outbreaks. The majority of cases have occurred in Africa (Bruce 2002). It is found in forests in rainy season, low socioeconomic status areas, and areas with limited health-care services.

- Incubation is 2 to 21 days, with the majority evident within 5 to 12 days of exposure
- Hemorrhage within 5 to 7 days of onset and death within 7 to 14 days
- Spread by close contact, contact with clothing, blood, stool, saliva, and possibly sweat
    — Those caring for the dead may also contract Ebola from contact
- No treatment, cure, or vaccination for this virus.

Ebola HF

Virus: Ebola hemorrhagic fever

Signs and Symptoms: rapid rise in temperature within hours, diaphoresis, shivering; at 48 hours pain with movement of the eyes, jaw, and head; 5 to 7 days hemorrhage from every orifice, abnormal platelet function

(Continued)

Ebola HF (*Continued*)

Recovery: slow improvement by week 2; palmar and plantar desquamation, gradual disappearance of rash; Long-term effects hepatitis, uveitis, orchitis

PPE: Formidable Epidemic Disease Pack—all isolation gear until 2 blood cultures, 24 hours apart are both negative; standard and contact isolation precautions

Treatment: maintenance only with oxygen, hydration, hemostasis with replacement of clotting factors and platelets

Tularemia

Tularemia (*Francisella tularensis*) is a Gram-negative coccobacillus and is currently one of the most infectious bacteria identified (CDC 2008).

- Transmitted by direct contact with infected animals, infected food, handling infected carcasses, insect bites, or can also be aerosolized as a weapon
- Cannot be transmitted human to human
- Onset is typically in 3 to 5 days but can take up to 14 days
- Mortality rate is ~2% usually caused by pneumonitis in inhalation cases
  — Pneumonitis presents with hemoptysis, purulent sputum, respiratory insufficiency or failure, sepsis, and shock.

Tularemia

Bacteria: *Francisella tularensis*

Signs and Symptoms: abrupt onset of fever, chills, headache, fatigue, malaise, backache, rigor, dry cough, sore throat without adenopathy; progressive diaphoresis, weakness, and anorexia, weight loss

Recovery: good; prevention by wearing insect repellent, hand washing

PPE: standard barrier precautions; clothing and linens can be laundered with standard protocol

Treatment: streptomycin or gentamycin, aminoglycoside for 10-14 days; with mass casualties doxycycline or ciprofloxacin; inhalation tularemia requires treatment within 48 hours of exposure; exposure only tetracycline or doxycycline for 14 days

Botulism

Botulism (*Clostridium botulinum*) is caused by bacteria that work directly by blocking acetylcholine from fusing with terminal membranes of neuronal end plates, resulting in flaccid paralysis (CDC 2008).

- Transmitted by direct contact and is not spread human to human
- Onset is within 6 hours to 2 weeks (typically 12-36 hours) for foodborne exposure
- Mortality is ~5% and is related to respiratory failure, inadequate tidal volume, and airway obstruction

Botulism

Bacteria: *Clostridium botulinum*

S&S: GI—abdominal cramps, nausea, vomiting, diarrhea; fever, symmetric descending flaccid paralysis including respiratory muscles, cranial nerve palsies, diplopia, dysphagia, dry mouth; possibly ptosis, blurred vision, dysarthria, dysphonia

Recovery: good but may require weeks to months of supportive care

PPE: standard barrier precautions; skin exposure should be washed with soap and water or 0.1% hypochlorite solution

(Continued)

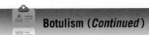

Botulism (*Continued*)

Treatment: Support ventilation, equine antitoxin minimizes subsequent neuronal damage (anaphylaxis can occur prepare with diphenhydramine and epinephrine), nutrition, fluids, prevent complications of paralysis; Aminoglycosides and clindamycin contraindicated due to exacerbating neuromuscular blockade

Plague

Plague (*Yersinia pestis*) has resulted in widespread mortality in the past and continues to have ~2 to 3000 cases each year throughout the world. Approximately 5 to 15 cases are in rural western United States (CDC 2008). Pneumonic plague is easily spread by droplet through coughing or sneezing whereas bubonic plague requires the bite of an infected insect. Untreated bubonic plague can spread to the lungs resulting in a secondary pneumonic plague.

- Pneumonic plague symptom onset is from 1 to 6 days
- Treatment should be initiated within 24 hours of onset of symptoms
- 100% mortality if untreated within 24 hours
  - Lab diagnosis of plague can occur within 2 hours with confirmation at 24 to 48 hours
- Bacteria is destroyed by sunlight and drying but can remain active when aerosolized for up to 1 hour

Plague

Bacteria: *Yersinia pestis*

Signs and Symptoms: Pneumonic—bronchospasm, dyspnea, chest pain, cough, hemoptysis; Bubonic—fever, chills, swollen tender lymph nodes groin, cervical, and axilla (buboes), weakness, sepsis, shock; Primary septicemic—DIC, small vessel necrosis, purpura, gangrene of digits and nose (black death)

Recovery: no vaccine; pneumonic—death if treatment delayed >24 hours

PPE: isolation barrier precautions with full face respirators; patients should wear a mask; terminal cleaning of the room; clothing and linen standard laundering; routine precautions in death

Treatment: streptomycin or gentamicin for 10 to 14 days; alternatively tetracycline or doxycycline; close contact exposure doxycycline prophylaxis

Anthrax

Anthrax (*Bacillus anthracis*) is a Gram-positive encapsulated rod bacterium that is naturally present in the soil throughout the world. It is infectious in the spore form only. Transmission is through contact with the spores by inhalation or direct contact with infected raw meat. There is no human-to-human transmission. Anthrax spores can travel a great distance therefore infecting patients far from the release site. It is the most likely to be weaponized bacterium. There were 22 cases of anthrax inhalation or skin exposure in the United States in 2001, resulting in 7 deaths (CDC 2008).

- Exposure is through food, skin contact, or inhalation
- Incubation is approximately 1 to 6 days
  - Inhalation anthrax can incubate for 42 days and manifests itself with flu-like symptoms, followed by a brief recovery period and then a more severe respiratory phase (Spencer 2001)
  - Typically presents during the second phase
- Mortality after inhalation anthrax can reach nearly 100% after the onset of severe respiratory distress
- Medical examiners and morticians need to use caution in examining the bodies of anthrax victims as the spores can survive for decades after the patient's death

Anthrax

Bacteria: *Bacillus anthracis*

Signs and Symptoms: Skin—edema with pruritis, macules or papules and ulceration; GI—nausea and vomiting, abdominal pain, bloody diarrhea, fever, and occasionally ascites, sepsis; Inhalation—first stage mimics the flu—cough, headache, fever, vomiting, weakness, chills, dyspnea, syncope
Second stage, respiratory distress, stridor, hypoxia, cyanosis, diaphoresis, hypotension and shock; >50% have hemorrhagic mediastinitis; can progress to meningitis with subarachnoid hemorrhage

Recovery: Skin—painless eschar falls off in 1 to 2 weeks; Inhalation—mortality within 24 to 36 hours after the onset of respiratory distress; antibiotics within 24 hours of exposure prevents death

PPE: standard precautions as the patient is not contagious; standard laundering of linens; cremation recommended

Treatment: penicillin sensitive; recommend penicillin or erythromycin, gentamicin, or doxycycline for 60 days; mass casualty—ciprofloxacin or doxycycline; exposure without signs or symptoms—ciprofloxacin or doxycycline prophylaxis for 60 days; GI—with excessive diarrhea, manage fluid volume; Inhalation—optimize oxygenation, ventilation, hemodynamic support

Anthrax treatment is typically ciprofloxacin which is not approved for children <18 years. Doxycycline, the alternative to ciprofloxacin is contraindicated <8 years. There is not yet a vaccine for anthrax where safety and efficacy has been evaluated <18 years.

Smallpox

Smallpox (variola) is a DNA virus. Transmission is through direct contact, contact with clothing, or droplet human to human when the rash phase has begun. Widespread dissemination could occur through aerosolization of the virus. The virus was declared eradicated in 1977 with the last person vaccinated world-wide in 1980. The last child vaccinated in the United States was in 1972 (CDC 2008).

- Smallpox can survive up to 24 hours in a cool temperature and low humidity environment
- Incubation is ~7 to 17 days
- Extremely contagious once the rash appears and until the scabs fall off
  — May be infectious during the prodrome
- Variola major is the most common form and results in high fever and extensive rash.
- Mortality rates ≥30%
- Hemorrhagic smallpox also exists and includes erythema and petechiae or frank hemorrhage of the skin and mucous membranes with death in 5 to 6 days
- Medical examiners and morticians must be careful as the virus can survive in the scabs for up to 13 years

Smallpox

Virus: *Variola*

Signs and Symptoms: Prodrome (2 to 4 days)—high fever, malaise, body aches, headache; Rash (infectious phase 5 to 6 days)— red spotted rash first on face, mouth, pharynx, forearms developing at same rate breaking open and releasing virus into mouth and throat, then progresses to trunk, fever decreases and becomes bumps on day 4 with depressions in the center, fever rises again until scabs form over pustules; Scabs (6 days)—after scabs fall off, no longer contagious (Veenema 2003)

Recovery: dependent upon supportive care

(Continued)

Smallpox (*Continued*)

PPE: transmission precautions and isolation; laundry and all biologic waste containers must be autoclaved, then washed with hot water and bleach; standard room decontamination; cremation recommended

Treatment: no specific treatment except supportive care; retrovirals may assist with symptoms; face-to-face contact or exposure after the onset of fever requires vaccination within 4 days to prevent infection

Currently in the United States, children are not immunized against smallpox, making 100% of children and ~80% of adults susceptible to smallpox, which may be mistaken for varicella. Figure 15-2 demonstrates the rash pattern of variola in comparison with varicella. Smallpox vaccination within 3 to 4 days of exposure can prevent death. Retrovirals may help mitigate symptoms but there is no approved pediatric dosage.

Chemical Agents

Chemical agents are more overt than biologic agents because the signs and symptoms of chemical agents are more readily evident and occur more rapidly than biologic agents. Many chemicals are readily available as they are used in industry and are transported on roadways and rail. Chemical events can result in mass casualties with chemical exposure by a collision or derailing. It is necessary to understand the types of chemicals to prepare for the patient symptoms as well as decontamination needs (Martin 2003). Management includes evacuation and decontamination usually with soap and water. PPE are worn for the decontamination procedures and the runoff is collected and contained for disposal.

Characteristics of chemical agents that affect care include volatility, persistence, toxicity, and latency. These characteristics determine the effect of the chemical on the victim.

- Volatility—tendency of the chemical to become a vapor; most volatile are phosgene and cyanide; most chemicals are heavier than air and stay low to the ground

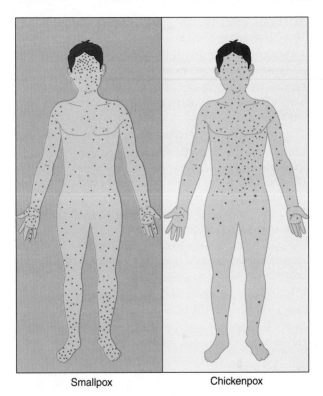

Smallpox   Chickenpox

Figure 15-2   Variola vs varicella rash distribution. (Adapted from http://emergency.cdc.gov/agent/smallpox/diagnosis/pdf/spox-poster-full.pdf. Accessed May 8, 2008)

- Persistence—chemical that is less likely to vaporize and disperse; most industrial chemicals are not persistent; persistent chemicals are more likely to penetrate skin and mucous membranes; penetration can result in secondary exposure
- Toxicity—potential for the agent to result in injury
  — Concentration time—amount released multiplied by time exposed

— Median lethal dose (LD_{50})—amount required to result in 50% mortality of those exposed

— Median effective dose (ED_{50})—amount required to result in signs and symptoms in 50% of those exposed

- Latency—time from absorption to appearance of signs and symptoms; vesicants, nerve agents, cyanide have short latency (rapid onset); sulfur mustard and pulmonary agents have long latency

  Special considerations for children exposed to chemicals include

- Children are lower to the ground, positioning them at the level where chemical (heavier than air) agents accumulate (Bernard 2001). This results in increased exposure from both positioning and a higher respiratory rate.

- Use warm, moist air or oxygen to treat respiratory exposures, especially chlorine or ammonia gas

- Phosgene is also heavier than air but affects the bronchioles directly causing serum leak and volume depletion

  — Puts the child at increased risk of shock

- Exposure to mustard gas, children demonstrate cough, vomiting, and bullae development earlier than adults

- Atropine dosing for sarin gas treatment must be adjusted to children based upon age greater or less than 2 years

Nerve agents

Nerve agents are the most toxic chemical agents available that can and have been weaponized. These agents include sarin, soman, VX, and organophosphates (pesticides). These are easily dispersed, odorless, and colorless liquids or gases. Nerve agents bond with acetylcholine preventing it from being de-activated. The result is overstimulation. Organophosphates specifically inhibit acetylcholinesterase but ultimately spontaneously become unbound (Fruedenthal 2008). Unfortunately, new acetylcholinesterase must be formed before nerve function returns to normal.

- Effects can be seen from 30 minutes to 18 hours after exposure

- Intentional release is not the only method of organophosphate exposure

— Because of the easy access and use of organophosphates, especially malathion and sevin, can occur at home or on a farm

Note that with sarin gas exposure, the airway equipment will absorb the gas and result in continuous exposure to the agent. Other management specifics regarding atropine and pralidoxime are essential to reversing the cholinergic effects.

- Atropine is administered IV for up to 24 hours until anticholinergic activity returns
  — Indicated in the presence of bronchorrhea and other secretions
- Pralidoxime (2-PAM) is indicated in the presence of muscle weakness
  — Needs to be administered as soon as possible as its ability to function decreases with prolonged exposure
  — Does not treat the neurologic effects of the exposure
- Avoid drugs that increase the effects of exposure—morphine, caffeine, theophylline, succinylcholine, loop diuretics

Nerve Agents

Absorption: inhalation or percutaneous

Action: Inhibit cholinesterase

Signs and Symptoms: increased secretions, increased GI motility, diarrhea, bronchospasm, sweating, myosis, visual disturbances, fasciculations, incontinence, bradycardia, atrioventricular block, insomnia, forgetfulness, impaired judgment, irritability

Lethal dose: loss of consciousness, seizures, apnea, flaccidity, copious secretions, fasciculations

Decontamination: copious amounts soap and water for 8-20 minutes; blot to dry; 0.5% hypochlorite solution can be used

Treatment: maintain airway, breathing, circulation; benzodiazepines for seizures, pralidoxime, atropine

Vesicants

Vesicant agents are incapacitating agents with minimal death but large numbers of ill. Common vesicants include lewisite, sulfur mustard, nitrogen mustard, and phosgene. Liquid sulfur mustard is the most frequently used (Davis 2001). It has a garlic odor, penetrates skin, and has long latency. The skin damage is irreversible.

- Skin presents as stinging and erythema for 24 hours followed by pruritis, painful burning, and vesicle formation.
- Vesicles form large bullae by coalescing
- Immediate pain if exposed to lewisite and phosgene
- DO NOT scrub and/or use of hypochlorite solution as it results in deepening the injury
- Dimercaprol is administered IV or on skin lesions from exposure to lewisite
- Monitor patients for a minimum of 24 hours, especially after sulfur mustard exposure

Vesicants

Absorption: percutaneous

Action: blistering agent

Signs and Symptoms: superficial to partial thickness burns perineum, axillae, antecubital spaces; conjunctivitis, lacrimation, photophobia, corneal ulcer

Lethal dose: respiratory exposure, hematopoietic suppression, pneumonia, bronchitis, purulent fibrous pseudomembrane discharge within the airways, nausea, vomiting, upper GI bleed

Decontamination: copious amounts soap and water; blot to dry; DO NOT scrub or use hypochlorite solution

Treatment: maintain airway, breathing, circulation; benzodiazepines for seizures, pralidoxime, atropine

Pulmonary agents

Pulmonary agents disrupt the pulmonary membrane preventing alveolar-capillary oxygen exchange and causing capillary leak. Typical pulmonary agents include phosgene and chlorine which vaporize rapidly.

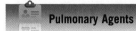

Pulmonary Agents

Absorption: inhalation

Action: Inhibit alveolar-capillary gas exchange by separating the alveoli from the capillary bed, causing capillary leak

Signs and Symptoms: pulmonary edema, bronchospasm, shortness of breath especially with exertion, hacking cough, frothy sputum

Decontamination: Airway management; healthcare personnel should wear masks

Treatment: maintain airway, ventilator support, bronchoscopy

Blood agents

Blood agents directly affect cellular metabolism, resulting in asphyxiation. Common blood agents include cyanide and cyanogen chloride. Cyanide is known as a suicide agent, however less known is that it is widely used in plastics, mining silver and gold, and dye industries. Cyanide can also be inadvertently released during a house fire because of its presence in everyday items such as furniture, carpeting, and other materials. House-fires also result in the release of carbon monoxide, which affect the blood's oxygen-carrying ability by binding more readily to hemoglobin than oxygen. Cyanide release has the odor of bitter almonds.

Blood Agents

Absorption: inhalation, percutaneous, ingested

Action: disrupts cellular aerobic metabolism

Signs and Symptoms: tachypnea, tachycardia, coma, seizure, respiratory failure/arrest, cardiac arrest

Lethal dose: respiratory arrest, cardiac arrest

Decontamination: administer cyanide reversal agents

Treatment: maintain airway, breathing, circulation; sodium thiocyanate, amyl nitrate, hydroxocobalamin

The treatment of cyanide exposure is a specific regimen to counteract the effects of the cyanide at the cellular level.

- A hyperbaric chamber increases oxygenation through saturation of the serum regardless of hemoglobin's inability to carry oxygen
  — Allows for oxygenation while the "cyanide kit" is delivered to the patient
- Amyl nitrate pearls are crushed and placed in the ventilator reservoir
  — Induces methemoglobinemia; methemoglobin binds with cyanide at a 20% to 25% higher affinity than hemoglobin
- Sodium nitrate is given next via intravenous (IV) as its affinity for cyanide is even better than methemoglobin
  — Sodium thiocyante can be excreted through the kidneys
  — Cyanomethemoglobin is detoxified in the liver
- Monitor the patient for hypotension, vomiting, psychosis, and joint or muscle pain
- Hydroxocobalamin (vitamin B_{12}a) is an alternative method of treatment that binds with cyanide to form cyanocobalamin (vitamin B_{12}) (Sauer 2001)

— Requires large doses

— Mucous membranes, skin, and urine may turn pink

— Transient hypertension and tachycardia also may occur for ~48 hours

If the patient also has high carboxyhemoglobin levels (eg, a victim of a house fire), induction of methemoglobinemia is contraindicated. The hyperbaric chamber is useful in oxygenating the patient, as well as forcing the release of the carbon monoxide.

Radiation Exposure

Radiation exposure can occur from many sources. A "dirty bomb" includes such radioactive material. A radioactive weapon disperses radioactive material when it explodes. A nuclear weapon requires a complex fission reaction, not simply the carrier of radioactive materials. A radioactive specimen could be placed in a public place, exposing many people to the radiation and then to everyone with whom they come in contact.

Different types of particles exist with differing effects on the body. In general, protons, neutrons, and electrons, reside in balance or element stability within atoms that then make up molecules. An imbalance in the nucleus where there are too many neutrons, results in radioactivity. Particles are ejected as the nuclide attempts to stabilize itself.

- Alpha particles—low-level radiation; cannot penetrate skin and can be prevented from contact through a single layer of clothing or paper; entry occurs through a wound, ingestion, inhalation resulting in localized injury

- Beta particles—high-energy radiation; able to penetrate skin to the cell production layer; injury is caused if exposure is prolonged

- Gamma particles—short-wave electromagnetic energy; deep penetrating particles; difficult to shield; often accompanies alpha and beta particle emission

To understand the effects of radiation and decontamination, it is necessary to discuss measurement of radiation.

- Rad: equals one joule of energy per kilogram of tissue
- Rem: reflects the degree of potential damage based upon absorption
  — On average, a person is exposed to 360 millirem (mrem)
- Mild radiation sickness occurs with 200,000 mrem

Half-life reflects the amount of time it takes for a sample to lose half of its initial radioactivity. Levels of radiation must be measured to determine exposure. Typically a Geiger counter is used to measure background gamma radiation as well as some beta radiation. Other tools that can be used include an ionization chamber, alpha monitors, and personal dosimeters which are worn by radiology personnel.

Exposure results in injury. Length of exposure, distance from the source, type of source, and any shielding affect the ultimate depth of penetration. Injury is inversely proportionate to distance. Sequelae of serious radiation contamination or incorporation may not be evident for years. Radiation injury is of three types.

- External—radiation has penetrated and passed through the body; irradiation means that the patient is not radioactive as there are no particles within the body since the radiation only passed through
- Contamination—exposure has occurred either externally or internally; immediate medical treatment is necessary especially if the exposure was internal where the particles can become deposited within the body; radiation is present
- Incorporation—the exposure to radiation by contamination has resulted in uptake of particles by the body into tissues; most commonly these are the kidneys, liver, thyroid, and bone

As with all hazardous materials exposures, decontamination should occur first at the scene. It is essential that it is done outside of the hospital and by personnel with appropriate PPE to prevent cross-contamination. Hospital lockdown is important with the ability to decontaminate victims outside the emergency department.

- Floors should be covered to prevent tracking
- Strict isolation is needed
- Air ducts need to be sealed

- PPE includes water-resistant gowns, double gloves, booties, masks, and goggles
  — Dosimeters are worn by everyone in contact with the victims
- Incoming patients are surveyed for radiation levels before entry into the hospital in case secondary decontamination is necessary
  — If proper PPE are worn and dosimeters are monitored, there is minimal risk to staff

Acute radiation syndrome

Acute radiation syndrome (ARS) occurs after radiation exposure. The degree of reaction to the exposure is dependent upon the dose received (>100 rad). Penetrating radiation and the rate of exposure also affect the outcome. There are differing affects throughout the body and there are distinct phases of response to the exposure. Table 15-2 describes the effects of radiation on the body systems.

The hematopoietic system response is a good predictor of long term outcome. Lymphocyte counts of 300 to $1200/mm^3$ within the first 48 hours are indicative of significant exposure. Each cell responds in its own time such that neutrophils decrease within 1 week, platelets within 2 weeks, and red blood cells within 3 weeks. This patient should have barrier precautions to prevent infection.

Table 15-2   Radiation Effects

Body System	Effects
Hematopoietic	Decreased lymphocytes, granulocytes, thrombocytes, reticulocytes; fever, opportunistic infection, sepsis
Gastrointestinal	Nausea and vomiting, fluid and electrolyte imbalances, bloody diarrhea
Neurologic	Cerebral edema, headache, increased intracranial pressure
Cardiovascular	Collapse, hypotension, cardiac failure
Skin	Erythema, desquamation, necrosis

The gastrointestinal (GI) system is made of rapidly reproducing cells and therefore is also seriously affected by radiation exposure. GI symptoms occur rapidly. Within 2 hours, nausea and vomiting occur. A high fever with bloody diarrhea heralds high mortality and can occur within ~10 days. Neurologic symptoms occur after an exposure of 1000 rad. Increased intracranial pressure (IICP) is also a sign of mortality caused by irreversible injury.

The skin is the visible component of radiation injury. Exposure levels of 600 to 1000 rad result in erythema whereas desquamation will occur with exposure >1000 rad. If the exposure is >5000 rad, necrosis will occur from days to months later. In addition to radiation exposure itself, other trauma injuries may occur. These are treated in the usual fashion with attention to airway, breathing, and circulation first (Chapter 2). After the immediate life-threatening injuries are managed, subsequent surgeries must be delayed due to infection risk and delayed healing.

The likelihood of survival is dependent on the exposure. Scene and hospital triage are the same as for any mass casualty incident. Minimal symptoms that resolve within a few hours are probable survivors.

• If nausea and vomiting persists >24 to 48 hours, the patients have had a significant enough exposure to warrant monitoring over time

• Supportive treatment to prevent infection and stabilize cell counts is needed to protect the patient through the latent and illness phases

— Improbable survivors have been exposed to >800 rad with total body penetration

— Initial symptoms include vomiting and diarrhea, shock

— Any neurologic symptoms are indicative of a nonsurvivable dose of radiation

— However, not all patients have neurologic symptoms and present much like a high percentage burn with shock and instability, but a normal neurologic state

— In most cases death is rapid caused by shock

— In a mass casualty situation, these patients are classified "black" and are provided comfort measures after decontamination to protect the other victims and caregivers

Phases of Injury after Radiation Exposure

Prodrome: 48 to 72 hours after exposure; nausea and vomiting, diarrhea, fatigue, loss of appetite; high dose—fever, respiratory distress, increased excitability

Latent: symptom-free period after prodrome lasting up to 3 weeks (less if high dose); decreasing lymphocytes, leukocytes, thrombocytes, and red blood cells (RBC)

Illness: follows latent phase; complications—infection, fluid/electrolyte imbalances, diarrhea, bleeding, altered consciousness, shock

Recovery: follows illness; can take weeks to months to fully return to normal

Death: IICP and/or bloody diarrhea signs of impending death

Decontamination

The first step toward decontamination is the removal of the clothing. Decontamination involves showering the patient with soap and water in an area with a collection device.

- Shower from head to toe to prevent recontamination of an area of the body already washed and decontaminated
- Waste water from decontamination is collected and double-bagged
- Paper gowns are provided
- After the shower, patients are resurveyed for radiation levels
  - Biological samples must be taken as well to determine internal exposure such as nasal and throat swabs
  - Lab work such as complete blood count (CBC) and differential provide a baseline

— Any wounds should be irrigated before decontamination and covered with water resistant dressings

— If internal decontamination is needed, it is accomplished through cathartics, gastric lavage, and chelating agents

— Samples of stool, gastric contents, and urine are taken to identify continued levels of radiation

- Pediatrics

  — Have a relatively large total body surface area in comparison with adults

    ■ Results in rapid cooling during decontamination procedures as well as increased body surface chemical/radiation agent absorption through the skin

  — Skin is also thinner increasing both thermal and chemical burns

  — Warm water is needed for decontamination to prevent hypothermia

  — Water pressure may also need adjustment to prevent injury to a child

SPECIAL SITUATIONS

Every mass casualty situation involves people of all varieties. There are age extremes, extensive past medical histories, disabilities, language barriers, and more. These differences need to be taken into account and anticipated in the emergency operations plan (EOP). Designated people are assigned to manage the needs of the disabled, medications, language issues, and children.

Pediatrics

Pediatrics is not exempt from being involved in a disaster situation. There are special considerations for children beyond the usual steps taken for pediatric trauma (Fendya 2006). One of the first situations to take into account in community EOP is that there are ~1.6 million children aged 5 to 14 years who are home alone (Phillips and Hewett 2005). These children average 5 to 10 hours each week in unsupervised situations at home. The EOP should include age-appropriate training for these children that is repeated every 4 to 6 months and include parent training manuals as well.

Equipment of all sizes, pediatric and adult, as well as medications in dosages appropriate for children are needed. Children are part of a family therefore the EOP must be prepared to manage not only a child, but the family as well.

Geriatrics

Geriatric patients are more susceptible to injury because of osteoporosis, thinner skin and loss of subcutaneous tissue. Past medical history also affects the ability to combat a contagion or manage a chemical or radiation exposure. Blast injuries as with any trauma exacerbate these concurrent medical problems. Medications can also mask injury, eg, preventing tachycardia, missing a shock presentation. Low bone density increases the risk of fracture during a blast or the aftermath of a disaster situation. Elderly patients have less pulmonary reserve, which increases the risk of respiratory complications from injury, chemical, biological, or radiation exposure.

Decontamination can result in hypothermia, thus water temperature needs to be adjusted. Access to decontamination areas may also need adjustment to manage walkers, and other assistive devices.

Specialty populations

Consideration needs to be taken for the pregnant patient. In the case of a blast event, the placenta is highly susceptible and can result in abruptio placenta. The pregnant patient presents two patients for consideration in all disaster situations with the primary care delivered first to stabilize the mother (Chapter 11).

Patients with disabilities also need special consideration during a mass casualty situation (American Red Cross 2001). These patients may have extensive medical histories and medication and oxygen needs similar to the elderly. In addition, specialty equipment may be needed that was lost or damaged in the event. A plan in the community for evacuation assistance for the disabled is essential and it must include the service animals that may accompany the patient. Both communication and mobilization devices will be needed. Sign language experts are very useful at shelters and hospitals.

Language experts should also be part of the plan, especially the languages most often spoken within a region. There is a significant population of community members who may need language assistance as they do not speak English and are separated from English-speaking family members.

POSTRESUSCITATION MANAGEMENT AND REHABILITATION

Critical incident stress management (CISM) is an essential component of the EOP. CISM has two components, debriefing and critique. During the critique component, the technical aspects of the event are discussed, system and other issues are reviewed and areas of improvement are identified. The debriefing or defusing component allows for staff to express feelings and thoughts of stress, discomfort, difficulties sleeping, somatization, conflict, and other issues. Prior to a MCI, disaster preparedness education should include the CISM process, identification of symptoms of stress, and coping strategies. The CISM process incorporates these after the event to assist staff with processing the experience. The process is useful for local level events as well, not only large regional or national events.

 Critical Lifesavers

- **Children are lower to the ground, positioning them at the level where chemical (heavier than air) agents accumulate**
- **Any neurologic symptoms are indicative of a nonsurvivable dose of radiation**
- **With sarin gas exposure, the airway equipment will absorb the gas and result in continuous exposure to the agent**
- **Small pox presents with red spotted rash first on face, mouth, pharynx, forearms developing at same rate**
- **A "dirty bomb" includes radioactive material within the bomb**
- **Self-evacuation usually precedes the arrival of emergency medical personnel, which makes the hospital part of the scene**

REFERENCES

American Red Cross Disaster Services. (2001). *Disaster preparedness for people with disabilities.* Available at: http://www.redcross.org. Accessed May 8, 2008.

Bernard LM. Pediatric implications in bioterrorism part I: physiologic and psychosocial differences. *Int J Trauma Nurs.* 2001;7(1): 14-16.

Bruce J, Cur B, Brysiewicz P. Ebola fever: the African emergency. *Int J Trauma Nurs.* 2002;8(2):36-41.

CDC. *Bombings: Injury Patterns and Care.* Available at: http://www.bt.cdc.gov/masscasualties/blastinjury/ems.asp. Accessed May 8, 2008.

CDC. Anthrax. Available at: http://www.emergency.cdc.gov/agent/anthrax/needtoknow.asp. Accessed May 8, 2008

CDC. Botulism. Available at: http://www.emergency.cdc.gov/agent/botulism.facts.asp. Accessed May 8, 2008.

CDC. Plague. Available at: http://www.emergency.cdc.gov/agent/plague/faq.asp. Accessed May 8, 2008.

CDC. Smallpox. Available at: http://www.emergency.cdc.gov/agent/smallpox/overview/diseasefacts.asp. Accessed May 8, 2008.

CDC. Tularemia. Available at: http://www.emergency.cdc.gov/agent/tularemia.facts.asp. Accessed May 8, 2008.

Centers for Disease Control and Prevention Strategic Planning Workgroup. Biological and chemical terrorism: Strategic plan for preparedness and response. *MMWR Recomm Rep.* 2000;49 (RR-4):1-14.

Centers for Disease Control and Prevention. (2004). Severe acute respiratory syndrome (SARS). Available online: http://www.cdc.gov/ncidod/sars. Accessed June 26, 2006.

Currance P, Bronstein AC. *Hazardous materials for EMS: Practices and Procedures.* St Louis, MO: Mosby; 1999.

Davis KG, Aspera G. Exposure to liquid sulfur mustard. *Ann Emerg Med.* 2001;37(6):653-656.

Department of Homeland Security (DHS). Homeland Security Advisory System: Current Threat Level. Available at: www.dhs.gov/xinfoshare/programs. Accessed September 5, 2008.

Fendya DG. When disaster strikes- care considerations for pediatric patients. *J Traum Nurs.* 2006;13(4):161-165.

Fruedenthal W. Toxicity, Organophosphates. 2008. Available at: http://www.emedicine.com/ped/topic1660.htm. Accessed September 5, 2008.

Garner A. Documentation and tagging of casualties in multiple casualty incidents. *Emerg Med.* 2003;15(5):475–479.

Grigg E, Rosen J, Koop CE. The biological disaster challenge: why are we least prepared for the most devastating threat and what we need to do about it. *J Emerg Manag.* 2006;4(1):23-35.

Kluger Y, Nimrod A, Biderman P, et al. The quinary pattern of blast injury. *J Emerg Manag.* 2006;4(1):51-55.

Martin T, Lobert S. Chemical warfare. *Crit Care Nurse.* 2003;23(5):15-20.

Newport Beach Fire Department. START triage protocol. Available at: www.START-triage.com. Accessed September 5, 2008.

Nicholson WC. The role of the incident command system. *J Emerg Manag.* 2006;4(1):19-21.

Phelps S. There is no cold zone: the hazardous materials zone model and mass terrorism chemical weapon events. *J Emerg Manag.* 2006;4(2):52-56.

Phillips BD, Hewett PL. Home alone: disasters, mass emergencies, and children in self-care. *J Emerg Manag.* 2005;3(2):31-35.

Ritenour AE, Wickley A, Ritenour JS, et al. Tympanic membrane perforation and hearing loss from blast overpressure in Operation Enduring Freedom and Operation Iraqi Freedom wounded. *J Trauma.* 2008;64(2):S174-178.

Romig, L. JumpSTART triage protocol 1995. Available at: http://www.jumpstarttriage.com. Accessed September 5, 2008.

Sauer SW, Keim ME. Hydroxocobalamin: Improved public health readiness for cyanide disasters. *Ann Emerg Med.* 2001;37(6);635-641.

Spencer DA, Whitman KM, Morton PG. Inhalational anthrax. *Med Surg Nurs.* 2001;10(2):308-312.

Veenema TG. Diagnosis, management, and containment of smallpox infection. *Disaster Manag Response.* 2003;1(1):8-13.

Waugh WL. The principles of emergency management. *J Emerg Manag.* 2007;5(3):15-16.

Index

Page numbers followed by *f* or *t* indicate figures or tables, respectively.